D1522707

Local Hospitals in Ancien Régime France
Rationalization, Resistance, Renewal, 1530–1789

At a time when governments are obsessed with cutting back the social network and encouraging private charities to meet the needs of the poor and the sick, Daniel Hickey provides a timely look at retrenchment strategies in local hospitals in Ancien Régime France. He explores two opposing campaigns to reform poor relief and aid to the sick: attempts by the French Crown to centralize social services by eliminating local institutions and initiatives taken by the local population to revitalize those same institutions.

During the sixteenth and seventeenth centuries the French Crown, supposedly acting in the name of efficiency, better management, and elimination of duplicate services, closed down thousands of local hospices, *maladreries*, and small hospitals that had been refuges for the sick and poor. Its true motive, however, was to expropriate their revenues and holdings. Hickey shows how, in spite of government efforts, a countermovement emerged that to some degree foiled the Crown's attempts. Charitable institutions, churchmen inspired by the new message of the Catholic Reformation, women's religious congregations, and community elites defied intervention measures, resisted proposed changes, and revitalized the very type of institution the Crown was trying to shut down.

Hickey's conclusions are supported by a study of eight small hospitals, which allows him to measure the impact of Crown decisions on the day-to-day functioning of these local institutions.

Challenging the interpretations of Michel Foucault and other historians, Hickey throws new light on an important area of early modern French history.

DANIEL HICKEY is professor of history, Université de Moncton.

McGill-Queen's/Hannah Institute Studies in the
History of Medicine, Health, and Society

Series Editors: S.O. Freedman and J.T.H. Connor

Volumes in this series have been supported by the
Hannah Institute for the History of Medicine

Local Hospitals in Ancien Régime France

Rationalization, Resistance, Renewal 1530–1789

DANIEL HICKEY

McGill-Queen's University Press
Montreal & Kingston • London • Buffalo

© McGill-Queen's University Press 1997
ISBN 0-7735-1540-2

Legal deposit second quarter 1997
Bibliothèque nationale du Québec

Printed in Canada on acid-free paper

This book has been published with the help of a grant
from the Humanities and Social Sciences Federation of
Canada, using funds provided by the Social Sciences and
Humanities Research Council of Canada.

McGill-Queen's University Press is grateful to the
Canada Council for support of its publishing program.

Canadian Cataloguing in Publication Data

Hickey, Daniel
    Local hospitals in Ancien Régime France : rationalization,
resistance, renewal, 1530–1789
    (McGill-Queen's/Hannah Institute studies in the history
of medicine, health and society ; 5)
    Includes bibliographical references and index.
    ISBN 0-7735-1540-2
    1. Hospitals – France – History. 2. Medical policy –
France – History. I. Title. II. Series.
    RA989.F8H53 1997   362.1'1'094409   C96-900927-5

Typeset in Adobe Caslon 10.5/13
by Caractéra inc., Quebec City

Contents

Maps, Tables, and Figures

TABLES

FIGURES

Preface

The idea for this book first came to me during the summer of 1975. Working on tax records in the sleepy little town of Étoile-sur-Rhône, I came across a pile of local hospital documents that extended back to the sixteenth century: among them were the institution's charter, its financial accounts, lists of the poor eligible to receive free bread or grain, and slips signed by town notables granting admission for men and women from both inside and outside Étoile. Pursuing my work on tax structures and absolutism in other early modern French towns, I found that a good number of them also had hospital archives. By 1986 I had begun to examine these papers in more detail, and they opened up to me a whole new world of complex relationships between the poor who frequented these institutions and the local elite who contributed time and money to ensure their operation. To better understand the context of these relationships, I followed up leads to the Archives Nationales, eight departmental holdings, two hospitals, and three religious communities. While I was carrying out this research and the subsequent writing of this book, many colleagues, students, and archivists came to my aid. I would like to thank several of them whose advice was particularly important at different stages in my research.

Many colleagues have heard perhaps more than they would have liked about the problems of small hospitals, the entry of women's religious orders into charitable work, and the role played by town notables in local relief efforts. In France, from the very beginning of the project, Jean-

Pierre Gutton, the leading French scholar on early modern poor relief, and his wife, Anne-Marie, a specialist on confraternities, have regularly welcomed me into their home, discussed my hypotheses, suggested new approaches, and kept me up to date on recent new theses and papers on the subject of hospitals and charity. In Brittany, Jean-Luc Bruzulier and his wife, Guylaine, both of whom are preparing theses on early modern hospitals, took the time to meet with me to discuss sources on western French institutions and the particularisms of Breton hospitals. They have replied regularly to my questions, sent me material, and facilitated my work in a province outside the regions I have traditionally studied. In England, Colin Jones of Exeter University, another important scholar of early modern charity and hospitals, has been particularly helpful, reading my papers and suggesting new avenues of research or new sources for my work. At home in Moncton, my colleagues Chungchi Wen, Phyllis LeBlanc, and Jacques-Paul Couturier have more than once listened to my problems and suggested solutions.

Among archivists, my work was particularly aided by Mme Nathan-Tilloy and her staff at the Archives Départementales de la Drôme, by Vital Chomel, Yves Soulingeas, and Janine Lucet of the Archives Départementales de l'Isère, and by Claude Hohl and the personnel of the Archives Départementales de la Seine-Maritime. All of them transferred mountains of documents for me to study in France or microfilmed series to be analysed. Some of the records were still in local hospitals, and in those cases Christian Roquet and Louis Oriol, directors respectively of the hospitals at St-Vallier and Savenay, facilitated my access to early modern papers and documents. For the archives still in the hands of religious orders, Sister Stanislas Kostka of the Sisters of St-Thomas de Villeneuve kindly furnished me with records from the holdings of her congregation. Sister Marie-Thérèse Lauraine guided me through the papers of her order, the Sisters of St-Joseph of St-Vallier, and Sister Thérèse de l'Enfant Jésu provided me with documents from the archives of the Sisters of the Holy Sacrament of Valence.

A research team was organized around this project with assistants in France and Moncton. In France, Danielle Courtemanche, then a doctoral student at the Université de Montréal, and Laurent Grima, who had just terminated his *maîtrise* at the Université de Paris iv, copied documents, analysed archival series, and suggested new sources to be microfilmed for the project. In Moncton, Marc Pitre and Marc Robichaud proceeded to analyse the microfilms, compile their data, and suggest ways to integrate the most important findings into my text. Guy Lavoie, a recent graduate of our Département de Géographie, worked with us to express our statistical findings in the graphs and maps that illustrate the different chapters. With Marc Pitre and Marc Robichaud working on theses in complementary subject areas, a certain synergy developed around the question of early modern hospital reform, a dynamism that I have tried to express in the pages of this book.

The process of writing, revising, and rewriting has been long and solitary, taking up precious summers and many long weekends. I would like to thank different friends who have been kind enough to give up their spare time to read and criticize the different versions of my chapters. Manfred Winter of our English Department and Robert Michel, a former archivist at McGill University, who has remained in contact with me since our graduate student days, both read the entire manuscript, telling me when I was being redundant, when an idea was incomprehensible, and when sentences or paragraphs had to be modified. Maurice Basque, Chantal Hickey, and Andrée Courtemanche all read selected chapters and provided me with useful feedback. I would also like to thank Elizabeth Hulse, who copy-edited the manuscript, picking up numerous errors and oversights.

The project, of course, received very necessary financial backing. The Social Sciences and Humanities Research Council of Canada awarded me a first grant in 1987–89, including a very useful research-time stipend that allowed me to spend the year 1987–88 in France. A second grant, extending from 1992 to 1995, began just as I returned from a sabbatical year there, and with it I was able to order the necessary microfilms and select research assistants to carry out the remaining analysis and research. The Université de Moncton also provided me with aid and support. The 1990–91 sabbatical year and regular research-time stipends were provided to me by the Faculté des Arts, and the Faculté des Études Supérieures et de Recherche voted me regular financial aid to supplement my SSHRCC grants. Finally, the scholarly publications program of the Humanities and Social Sciences Federation of Canada accorded my work a grant to facilitate publication. I would like to express my appreciation to all these institutions for the aid that they have accorded me, particularly in this difficult time of academic and budgetary cutbacks.

Finally, this project has disrupted our family life for over a decade. My wife, Hélène, and my children, Chantal, Eric, and Jean-Pierre, all had to break off personal and school ties twice to follow me on the road to local French hospitals. They have had to put up with my tensions and frustrations in the face of hypotheses that proved wrong or arguments that I just could not get right. To all of them I dedicate this book.

Glossary of French Terms

Whenever possible, I have tried to translate French terms into English or explain them within the text. In the cases where the names of institutions or terms made no sense in a direct translation, had no English equivalents, or unnecessarily complicated the text, I have kept them in French. The principal ones appear below.

BAILLAGE
A district created in the twelfth century either as a *baillage* or a *sénéchaussée* and placed under the authority of a *bailli* or *sénéchal*. Named by the king from among the nobles of the sword, these officials contributed to increase royal power at the expense of seigneurial, ecclesiastical, and municipal justice. The creation of governors and then intendants eventually reduced their role. The tribunal of the baillage or sénéchaussée was an intermediary judicial instance between the seigneurial judges on the one hand and royal presidial courts and *parlements* on the other. It heard cases in first instance relating to the appointment of nobles to ecclesiastical livings, some criminal affairs, and cases in appeal relating to policing. The baillis and sénéchaux also published royal ordonances and had authority over fairs and markets.

CHÂTELAIN
The holder of a fief accorded by the crown on which a chateau had been built. Synonymous with seigneur, the *châtelain* possessed property rights

over landholdings (*domaine*) – exploited directly or indirectly – and judicial rights over his lands and their inhabitants. By his oath of allegiance to the king, he recognized that he held his fief from the sovereign, from whom he received the right to dispense superior, intermediary, and low justice on his lands. Such a right was a guaranty for the payment of the seigneurial dues (*cens*) owed to him by the inhabitants of his lands.

Consul

A chief magistrate elected or co-opted in the southern towns and cities of the kingdom. Most communities had two consuls, the *consul moderne*, a newly elected magistrate, and the *consul ancien*, the one previously elected, who presided over city and town consulates made up of representatives of the corporate groups of the community: officials, bourgeois, merchants, artisans, workers, and agricultural workers.

Commanderie

Commander of one of the district regions of a military-religious order (Knights of Malta, Knights of the Temple, Order of St-Lazare, etc.). In the case of the efforts by the Order of Mount Carmel and St-Lazare to suppress and expropriate the holdings of the hospitals that were not respecting their charter obligations, it was up to the regional *commanderies* to redirect the funds received to the different local officers of the order.

Controller general

The function of controller general of finances can be traced back to François I, who by an ordinance of 1527 created two *auditeurs des comptes* to treat incoming revenues. By 1547 these officials had received the title *controlleurs généraux*, and they accounted for the income and expenses of the royal treasury (*épargne*). The number of these positions fluctuated during the seventeenth century, with as few as one controller and as many as four. In 1661 control over the royal treasury was given to Jean-Baptiste Colbert, who became the new controller general. From his adminsitration until the end of the Ancien Régime, the controller general took charge not only of the finances of the kingdom, but also of all that affected its economic administration.

Décime

Imposition voted by the national assemblies of the clergy and levied upon each diocese. Following the apportionment carried out in 1516, each diocese was asked to pay its part and to distribute its quota to the different clerical groups (holders of clerical livings and regular and secular clergy). Payments were to be made to diocesan *receveurs* (collectors) to be transferred to the *receveur général* of the French clergy, a commissioner named by the Assembly of the Clergy.

Dépôt de mendicité

Institution created by Controller General Laverdy in 1764. In the face of what they saw as a lack of collaboration by French hospitals with the attempt by the crown in 1724 to intern beggars, royal officials argued that hospitals should receive only the sick and the handicapped and that new institutions (*dépôts*) should be set up to intern and reform the poor and the vagabonds. The royal intendants in each *généralité* were to oversee the eighty-eight dépôts that were established in order to control their costs, intern the largest possible number of inmates, and organize them into detachments in order to instil in them a work ethic and pay the costs of their internment. The resulting institutions were somewhere between a workhouse and a prison, but the experiment was generally unsuccessful: it cost far more than planned, and the work detachments were never able to produce sufficient revenues. Controller General Turgot suspended the operation in 1775 and then authorized a limited number of dépôts to be reopened a year later. His successor, Necker, tried to reinstitute the dépôts on a more limited scale in 1780, but they were all closed by the beginning of the Revolution.

Dévot

In the first half of the seventeenth century, this term designated a partisan of an ultra-Catholic policy directed against Protestants within the kingdom and favourable to a Spanish alliance outside it. The *dévots* advocated respecting the traditional liberties and privileges of intermediary officials (parlements, estates, provincial bureaucracy) and were hostile to the centralizing agents of royal absolutism (intendants and commissioners). Despite their failure to impose their policies under Cardinal Richelieu, the influence of the dévots remained considerable, especially through the Company of the Holy Sacrament, founded in 1627. This pious, charitable, and moralizing organization of nobles and notables became a very powerful lobby under the queen mother, Anne of Austria. Up to the time of its disbanding by royal order in 1666, it influenced magistrates, city councillors, and provincial and royal officials.

ÉLECTION
Local financial district. In the fourteenth century, the crown created a
tax system based on local districts supervised by an official (*élu*), initially
elected but thereafter appointed. He gave his name to the district he
supervised, the *élection*.

FEU
Literally a hearth. It was the community basis of the fiscal assessment
of the royal tax, or *taille*, paid by all commoners. The real assessment
varied from province to province. Sometimes, as in Dauphiné, the
calculation included the soil quality in a village along with the number
of hearths. In other provinces, such as Brittany, the average fourteenth-
century *feu* counted three real households.

GÉNÉRALITÉ
Regional financial district. The districts took their name from their chief
officer, the *général*. Most *généralités* had a large complement of officers
organized into a *bureau des finances*. They were responsible for receiving
tailles, *aides*, and the *gabelle*. From the entry of France into the Thirty
Years War, the crown dispatched *maîtres de requêtes*, commissioners, and
finally intendants into the généralités to carry out its orders. From 1637
the intendants took up residency in the capital of each généralité, and
after 1680 they became the principal officers responsible for justice,
policing, and finance.

HÔPITAL-GÉNÉRAL
A hospital created during the seventeenth century to intern vagabonds,
beggars, and marginals. The first of these institutions, La Charité, was
built in Lyon in 1622, and an *hôpital-général* was created in Paris in 1656.
A royal edict issued in 1673 asked all the major cities of the kingdom to
establish such hospitals, in which their beggars and marginals could be
confined, organized into work groups, and exposed to religious and
moral lessons designed to "rehabilitate" them. Going a step further in
1724, the crown ordered all beggars and vagabonds in the kingdom to
be arrested and confined in 156 designated hôpitaux-généraux.

HÔTEL-DIEU
A hospital in a larger city that tended to eliminate its service to the poor
and the vagabonds in order to concentrate on caring for the sick, injured,

and dying. During the course of the seventeenth century, these institutions began to sign contracts with doctors and surgeons to ensure that they visit and treat patients, although few of the hospitals had regular medical services available within their walls before the end of the eighteenth century. The personnel of these *hôtels-Dieu* also changed during the late seventeenth and early eighteenth centuries with the creation of numerous women's religious congregations founded to nurse the sick and the injured. Despite these modifications, the hôtels-Dieu were still described in Diderot's *Encyclopédie* as dens of contageous disease – institutions for which reforms had often been proposed but never carried out.

LIVRE
French pound; known as the *livre tournois*, or the pound of Tours. The livre was an amount of money, not an actual coin. In equivalency, 1 livre=20 sous, and 1 sous=24 deniers.

MAISON DE FORCE
A hospital that took in *correctionnaires*, people whose internment was requested by their family. This practice was carried out between the 1740s and 1789 through the use of *lettres de cachet*, royal orders of confinement obtained by a family member. Most of the men and women locked up were "inadapted" individuals from relatively well-to-do families: alcoholics, the mentally deranged, gamblers who put the fortunes of the family at risk, or over-rebellious young people. The family of the detained patient was responsible for paying the cost of the internment, and many institutions took in substantial revenues from this practice.

MAÎTRES DE REQUÊTES
Justice officials who presided over the Chambre des requêtes, one of the four chambers of the Parlement of Paris. They heard pleas and granted letters permitting clients to present their cases before the other chambers (Grand' Chambre, Chambre des Enquêtes, and Tournelle Criminelle). These officials were frequently sent on missions throughout the kingdom to counsel the crown on difficult issues.

MALADRERIE
A small house that indiscriminately took in the poor, the itinerants, the sick, and the dying. The particularity of these institutions was the fact that they had originally been founded in the late Middle Ages to care

for lepers; with the decline and virtual disappearance of leprosy in the fifteenth century, most of them were converted into local hospitals.

Oblat

A practice by which the crown claimed the right to appoint former army officers and handicapped soldiers to places in abbeys and monasteries. It dated back to vague precedents in the twelfth century, although the actual naming of old soldiers to these *oblats* was most apparent towards the end of the fifteenth century. The Concordat of 1516 officially recognized the right of the sovereign to name former army officers to live in abbeys founded under royal charter, that is, institutions where the king could name the abbot. However, the crown claimed subsequently to have the right to name these old and often handicapped officers to any abbey in the kingdom headed by an elected abbot.

Passants

Itinerants or vagabonds who were to be granted asylum in most hospitals during the early modern period. This function dates from the Middle Ages, when these institutions welcomed pilgrims and travellers. During the early modern period, most of the hospitals still made a distinction between the honourable people, whom they often lodged in single reserved rooms, and the others, who were placed in open dormatories.

Recteur

The director of poor relief in a city or town. In the southeastern towns he headed the bureau of the poor (*bureau des pauvres*), which oversaw the distribution of bread to the poor and the supervision of the hospital, whereas in the northwestern towns he was in charge of the hospital as such since the other functions of poor relief were left to the parish priest (curé).

Sénéchal

See under *baillage*

Sénéchaussée

See *baillage*

Subdélégation

Confronted with the multiplication of their responsibilities, the royal intendants, installed in most provinces by the end of the seventeenth century, divided their jurisdictions (généralités) into *subdélégations* headed by *subdélégués*. The latter were initially named and revoked at will by the intendant. For purely fiscal purposes, the position became venial through a 1704 edict, but by 1715 this measure had been abandoned and the nomination of the subdélégués was once again dependent on the intendant.

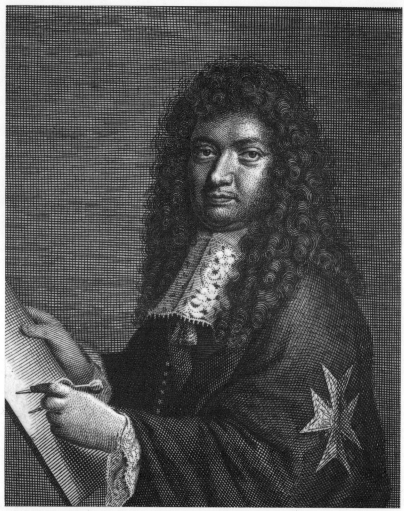

François-Michel Le Tellier, Seigneur de Chaville, Marquis de Louvois. The son of Michel Le Tellier, *chancelier* de France under Louis XIV, Louvois was named secretary of state for war in 1662. He was responsible for creating the Order of Notre-Dame of Mount Carmel and St-Lazare to oversee the "reform" of local hospitals. He is shown here in the ceremonial dress of the order. (BN, Dépt des Estampes, C 121 929)

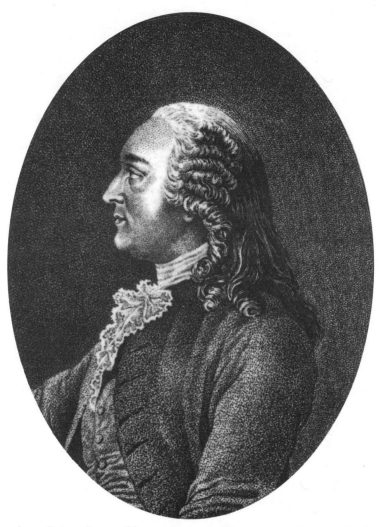

Anne-Robert-Jacques Turgot, Baron de l'Eaune, controller general of France, 1774–76. Turgot was linked to the physiocrats and was particularly interested in fiscal and welfare reform. As controller general he initiated a wide-ranging attempt to restructure charitable institutions in 1774. (BN, Dépt des Estampes, B55 461)

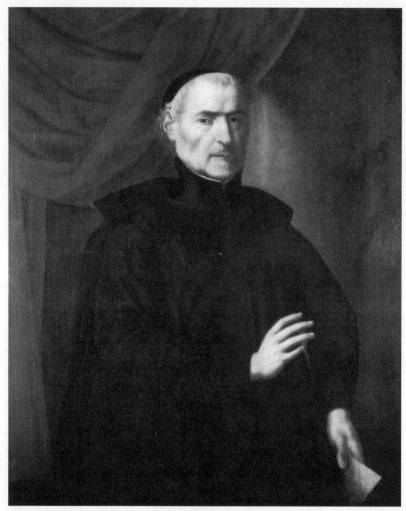

Father Honoré Chaurand, a Jesuit priest who was among the most active supporters of new structures of poor relief. From 1677 on, he visited cities and towns preaching and counselling elites to create new *hôpitaux-généraux* to reform and retrain the local poor. He worked hand in hand with two other Jesuits, Fathers Dunod and Guevarre, and with a minor nobleman from Brittany, Sieur Gabriel Calloët-Querbrat, who called himself the "avocat général des pauvres." (Musée Crozatier, Ville du Puy-en-Velay)

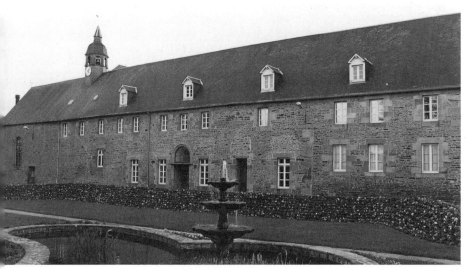

A wing of the Hôpital St-Antoine de la Charité in Pontorson. Built between 1715 and 1723, this addition was to house a chapel, a dormitory for patients, an apothecary shop, and six rooms for the Brothers of Charity.

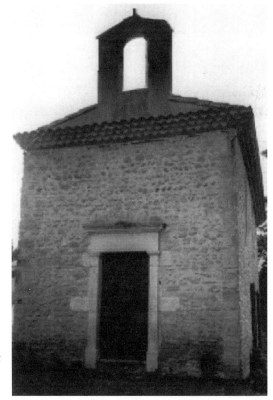

The sixteenth-century chapel of the hospital at Étoile-sur-Rhône re-established by a 1543 grant from Guillaume de Poitiers and by subsequent grants from his daughter Diane de Poitiers.

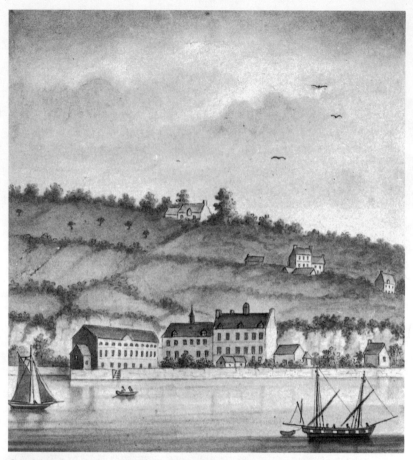

Caudebec hospital on the bank of the Seine. The drawing shows the
institution in 1827 with the 1725 construction facing the Seine on the left, the
1765 building located between the Seine and the rue de l'Hôpital on the far
right, and the original 1689 hospital structure in the middle. (Abbé Miette,
"Monuments civils et religieux et maisons particulières de Caudebec," BM
Rouen, MS Y8, vol. 1, f. 52vo)

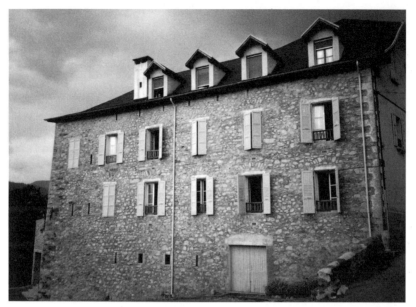

The hospital at Seyne-les-Alpes. This structure was built in 1680 as a result of the merger of the Hôpital St-Jacques and the Hôtel-Dieu.

Local Hospitals in Ancien Régime France
Rationalization, Resistance, Renewal, 1530–1789

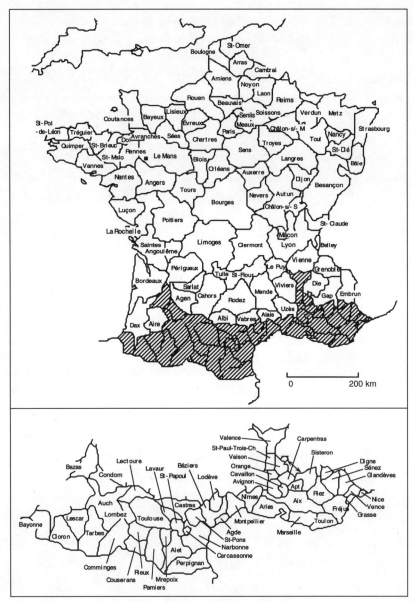

Map 1   Dioceses in France in the eighteenth century

Introduction

Small charitable institutions dotted the French kingdom at the end of the Middle Ages. Every region and most towns and villages had hospices, *léproseries*, and "hospitals." Developed out of the Christian tradition of *caritas*, these institutions had two distinctly different roots. In the cities, they had been created using the alms collected by cathedrals and episcopal seats; in the countryside, similar institutions found their origins either in the "hospitality" offered to pilgrims and travellers by abbeys and monasteries or in the efforts of communities to set up houses where lepers could be isolated from society.[1] The resulting establishments formed the basis of the hospital network that is discussed in this book.

Far from today's image of institutions aimed at healing sick patients, the different types of early modern hospitals continued to serve a disparate clientele inherited from earlier efforts to aid the poor and the sick. They offered shelter to travellers and pilgrims and assistance to different groups in need: orphans, old people, handicapped, and poor villagers, as well as the sick and dying. However, by the eighteenth century a considerable number of these hospitals, hospices, and léproseries had disappeared. Large French cities had almost all established the new *hôpitaux-généraux* where the poor, the beggars, and the undesirables were confined, or *hôtels-Dieu*, which treated the sick and the handicapped. With the creation of these new institutions, many of the smaller city, town, and village hospitals became victims of a fundamental transformation in societal values and priorities. To justify their closure, charges of corruption and inefficiency were regularly levelled at small, local hospitals by crown officials. It became more and more obvious that the rationale of centralizing services to the sick and the poor in the name of efficiency became the leitmotif in the creation of the large urban establishments.

This transformation of assistance to the poor and the sick from small, local hospitals to large urban institutions has been treated in ground-breaking research since the 1960s, but always from the point of view of the new large hospitals and centres of internment that had been created. Among the first to revise the nineteenth-century work on charity and hospitals was Michel Foucault, whose studies concentrated on the great confinement movement (*le grand renfermement*), an initiative that he traced to the "absolute monarchy" and the "urban bourgeoisie." The collaboration of these two elements produced the edict of 1656, which created the Hôpital-Général de Paris.[2] Foucault argued that through such initiatives, authorities sought to arrest and intern the mentally ill and the handicapped along with vagabonds, beggars, and all groups whom the bourgeois saw as marginal. This attempt to "exclude" and virtually imprison all the so-called deviants necessitated the creation of a network of large hôpitaux-généraux to house these groups. Once they had been interned, the personnel of these institutions sought to "reform" their new inmates according to the values of bourgeois society, instilling in them basic religious doctrines and a certain work ethic. Foucault described at length the horrors of such institutions.

His thesis has provoked considerable debate among historians. From a methodological point of view, his perceptions are seen as "revolution-ary," emphasizing historical explanation based upon practices rather than upon ideology, cultural representations, or political decisions. Concen-trating upon the practice of exclusion has led him to explore the objects of the practice, the political goals behind the movement, the relative power of different social groups, and changing economic relationships.[3] At the same time, other historians often accuse Foucault of being too selective in the construction of his arguments.[4] He is charged with losing sight of the fact that there were, in fact, two competing and often coexisting visions of hospital reform: the bourgeois-absolutist movement on which his *Folie et déraison* concentrated and also an older, more traditional approach rooted in Christian attempts to come to the aid of the poor and suffering. This latter vision was given renewed vigour by the *dévot* movement during the Catholic Reformation, but Foucault chose to ignore its influence.

Jean-Pierre Gutton, in his thesis and subsequent work, tries to integrate the two visions of reform, showing that the roots of the great confinement movement extended back to the reform-minded humanists of the sixteenth century, who built upon the medieval tradition. He argues that in 1614, long before the creation of the Hôpital-Général in Paris, the Hôtel-Dieu and La Charité in Lyon had adopted statutes regulating the internment of the poor and beggars of the city and had, in effect, begun the great confinement.[5] More recent work on the implementation of the movement in other city hospitals has been carried out, with Cissie Fairchilds working on Aix-en-Provence, Pascal Even looking at La Rochelle, and Patrice Cugnetti and Kathryn Norberg carrying out their studies of Grenoble.[6] None of this work has confirmed the horrors that have become associated with those institutions. The cold, dank cells and the "treatments" ranging from bloodletting to ice-cold baths have conjured up what Colin Jones refers to as the "black legend" of hospitals. The major elements of this discourse were developed in the eighteenth century, only to be resurrected by Foucault.[7]

Instead of confirming this "legend," recent studies have shown that hospitals took a very paternalistic approach to helping the poor and the sick, an approach strongly influenced by the charitable renewal of the Catholic Reformation. All of these studies have examined the seemingly contradictory philosophy of charity and internment, but in contrast to Foucault's arguments, they have shown that seventeenth- and eighteenth-century elites made personal sacrifices in their sincere attempts to improve the lot of the poor. These groups made donations, sought out new funds from city or crown authorities, supported the new religious orders that worked with the poor and the sick, and presided over expansions in education and charitable services.

The historiographical debate over motivations behind expanding services to the urban sick and poor has, however, lost sight of the fate of the older network of hospitals in the small cities and towns. What, in fact, happened to these small, local institutions as poor relief was transformed into urban internment? How were they affected by the great confinement movement and by the imposition of the new bourgeois moral and religious values described by Foucault? Since they were the apparent victims of crown efforts to centralize and rationalize poor relief, how did they respond to the attacks of royal officials? This book deals with the fate of these small hospitals and welfare institutions as the numerous edicts, inquiries, inspections, and reforms tried to shut down those that were viewed as redundant, corrupt, or inefficient.

In a number of different phases from the 1530s to the 1760s, crown officials concentrated, more or less successfully, on reducing the number of small hospitals. In 1266, under Louis VIII, over 2,000 leproseries alone were enumerated in the kingdom, while in 1791 a national inquiry "to determine the situation of the hôtels-Dieu, hospitals, hospices, and other institutions of charity" counted a total of 1,961 hospitals of all types in a much larger French territory than that of 1266.[8] Of the hospitals enumerated, 1,034 were in agglomerations of fewer than 2,000 inhabitants, and 768 contained ten beds or less.[9]

Although there was an evident decline in the small, local hospitals and charitable institutions operating in France, the number of them remaining in 1791 was nevertheless impressive. After two centuries of concentrated attempts to shut them down or make them accountable to regularly renewed national inquiries and reform movements, over a thousand of these hospitals were still operating. To explain in part their resistance to the attempts at closure, four recently developed historical themes will be integrated into my treatment. These themes rise out of new approaches to rural history, the Catholic Reformation, gender history, and absolutism.

The first of these revisionist themes argues that the thesis of the ineluctable and linear decline of small towns and rural areas in France has been overstated. Historians of almost every period of French history from the sixteenth century to the present have analysed the small-town and rural world in terms of the "decline," "stagnation," or "collapse" of small communities under the assault of centralization and urbanization.[10] They have described how emigration from the countryside to the cities led to the disappearance of small-town and village structures almost everywhere, and most have concluded that these changes foreshadowed the end of town- and village-based society.[11] Nevertheless, despite consistent attempts to rationalize and centralize local institutions such as hospitals and *maladreries* (institutions that grew out of léproseries), small communities continued to perpetuate social patterns and value systems different from those of the urban world.[12] Why did they do so? Given the stagnation in rural population and the progressive elimination of reinforcing structures, what explains the resistance of rural values to the assaults of centralization and urbanization?

This question forms the backdrop of the present study of charitable institutions in towns and villages. My work questions the linear "decline" of small towns and villages, arguing that their structures and institutions reacted individually to the assaults on them by agents of the central government and the cities. Their waning appears to have taken the form, not of a sudden disappearance or a long stagnation leading to a final collapse, but rather of a series of detached crises punctuated by periodic efforts at rebuilding and restructuring. The authorities of the crown and the cities directed three major centralized initiatives to shut down local hospitals, the first by using a royal commission in the period 1604–72, the second by giving a renovated hospitaller order the mandate to carry out such reforms in the years 1672–93, and the third by using crown officials to organize the fusion of small hospitals with larger institutions between 1693 and 1700. In response, community elites demonstrated great ingenuity, in some cases defying the intervention measures, resisting the proposed changes, or more often discretely continuing the old structures under new forms. Furthermore, town and village notables were not alone in this struggle, and their actions were frequently seconded by the secular and regular clergy.

The second theme that is expanded upon in this study concerns the Catholic Reformation and its role in reinforcing the church's infrastructure, including charitable services and, of course, involvement in the direction and management of local hospitals. Traditional historical work concerning the movement has emphasized the leadership of the bishops and the new missionary orders in making pastoral visits and initiating missions to "reconquer" the towns and villages of rural France.[13] As Jean Delumeau stated in the 1970s, the dynamic for change was essentially urban; both he and Alain Croix have emphasized the difficulties of the new Catholicism in penetrating the small towns and villages.[14] The charitable renewal, which became an integral part of the Catholic Reformation, began as an urban experiment frequently hostile to the more traditional approaches to poor relief practised in the local hospitals. It sought to transform the traditional custom of indiscriminate alms giving into more selective types of aid. Institutionalized assistance was seen as better suited for making the necessary distinctions between deserving and non-deserving poor, and the hôpitaux-généraux created in the cities of the kingdom became the backbone of this new policy. Despite St Vincent de Paul's initial reluctance to participate in the actions taken by this movement to organize services in the hôpitaux-généraux,[15] the Company of the Holy Sacrament and the ultra-Catholic urban dévots supported them enthusiastically. They donated time and money, lobbied for new taxes to fund the institutions, and often sought to expropriate small, local hospitals to expand their facilities.[16]

On the other hand, small-town and village benefactions were not totally forgotten by the new Catholicism. Charity was a fundamental message emphasized by the Lazarists and the new missionary orders created to evangelize small-town and rural France. In their missions, they promoted the foundation of local bureaux of charity and encouraged financial support for local relief institutions. Louis Châtellier, in his recent book, emphasizes the fact that the new orders saw the salvation of souls as inherently linked to the reduction of hunger and poverty. A fundamental aspect of the new message was to encourage parishioners to abandon the traditional indiscriminate and individual alms giving to the poor and support instead what was seen as the more efficient community institutions that had been founded to assure poor relief.[17] As far as hospitals are concerned, the new orders created by the Catholic Reformation often reinforced and reinvigorated declining local institutions; indeed, Colin Jones shows that over 60 per cent of the hospitals staffed and supported by the Daughters of Charity of St Vincent de Paul were small, local institutions.[18] Despite the urban-rural dichotomy that so many historians have perceived in the Catholic renewal, the charitable institutions of the small French towns were the clear beneficiaries of both the message and the actions of the new religious orders.

The third of the themes dealt with in this book comes from the recently developed field of gender history. In the course of the seventeenth and eighteenth centuries, the arrival of thousands of women in the public domain to work in charity and nursing provides new insights into the increasingly differentiated tasks of men and women. The period witnesses the creation of hundreds of new women's religious communities, which were encouraged by bishops, abbots, and missionaries to become involved in service in the hospitals and charitable agencies that grew up in cities, towns, and villages. Although the recent *histoire des femmes* has underscored the education of women and the opening of convent schools, its authors have practically ignored the fact that in the course of the eighteenth century in virtually every hospital in the kingdom, lay women became involved as patrons or volunteers and nuns were called in as managers or staff.[19] They replaced the men who had previously run these establishments as caretakers, wardens, or chaplains. The complex relationship developed between the missionaries, priests, and bishops who encouraged and aided the foundation of these new women's orders and the women who were drawn into them has been treated by Colin Jones for the Daughters of Charity and by Marguerite Vacher for the Sisters of St-Joseph.[20] I will be comparing their findings with case studies of two smaller orders, the Sisters of St-Thomas, founded in Brittany in 1661, and the Sisters of the Holy Sacrament, founded in the Ardèche in 1722. The virtual invasion of hospitals and charitable services by the women from orders such as these produced a new division of labour and authority for men and women in the field of charity and a considerable expansion in the services rendered to the poor and the sick.

The final revisionist theme, the centralization and rationalization of French institutions by agents of the absolute monarchy, is another of the factors mentioned by Foucault and is commonly used to explain the decline of local hospitals. It is true that the crown was at the root of most of the reform movements that sought to inspect and measure the functioning of local charitable services and to shut down and expropriate the revenues of those found to be corrupt or redundant. Christian Paultre and Léon Lallemand have underlined the leadership of the crown in determining the form and content of poor relief, and a rapid consultation of the numerous royal edicts dealing with assistance confirms the idea that the king and his officials did try to define new policies.[21] However, this context also seems to have been overemphasized, for, as Pierre Goubert has shown, the great majority of absolutist initiatives were never fully implemented. Although numerous, they were often ignored or applied half-heartedly by the myriad of local authorities in overlapping and frequently contradictory jurisdictions.[22]

In the field of hospital reform, Olwen Hufton showed that the generally ambitious crown reforms were totally unrealistic, having been proposed without considering the available financial resources or the practicability of the new structures.[23] While her criticism is often exaggerated, even the more balanced recent treatment of Jean Imbert shows that most of the centralized reforms, such as the great confinement, were difficult to implement since the establishment of the institutions was generally left to city and town governments.[24] In the welfare measures that punctuated the last half of the eighteenth century, controller generals Laverdy, Turgot, and Necker tried to strike a new balance in assistance to the poor. They played down the emphasis placed on the overambitious urban experiment, returning to the idea of locally based assistance and to the older tradition that local communities were responsible for their poor.[25] Their changes, however, conflicted directly with the ambitions of the large urban hospitals and the views of the judges, *parlementaires*, nobles, and officials who protected them. Most of the eighteenth-century efforts at hospital reform did recognize the primacy of local endeavours, but they did not resolve the problem of who was responsible for establishing priorities in such assistance, nor did they provide the funding necessary to carry out the new responsibilities given to local communities.

In presenting an analysis of the competing visions of local hospital reform, this book is divided into two parts. The first section treats the varying forms and relative successes of the long series of royal and provincial initiatives to close down redundant and corrupt local institutions. It discusses how they sought to redirect these resources to other, more pressing needs, either in support of the new hôpitaux-généraux and the growing urban medical institutions (the hôtels-Dieu) or as pensions to the aging and handicapped veterans of the French armies. The second section deals with the forces that resisted these closings and rationalizations. It examines how the enthusiasm of the missionary orders and the penetration of the message of the Catholic Reformation into the small towns and villages led to the rediscovered importance of charity that can be observed in the seventeenth and eighteenth centuries. Missionaries encouraged new forms of assistance to the poor and sick and revitalized the small hospital network. At the same time, attempts by the crown and the cities to suppress local hospitals were opposed by community elites inspired by the new Catholic message or by the fact that they had vested interests in the local poor-relief structures.

Accusations that local hospitals were rundown and poorly administered began to ring false with the arrival of the religious congregations created to staff the French hospital network. Finally, Laverdy, Turgot, and Necker, in the course of new welfare initiatives, looked into ways of reforming French poor relief in the 1760s and 1770s, distancing themselves from the great confinement movement, which they considered to have been both too costly and also unable to achieve its goals of ridding the streets of the poor. In place of this vast and unwieldy movement, the eighteenth-century reforms proposed more localized measures, better hospital structures for the sick, and workshops to put the able-bodied poor to work. They also placed greater pressure on town and village hospitals and bureaux of charity to keep the poor from leaving their communities.

These two contradictory tendencies – on the one hand, to shut down local hospitals and, on the other, to redress and rehabilitate them – will be analysed at the national, provincial, and local levels. At the national level, I have examined the available documents concerning the different crown initiatives to close local hospitals, hospices, and former leproseries or maladreries. They vary from the edicts of the sixteenth century instructing local judges to intervene to the voluminous series of closure decisions taken by the Chamber of Christian Charity (1606–10), and the Chamber of the General Hospital Reform (1611–72) and the appeals against these decisions heard by different royal tribunals. Just as abundant is the series of decisions rendered by the Chamber of the Arsenal (Chambre de l'Arsenal), created when the crown transferred the initiative for the suppressions to the Order of Mount Carmel and St-Lazare between 1672 and 1693. In addition, there are, of course, the numerous inquiries carried out by eighteenth-century commissions between 1724 and the end of the Ancien Régime.

It has been known for some time that royal edicts, inquiries, and initiatives were frequently blocked, suspended, or simply ignored at the provincial or local level. To better appreciate the effectiveness of crown attempts to close down and expropriate local hospitals, my study extends to the provincial and local levels, where I measure the impact of these decisions upon the actual functioning of local hospitals. To do so, I selected four provinces and eight local institutions. The choice was based upon a preliminary analysis of hospital closings in France under the Order of Mount Carmel and St-Lazare.[26] This examination showed that the province of Normandy, specifically the district, or généralité, of Rouen, was one of those most affected by the closure attempts and that Brittany was one of the least; both these provinces were retained as cases to be studied. Provence and Dauphiné were the two other généralités chosen because in the St-Lazare reform they both corresponded to about the normal range of closures attempted. In addition, Provence, in particular the diocese of Aix, was later cited by its intendant as having maintained exemplary local poor-relief structures.[27]

In each of these provinces, two local hospitals were selected for analysis. It was very difficult to locate small hospitals or hospices that had archives dating from the early modern period. Most of the smallest institutions were closed down during the seventeenth and eighteenth centuries, and while their legal titles and landholding records can frequently be found in the archives of the larger city hospitals that expropriated them, their financial accounts and deliberations and information about their day-to-day operations have almost all disappeared. A few towns and villages, however, did maintain their institutions in one form or another, and in these cases most of the original archives were preserved. The activities of the eight hospitals chosen will be studied in depth: four of them were in the small towns of Dauphiné and Provence in the southeastern part of the kingdom and the other four in Normandy and Brittany in the northwest (see Map 2).

For Dauphiné the study concentrates on the towns of Étoile and St-Vallier, which are both located in the plains of the Rhône valley. For Provence it analyses the functioning of Grignan, also in the Rhône valley, and the town of Seyne, high in the southern Alps. The population of these four communities varied between 1,000 and 2,000 inhabitants. About sixty kilometres to the south of Lyon, St-Vallier was estimated by Intendant Bouchu at 880 inhabitants, according to a 1698 report that he wrote for a new analysis of the *feux*, a hearth-tax census.[28] Étoile is located on the interior Rhône valley route linking Marseille with Valence and Lyon, and according to the 1699 *révision des feux*, it had roughly 2,000 inhabitants, including 350 commoner heads of family, 3 families of gentlemen, and 4 priests.[29]

Grignan, located lower down on the same highway, in reply to a 1726 ordinance by the intendant for Provence, claimed 263 commoner heads of family, 1 priest, 6 canons, and 11 dignitaries attached to the Chapter of St-Sauveur, for a total population of about 1,100.[30] Isolated in the southern Alps along a secondary commercial route linking Briançon with Digne and Cannes, Seyne listed 500 heads of families in the 1698 *affouagement*, or census, indicating approximately 2,000 inhabitants.[31]

In Normandy and Brittany the four hospitals retained for study were in towns of comparable size. Slightly larger than the southeastern towns was the Normandy centre of Caudebec-en-Caux. Situated between Le Havre and Rouen on the main road along the Seine towards Paris, the town counted 502 *feux* in 1713, 460 who paid the *taille*, the land tax levied on commoners by the crown, and 42 who were tax-exempt, representing the clergy and noblemen, for an approximate population of 2,259 inhabitants.[32] The second Normandy town, Pontorson, was at the southern extremity of the province on the main pilgrimage route leading from Brittany and the south towards nearby Mont-St-Michel. On the border of the two provinces, the town included a customs station and sixty-two houses, but the tiny bourg was dominated by the structures of the new and old hospitals and by the house of the Brothers of Charity, who ran the institution.[33] In 1713 Pontorson was evaluated at 182 *feux*, giving a rough figure of 819 inhabitants; by 1804 the population of the town had increased to 1,320.[34]

Located towards the middle of the Brittany peninsula was Malestroit, the seat of a *subdélégation* of the diocese of Vannes, which included fifteen

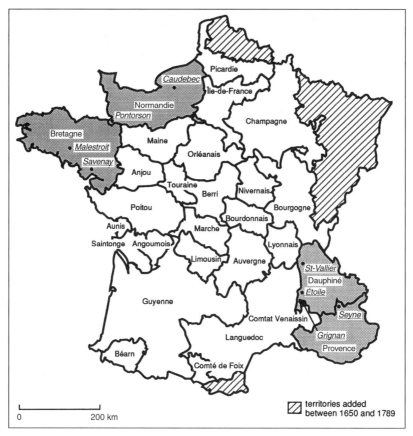

Map 2   French provinces in 1650 with the locations of communities and hospitals discussed in the text

parishes. Thirty-five kilometres from Vannes and sixty from Rennes, it controlled the highway that ran through Ploërmel and Redon to link the two larger towns. It counted 250 houses in the mid-seventeenth century, and in 1780 its mayor indicated that the town had 2,000 inhabitants.[35] Savenay, the smallest of the four northern towns, was in lower Brittany near Nantes on the route leading to Vannes. At the time that its hospital was founded in the 1450s, it had six beds, and it frequently housed pilgrims on the way towards Santiago de Compostela.[36] By 1741 the capitation rolls list 409 residents of Savenay, and by year two of the revolution (1793), this number had grown to 1,545.[37]

In analysing the evolution of poor relief at the national, provincial, and local levels, this book describes the ideological conflicts, procedural problems, and changing perspectives as the crown, the large hospitals, and the municipal governments attempted over two and a half centuries to alter the face of local poor relief. To a great extent, the attack on local hospitals came in response to increasing pressures upon the crown from both military and urban officials. The crown was anxious to solidify the support of the former for its policies by turning over to them numerous funds and holdings expropriated from the hospitals. The latter, who were attempting to deal with the increasing numbers of poor flocking to their gates, also claimed part of the spoils from the expropriated local institutions. Thus the small towns were caught in the middle. Through their efforts to maintain local institutions of poor relief, the towns illustrate the functioning of local power networks and value systems, which often took over and transformed urban poor-relief measures for their own ends. Frequently, as we shall see, these localized initiatives were the motors that provided small towns with the means to resist the closures and expropriations ordered by the king's officials, the royal commissions, and the crown edicts.

PART ONE

Beginning Hospital Reform

The welfare agencies inherited from the Middle Ages were many and varied. By the early sixteenth century, contemporary texts speak of these institutions as maladreries, hospices, almshouses, and hospitals. The maladreries had been founded between the tenth and the thirteenth centuries to confine and care for lepers; however, by the sixteenth century, the decline and virtual disappearance of leprosy had led these institutions to convert themselves to care for the local poor and handicapped. Most of the hospices had also been set up during the late Middle Ages. With the goal of housing pilgrims and travellers, they had originally been attached to monasteries or convents whose administrators saw their role as according hospitality to those in need. That role had been continued as the hospices gave shelter to itinerants as well as the local poor. The same monasteries and convents had been responsible for starting almshouses, which generally provided simple handouts to the poor. From the early Middle Ages the monasteries had received grants and legacies from which they distributed bread and money at their gates during Easter week, at Pentecost, and on certain weekdays during the winter months. The term "hospital" was less precise in its origins and had a tendency to encompass the functions of the other three types of foundations. Despite their differing origins, sixteenth-century officials tended to regroup all these institutions under the generic term "hospital," seeing them as essentially responsible for the poor and sick of the kingdom.

At the same time, one of the principal preoccupations of crown and municipal authorities had become the migration of peasants and vagabonds towards the major cities of the kingdom. Having left their villages behind, these individuals tended to become scapegoats for all the violence and disorder that occurred in the major cities. Nicolas Versoris, lawyer in the Parlement of Paris, expresses this perception in his analysis of disturbances in that city in 1524: "Because of the presence in Paris of bad boys [*mauvais garçons*] and large bands of adventurers, who committed innumerable minor crimes, stealing all that they could, and major crimes such as murders, illegal assemblies, looting, etc., on Monday 23 May and the day after the Trinity, the crier for the Court ... [announced] that within twenty-four hours all adventurers who did not want to earn their living honestly should leave Paris."[1] Similar decrees and edicts were published regularly in this period, indicating the increasing problem posed by immigrants, vagabonds, and marginals in large cities such as Paris.[2]

These urban difficulties led city and crown officials to examine more closely the institutions for the poor in small towns and villages. If, according to their charters, they were supposed to house and feed the handicapped and indigent population of their regions, why were so many of these groups flocking to the gates of the large cities? The officials began to wonder why the traditional safety net for the poor was not working. In the course of the sixteenth and seventeenth centuries, a number of inquiries were launched into the functioning of these local hospitals, and new orientations were given to charitable action.

1 Changes in the Organization and Direction of Town and Village Charity, 1540–1640

On 15 October 1548 an ordinance of the Parlement of Brittany gave the Hôtel-Dieu of Nantes supervisory rights over all the hospitals in the diocese of Nantes. Using those powers, the bureau of the Hôtel-Dieu ordered the Hôpital St-Armal in the town of Savenay to replace the priest in charge with a lay administrator.[1] Seven years later an order-in-council stipulated that the Savenay hospital was to be "united" with the Hôtel-Dieu of Nantes, thereby depriving the parish of its right to select the administrator. The text declared that in the future the institution would be governed by the *recteur*, the *sénéchal*, and the treasurer of the town. They were to submit their accounts to the directors of the Hôtel-Dieu.[2] However, these interventions produced limited results, for only during the next four years did the Savenay recteur actually present his accounts to the directors in Nantes, and from 1580 on, a priest was once again the recteur of St-Armal.

The attempt to place the St-Armal hospital under the control of the city of Nantes was typical of a wave of sixteenth-century initiatives aimed at strengthening urban charitable institutions that were besieged with demands for aid from peasants migrating to the cities in search of work or handouts. In Nantes the lack of space in the hospital forced the city council to look for new revenues in order to create an annex to house the increasing number of sick – victims of contagious diseases and epidemics. The expansion was eventually undertaken near the Ste-Catherine cemetery. At the same time the Parlement of Brittany gave the Nantes administration rights over the hospitals of Ancenis, Bouin, Bourgneuf, La Chappelle-Glain, Loroux-Bottereau, Plessé, Pontchâteau, Machecoul, St-Père-en-Retz, and St-Julien-de-Vouvantes, as well as Savenay. These transfers were an obvious attempt to provide the Hôtel-Dieu with the means to obtain the new funding that it needed, eventually by expropriating the holdings and funds of the smaller institutions.[3]

Cities of the kingdom were becoming particularly hostile to the traditional forms of charity that attracted vagabonds and beggars identified as possible carriers of disease and harbingers of social turmoil. They sought new means to centralize and reorganize poor relief; one way was to obtain greater control over the revenues and holdings of foundations such as the Savenay hospital. A debate started between those who defended traditional, indiscriminate alms and care to all needy – the type of aid dispensed by Savenay – and those who wanted to abandon indiscriminate handouts and concentrate upon the creation of more efficient institutions to serve the sick and needy poor who were flocking to the cities.

In most of the large cities such as Nantes, the dangers of periodic epidemics were exacerbated by memories of the role played by the poor in revolts and explosions of social violence. It was the combination of these factors that brought the cities of early modern France to adopt a new approach to social welfare. In 1531 Lyon set up a temporary agency to distribute bread to the needy in an attempt to avoid any more disturbances like the violent *grand rebeine*, a localized uprising two years earlier that had pitted the poor against the rich. This new agency, the Aumône Générale, became a permanent institution in 1534. Despite its goal of "nourishing the poor forever," the new assistance was offered only to registered city residents, and the Lyon councillors made a conscious threefold decision: to aid townspeople in difficulty, to refuse entry to beggars and vagabonds, and to evict those newcomers who merely sought handouts.[4]

Four years later neighbouring Grenoble sought to reorganize its assistance along the lines of the Lyon reform. Just as in that city, the initiative followed upon outbreaks of plague and two decades of efforts to drive out beggars and vagabonds. In 1538 it was decided that the city would take over the organization of assistance to the poor, that the three-hundred-odd poor beggars in Grenoble would be placed in a hospital, and that the four existing city hospitals would become integrated under the control of a central relief agency, the bureau of the poor (*bureau des pauvres*). Again in the face of an epidemic that broke out in 1544–45, a monthly tax was instituted to support the hospital as well as to aid the poorer inhabitants, and it was decided to prepare a street census of the city poor from which it could be determined who would be eligible for such relief and who would be driven out.[5]

In Normandy, Rouen too followed this pattern in reorganizing its poor relief, and in a 1534 city council debate, orators referred specifically to the Lyon experiment. Robert Billy, president of the Parlement of Rouen, argued for energetic measures to counter begging and vagrancy. Replying to the traditionalists who upheld the Christian notion of indiscriminate charity, he noted that many vagrants and common criminals pretended to be poor, but lived as parasites from thievery, robbery, and charity. They took the bread from the mouths of the true poor, those whom every community was committed to feed.[6] A basic principle of the early modern reform of assistance was spelled out in the Rouen debate when it was argued that if the phoney poor were rooted out, there would be sufficient funds to support those truly in need.

The assembly accepted this principle, and it was decided that within eight days all inhabitants of Rouen who were able to work, but who had neither a regular job nor other revenues, should either leave the city or enrol with a master. At the end of the eight-day period the bailiff was to order the arrest of all vagrants remaining in the city. They were to be chained together and forced to carry out public works to earn their daily bread. All public begging, even by the sick and handicapped, was to be forbidden. Commissioners in each parish were to establish lists of the poor who should receive public relief, and a treasurer, named by the city authorities, was to organize collections and distribute the funds received among those officially recognized as poor. This structure was set up in Rouen, and the first listing of those to receive assistance was carried out. It showed that there were over 7,000 truly poor and "miserable" and that only 532 able beggars and vagrants had been identified for expulsion. The finances of the city allowed it to support no more than about 150 of its poor; therefore, beyond trying to enforce its decrees against begging, even at this early stage Rouen clearly did not have the means to aid its deserving poor effectively.[7]

Besides the evident desire to limit the number of newcomers to the cities, control epidemics and plague, and restrict begging and vagrancy, what were the theoretical arguments proposed by the advocates for the reform of poor relief? Earlier historians often portrayed these reforms as "Lutheran" or Protestant-inspired, but Natalie Davis has shown that the fundamental influences upon the founders and upon the guiding principles behind Lyon's Aumône Générale came from humanist sources –

the idea expressed in Renaissance writings that human beings were inherently good and capable of being re-educated and reformed. The initiators of the Aumône sought to eliminate the causes of poverty and mendicity not only by supplying upkeep but also by aiming at a more permanent rehabilitation of the poor by providing education and stimulating the creation of jobs in the textile and silk trades. To do so, the Aumône Générale of Lyon followed the earlier example of Ypres and created a government body to centralize all charitable services. It discouraged handouts by private citizens or religious groups and demanded that all sums of money or aid traditionally distributed to the poor and sick by monasteries, parishes, or hospices be turned over to the administrators of the new central agency.[8]

The large city hospitals of the kingdom put forward global reforms that contrasted with the practices of traditional poor relief. For example, the charter of the small Savenay hospital encouraged the customary alms giving, even permitting its inmates to go from house to house begging for food.[9] Typical of the more traditional form of hospice that the reformers were seeking to eliminate, institutions such as Savenay continued to dispense alms indiscriminately and care for the "sick poor," the "mentally retarded" of the community, and poor itinerants. Such hospitals showed little interest in the humanist vision of rehabilitating the poor and instilling in them the basic Christian moral values and a work ethic.

A second preoccupation that is evident in the acts giving the Nantes hospital control over Savenay reflects another, larger debate over assistance in the kingdom. Municipal and royal officials viewed with increasing suspicion the control by priests or religious orders of charitable foundations, hospitals, and small centres of care (maladreries). For that reason, the 1548 ordinance directed Savenay to elect a lay administrator. Town officials in the nearby community of Vitré went before the Parlement in 1549 to take control of the St-Nicolas hospital from the Priory of St-Nicolas,[10] and in 1548 the city of Angers in Maine obtained control of its Hôpital St-Jean-l'Évangéliste from the Augustinians, who had directed the institution since its foundation in 1175.[11] By their actions, these towns were following a trend begun in the late fifteenth century when the city councils of both Paris and Lyon took over the administration of their hospitals from religious orders.[12]

Jean Imbert argues that this tendency of cities, towns, and villages to assume control of their charitable institutions does not really indicate their laicization, since the establishments generally remained staffed by religious orders. In some cases, the clergy even supported the takeover and reorganization by municipal authorities. For Imbert, this movement indicates a municipalization of poor relief, rather than an actual laicization.[13] His argument is consistent with Natalie Davis's position that humanist-inspired municipal leaders became more aware of the close links between immigration, criminality, and poverty. The takeover of poor-relief institutions by these towns and cities was generally carried out within the context of a fundamental reform designed to make the establishments more responsive to community needs.

Another important element in the desire of cities and towns to control their institutions of charity was the widespread belief that the resources devoted to charity were being badly managed in small traditional hospices. The order against the religious direction of the Hôpital St-Armal of Savenay illustrates this preoccupation, and it reflects the local application of a long series of royal edicts and decrees issued throughout the sixteenth century. In 1543 an edict from François 1 referred specifically to the widespread nature of this problem:

the great disorder present in the maladreries and leproseries of the kingdom founded by our predecessors, kings, dukes, counts, barons, and other lords as well as by other good, devout, and faithful Christians, towns, religious chapters, and communities, whose foundations have been usurped, titles and charters lost or stolen by absentee administrators and governors of maladreries, who ignored their mandates and leased out the fruits and revenues of their institutions, abandoning the buildings in ruin and decadence, starving and driving out the poor sick and lepers ... [who] desert their towns and become beggars in other cities and towns.[14]

The edict went on to order that the local circuit judges (*juges ordinaires*) visit the maladreries and leproseries of their jurisdiction, inspect their charters, titles, and financial accounts, look into their management, and determine when and to whom their accounts were to be presented. When irregularities were found, the judges were to discharge incompetent and dishonest administrators and replace them with two new governors from among the honest, solvent bourgeois, to be named or elected by the community. These new administrators were to take over management of the revenues of the institution and present their accounts annually to the officials of the town or village.[15]

A royal edict published two years later went even further and was specifically directed against hospitals controlled by religious orders; it contended that they were even more poorly directed than the majority of the smaller hospitals. The edict claimed that the administrators and prelates who governed these institutions often ignored the intentions of their founders and constantly tried to redirect holdings and funds towards themselves or members of their religious community. Under the pretext that they possessed the title to the endowment, the religious communities claimed that they could determine how it was to be used. According to the king, this attitude often led them to "defraud" the poor, refusing them the food and subsistence that was their due and driving them towards the cities of the kingdom, where collections had to be made to feed the hordes of new immigrants. Once again, he asked local justice officials to visit the hospitals in their jurisdictions and look into these abuses. In cases of corruption or refusal to collaborate, they were to name new administrators and place the hospitals under the control of town or village officials.[16]

A year later, in 1546, in an edict issued from Rochefort, the king asked local justice officials to appoint administrators for the small, local hospitals of each judicial district (*bailliage* and *sénéchaussée*), effectively removing religious officials from their positions of direction.[17] These decisions apparently provided the legal grounds for the Hôtel-Dieu at Nantes to take control of Savenay in 1555. However, as in the case of Savenay, justice officials in very few other areas seem to have carried out the royal edicts, and few local hospitals were actually affected by this municipalization movement.

All these edicts on hospital reorganization were repeated at regular intervals throughout the sixteenth century, an indication of the difficulties that the crown faced in reforming small, local hospitals.[18] The abuses referred to in these documents appear to have become a preoccupation of the church as well as of crown officials, and they were specifically addressed by the bishops assembled at the Council of Trent. At the twenty-second session of the council on 17 September 1562, it was decided that bishops should oversee all hospitals and ensure that they were well and faithfully governed by their administrators. And on 3 December the following year, the twenty-fifth session called on bishops to visit the hospitals of their dioceses in person; they should be presented with the financial accounts of the administrators of these institutions, who in cases of fraud or corruption should be called upon to repay the embezzled funds or face canonical censure.[19] As in the case of the royal edicts, these ringing declarations of the Council of Trent were aimed at improving ecclesiastical management of charitable institutions, but they were very rarely implemented and generally remained hollow declarations of intent.

The interventions of provincial, municipal, and town officials in the field of aid to the poor resulted in the most important structural changes to take place in sixteenth-century hospital jurisdictions. In addition to the reform of city charity, one of the clearest indications of these new initiatives was the creation of a tax, a twenty-fourth of the tithe (*vingt-quatrième partie de la dîme*), to aid the poor in the small towns and villages of the province of Dauphiné. Convinced that the church was not carrying out its role in helping the poor of the province, the Parlement of Grenoble on 29 April 1564 ordered that "a twenty-fourth of the goods and revenues of the clergy [the tithe] will be turned over and distributed to the poor of each parish annually, without any exception, and placed in the hands of able and competent individuals."[20]

As René Favier argues, this ordinance addressed both the particular context of Dauphiné and the general problem posed by the influx of poor town and village inhabitants in all the urban areas of the kingdom. Dauphiné had been hard hit by the initial outbreaks of violence that marked the beginnings of the French Wars of Religion. From 1562 on, rebel troops under the direction of the Baron des Adrets had conducted raids and sieges that had particularly devastated the villages in the Rhône valley. These raids and the insecurity of the exposed towns and villages led peasants to seek refuge in the walled towns and cities of the province, establishing a pattern that was repeated regularly during the following forty years of civil warfare.[21] Setting aside a twenty-fourth of the tithe to be distributed to the poor was one way to try to provide for the peasants in their villages and stem immigration to the cities.

This measure also corresponded closely to solutions envisaged by the crown for dealing with the exodus of rural poor in the kingdom as a whole. In the edicts ordering that local justice officials inspect small-town and village hospitals, it was implicitly understood that local communities should put their charities in order so that they could care for their own poor and sick inhabitants. Two years after the Grenoble initiative, this principle was clearly stated in the Edict of Moulins (1566). The king ordered that the funds of local and rural hospitals be "truly spent for the poor" and that "the poor of each city, town, and village should be fed and cared for by those of the city, town, or village of which they are natives and residents, so that they will not wander off and request aid elsewhere."[22] The text went on to state that the inhabitants of each community should contribute to feed their poor, each according to its ability, and that the collections should be carried out under the supervision of the mayors, councillors, consuls, and parish officials. If the poor needed treatment for their illnesses in town or city hospitals, they should obtain a certificate to that effect before leaving their village.[23]

The Dauphiné measure clearly conformed to the general intentions of the crown, but it went even further than the Edict of Moulins. Rather than establishing a general tax on all inhabitants, the Parlement of Grenoble placed the onus squarely upon the clergy to meet the needs of the poor. It is true that aiding the poor was a traditional obligation of the medieval church, a duty repeated in the deliberations of the Council of Trent. Besides, a twenty-fourth was far below the level of a quarter of the tithe, which had been recommended for the poor in canon law.[24] At the same time, the traditional obligations of the church towards the poor were probably no longer respected in most dioceses and parishes. The Wars of Religion were particularly devastating in Dauphiné since church lands and holdings were confiscated by Protestant and Catholic communities and by the "captains of war," the military commanders of both religious persuasions. In other cases, they were auctioned off to meet the heavy *décime* taxes that the crown levied on the church in the years 1578–95. The work of Ivan Cloulas illustrates how the dioceses of Die, Embrun, and Grenoble were among the most adversely affected by such operations.[25] Most parishes could not even meet the reduced level of support for the poor represented by the newly created twenty-fourth.

In the early seventeenth century, the province began a new campaign to try to enforce payment of the twenty-fourth. A ordinance issued on 13 May 1620 asked each community to establish a list of its poor and beggars and to distribute a pound and a half of bread to them each week up to the time of the harvest. The money for this distribution was to be taken from the revenues of the twenty-fourth, "which should have been distributed last year and in previous years and for this reason they [the clergy] should be forced to pay [arrears on these sums] for their ecclesiastics, farmers, and receivers."[26] Regulations concerning the payment and distribution of the twenty-fourth became more and more precise. The original 1564 ordinance had specified that "a twenty-fourth of the fruits and revenues of the clergy shall be turned over to and distributed to the poor of each parish every year without exception and placed in the hands of able and capable people."[27] The clause "able and capable people" led to the directive that in each parish, the priest, the consuls, and the *châtelain* should be charged with drawing up a list of the poor to receive aid and furthermore, that they should revise the list regularly.

Rather than bread, the aid generally took the form of grain, usually rye, which was supposed to be distributed in the presence of the priest, the consuls, and the châtelain.[28] These edicts were repeated and reconfirmed in 1626, 1648, and 1675, but the seventeenth-century intendants complained regularly that priests and villages were not living up to their obligations to distribute the twenty-fourth.

The charitable reforms of the early modern period tried to deal with two major preoccupations. First, there was an evident desire to come to the aid of the poor in the cities, small towns, and villages of the kingdom. The period witnessed considerable new interest in charitable institutions, and under the impetus of humanist values, municipal leaders tried to render them more efficient. The heart of the reform was the attempt to distinguish between the beggars who could work, what the Elizabethan poor laws in England were to term "sturdy beggars," and the real sick and disabled. The projects sought to eliminate assistance to the first group and to reorganize aid to provide more effective assistance to the second. These efforts to increase the efficiency of charitable interventions led authorities to look more closely at traditional forms of aid – maladreries, hospices, and periodic charities – as well as at the management of these institutions by religious orders. Secondly, the reforms were aimed at stemming the flow of migrants from the villages and towns towards the overcrowded cities of the kingdom. The onus was placed on small communities to restructure their welfare institutions in order to be able to provide for their own poor. Once again, the functioning of local charities came into question. The creation of the twenty-fourth part of the tithe for the poor in Dauphiné was a clear example of an initiative to shore up the welfare structures of the small towns and villages.

As innovative as the twenty-fourth may have been, it was an isolated gesture, and the vast majority of regions in the kingdom, including Dauphiné, continued to depend on the traditional charities – maladreries, hospices, hospitals, and almshouses – to support the poor and sick. Royal administrators tended to lump all these institutions together, targeting all of them as wasteful and outdated, monopolizing revenues that could be more effectively used elsewhere. This perception was deeply rooted, as was the increasing conviction that the local reform ordered in the numerous royal edicts had never been carried out. To what extent did this perception of corruption and redundancy correspond to reality in the small hospitals of the kingdom? Obviously, they were considered to be badly managed; at the same time, the crown felt that they possessed sizeable revenues and holdings that could put to better use. In fact, how did these small foundations function? Did they simply continue the medieval practices of indiscriminate charity, or was there a perceptible evolution in the services that they offered to the poor?

The variety of different institutions and the diverse approaches to charity in small, local hospitals has often been underscored.[29] Of the eight cases dealt with in this book, no two were exactly the same. The charitable organizations of the southeast tended to be more under the control of municipal governments. Each of the towns in Dauphiné and Provence had relatively similar poor-relief structures, and their charters reflected the medieval concept of indiscriminate charity and the multiple services that were to be rendered by these foundations. In each of the communities, a recteur, or director of services to the poor, was elected each year at the same time as the *consulat*, the governing body of the municipality. These recteurs presided over a group of the community elite who made up the bureau of the poor. In each town, such structures were supposed to assure four basic services to the poor: shelter, health care, food or grain distributions, and aid to poor girls and members of the elite who had fallen on hard times.

As to providing shelter, hospitals served both itinerants and the local population. To the poor vagabonds (*passants*), they were to offer hand-outs in the form of money or hospitality; sick vagabonds could be cared for in the hospice for four or five days before being sent or carried away. For the local poor, the institution was to offer shelter to the sick and needy, generally to abandoned or illegitimate children and sick or dying women. In the early period, health services rarely extended beyond providing shelter and elementary care for the sick and dying – bringing in a doctor when needed and preparing herb teas and broths – but later some of the hospitals would expand this function. As for providing food or grain, the administrators of the institution were to draw up lists of the local poor who should benefit from such distributions during the winter and spring months or, as in the case of Grignan, twelve months a year. Finally, as concerned aid to poor girls and what they saw as the honourable poor (*pauvres honteux*), they sought to furnish money for the dowries that would allow girls to marry who otherwise might turn to prostitution and to assist secretly those families who had always been self-sufficient but who, as a result of crop failure or other problems, had fallen into debt and poverty.

To provide these services, each of the hospitals had buildings, endowments, and property. The hospital in Étoile, La Charité, had been receiving the poor since the 1300s, but its modern foundation dated from a grant in 1545 of 356 ecus from Comte Guillaume de Poitiers; it was to be used for the internment of thirteen sick poor, for whom care was calculated at 18 deniers a day.[30] His daughter Diane, Comtesse d'Étoile, the mistress to Henri II, added another 500 livres to the hospital endowment in 1564.[31] In 1724 the Étoile hospital consisted of an old, two-storey house with a kitchen, a room for the caretaker, two bedrooms – one for the men, the other for the women, each with six beds and a fireplace – and a third small bedroom with a fireplace for passing ecclesiastics or distinguished poor. In addition to this building, La Charité owned a chapel, a courtyard, and a garden, all located outside the bourg.[32]

Similar facilities existed in Grignan. The town had possessed a medieval hospital and a leproserie, but the seventeenth-century hospital had been re-established, like that of Étoile, through a later grant. In 1444 Dame Alix Auriol had bequeathed a dwelling in the bourg near the old oven to house the poor.[33] By 1588 the foundation had received enough grants to build a new hospital outside the walls of the town to replace the 1444 house, which had become too small. Just as in Étoile, the local nobles were the principal benefactors, and each generation of the counts of Adhémar donated considerable sums of money to the Grignan hospital.[34] Louis d'Adhémar, Comte de Grignan, himself served as *recteur des pauvres* from 1662 to his death in 1668, and under his direction a permanent caretaker was hired.[35] Nevertheless, the Grignan facilities seem to have been more primitive than those at Étoile, and the 1665 accounts note the purchase of blankets and four straw mattresses, which the bishop of Die had ordered the hospital to acquire during his pastoral visit to the town the previous year.[36] In 1676, when new rules and regulations for the institution were adopted, there were still only four mattresses, two in the upstairs rooms and two downstairs for vagabonds.[37]

The hospital structure in Seyne illustrates one of the problems inherent in individual and indiscriminate charity. At the beginning of the seventeenth century, the town actually supported two welfare structures: the Hôpital St-Jacques, whose origins could be traced back to a 1293 grant, and the Hôtel-Dieu, which had been founded prior to the fifteenth century. Each of these institutions had separate administrations and frequently duplicated services to the poor. In 1656 the town council convened a general assembly to unite the two institutions, and in 1680 the councillors approved the construction of a new hospital building.[38]

These three southeastern institutions clearly fit into the context of "municipal" charitable organizations, where the towns maintained control over the internal functioning and management of hospital lands and revenues, as well as over the distribution of charity and aid to the sick and poor. The members of the town council selected the recteur of the poor from among the town elite, and he in turn presided over the leasing out of hospital lands and the purchasing of grain from the townspeople for distribution to the poor. The whole operation was financed from landholdings and funds that had been donated to the hospitals by noble families and ordinary townspeople. It is evident that the hospitals benefited considerably from the increased generosity that resulted from the activity of disciples of the Catholic Reformation in the middle and late seventeenth century.

The St-Vallier hospital, the fourth of the southeastern institutions to be examined, was founded later and was a direct result of the renewed interest in charity that characterized religious revival during the Catholic Reformation. St-Vallier had had a maladrerie, La Maison St-Antoine, outside its walls to house victims of the plague and lepers, but by the end of the sixteenth century, the institution seems to have died out, even though a 1607 document in the hospital archives recalls the obligation of the prior of St-Ruf to provide substantial alms payments to the poor of the town.[39] The renewed interest in charity can be traced to a mission in the town in 1639 by a Lazarist priest, Abbé Gernus. He grouped together a number of young women from St-Vallier into a charitable confraternity (Confrérie de la Charité) similar to the one founded twenty years earlier at Châtillon-les-Dombes by his mentor, St Vincent de Paul. After electing a president and a treasurer, this confraternity began taking up regular collections in St-Vallier, investing a certain amount of its revenues and starting regular distributions of food and money to the poor.[40]

Building upon this organization in 1670, Abbé Jean-Antoine de Bret, superior of the Priory of St-Vallier, turned over to the confraternity an annuity of 2,000 livres, producing an annual revenue of 100 livres.[41] This money was used to reconstruct a building that would serve as a hospital on the banks of the Galure river, but a document from the group noted that the finances of the institution were still insufficient because "not only do they [the poor] not have beds, or even straw mattresses to sleep on, but the building is open on all sides ... they have no one to attend to them and distribute at regular times the food that is donated by the ladies of the town."[42] This situation changed after 1675 when the successor to Abbé de Bret as prior, Jean-Baptiste de Lacroix-Chevrières, took an intense interest in the hospital. From the archbishop of Vienne, he obtained two Sisters of St-Joseph, to whom he personally furnished an annual revenue of 150 livres. In 1683 he presided over a confraternity meeting, setting up new rules and regulations for the hospital.[43] Having been named bishop of Quebec in 1685, Mgr de St-Vallier gave another grant of 2,000 livres to the hospital before leaving for New France. He and his family continued to support the financial needs of the institution.

The charitable structures of the four towns in Normandy and Brittany that have been analysed differed considerably from their counterparts in Dauphiné and Provence. Although the services to the poor and sick offered by the four northwestern hospitals were similar in nature, these institutions were organized differently and were less controlled by their respective municipal governments. They depended far more upon sporadic collections by charitable associations for the financing of their operations. These differences are evident at Caudebec, where the 1612 returns of the hospital indicate that the revenues and expenses of three separate institutions had been combined into one account. The Ste-Anne hospital, officially recognized by the Parlement of Rouen in 1538, had been founded through a grant made in 1533 by Jehan Houel, one of the *élus* for the *élection*, or administrative district, of Caudebec. At that time, he gave the town a parcel of land containing a mansion, houses, courtyard, gardens, and other buildings near the fort of the Mordière, bordered on one side by the walls of the town and on the other by the Ambion river. The grant stipulated that the buildings be used to found a hospital for the sick poor and that a chapel be built on the premises, where a mass was to be said every Sunday for the soul of the donor. Besides Houel, Maître Guillaume Letraulles, lieutenant of the *vicomté* of Caudebec, Guillaume Leroux, lieutenant for the seigneur of Caudebec, and the *bailli* of Caux had participated in founding the Ste-Anne hospital.[44] It retained a certain autonomy until the sale of its buildings in 1753, but after 1616 its financial accounts were united under a single treasurer named by the town consuls. He became responsible for the financial accounts of the chapels of St-Pierre and St-Maur, the St-Julien hospital, and the bureau of the poor.[45]

If Ste-Anne had been founded as a municipal hospital to cater principally to the poor of the town, the oldest of the Caudebec institutions, St-Julien, was in the hands of religious authorities in the sixteenth century. These authorities named a prior to direct the institution. The hospital seems to have dated from a donation made in 1200 by Sieur Rochard de Villequiet, Marquis de Bebec, and from an act by Henry, king of France and England, in which the institution was accorded rights over "dead wood" in the forests to provide heat for the poor and rights to pasture land for hospital livestock.[46] The treasurer (*contrôleur*), who administered the institution, was named by the prior and approved by the town's judges and councillors. Resentment against the control exercised by religious authorities may have been one of the reasons that the Parlement, in approving the charter of Ste-Anne, specified in 1538 that the new hospital was not to be placed in ecclesiastical hands. When the buildings of St-Julien burned down in 1562, an act had to be issued to force the prior or chaplain of the institution to continue distributing alms to the poor from its revenues, supplying straw for the poor to sleep on in the chapel, and providing them with wood from the forests. The buildings of the hospital were not rebuilt until 1614, under the administration of Maître Denis Arouel.[47]

The third institution, the bureau of the poor, dated from early in the seventeenth century and was founded to aid itinerants who were refused by both the town hospitals. It consisted of only a *caisse*, a fund managed by the town curé, and was made up of money collected by the Dames de Charité outside the parish church for distribution to the needy.[48] After the 1685 reconstruction and enlarging of the St-Julien hospital on the rue des Capucins, the majority of the poor and sick were housed there, and the buildings of the Ste-Anne hospital were rented out and eventually sold in 1755.

The organization of the two principal Caudebec hospitals demonstrates a mixture of private and municipal initiatives in their founding. Although St-Julien remained nominally in the hands of a prior throughout the sixteenth century, municipal authorities intervened increasingly to ensure its proper functioning. Besides ordering him to continue services to the poor in 1538, the town councillors obtained an order from the Parlement in 1614 giving them the right to inspect the accounts of the hospital and to confirm the nomination of its treasurer.[49] These new powers seem to have led to the appointment of a single treasurer for the two hospitals in 1616 and to the consolidation of the financial accounts of the institutions.

At the same time that the functioning of the hospitals in Caudebec illustrates a mixture of private and municipal initiatives both in the management and in the financing of services to the poor and sick, the St-Antoine hospital in Pontorson faced a clear takeover by a religious order. Founded in 1115 by the bourgeois from the town, it received several substantial donations during the eleventh and twelfth centuries. In 1347 a town meeting, which turned over another 1,200 livres to the institution, set up a governing structure in which a prior-chaplain, as at St-Julien in Caudebec, was charged with overseeing the distribution of alms in return for an annual stipend of 200 livres.[50] The building and holdings of the hospital suffered badly during the Hundred Years War, and the sixteenth-century register listing hospital property was never completed. In 1644 the holdings that remained were worth only about 800 livres, and according to a 1503 agreement, the institution was to be placed in the hands of a prior, a "worthy person," approved by both the bourgeois of Pontorson and the bishop of Dol.[51] From 1503 to 1644 the prior was always a priest who received a stipend for his position and usually engaged a caretaker to run the institution.

The minutes of an inspection of the hospital on 25 October 1644 by Vicomte Louis Bodin, mayor and judge of the town, René Mynier, treasurer, and Pierre Gervais, clerk, show that town authorities felt that the management of the hospital had deteriorated and that the institution had become a simple refuge frequented "night and day" by "large numbers of delinquents, such as soldiers who had deserted their companies pretending to be crippled and also numerous indolent men, vagabonds, and escapees accompanied by prostitutes, in whose company under the pretext of asking for alms as poor outsiders, they enter the hospital with the above-mentioned women and spend the night drinking, singing, dancing, and leading depraved lives."[52] It was also noted that the prior and caretaker passed their time quarrelling over whose cider should be sold to inmates of the hospital and to the public. The caretaker had begun selling a cheaper, competing cider, but the prior claimed that he possessed rights over all sales made in his institution.

The report on the inspection also described the physical condition of the hospital. The caretaker lived at the institution with his family and received 20 livres a year for his services. The building over which he presided consisted of three rooms, two of which were reserved for the poor. The first of these contained five old beds without curtains, sheets, or blankets and covered only with straw. The second held three beds made of poor-quality wood that were just as uncomfortable as the other five. The third room housed the caretaker and his family. During their visit, the delegation found a poor fifteen- or sixteen-year-old boy sick with fever and covered with straw in the first room; in the second were two men and a woman who claimed to be from Picardy.[53]

This inspection of the hospital buildings, with its emphasis upon the deplorable state of the institution, was made a few days after the town government of Pontorson had concluded an agreement with the Brothers of Charity of St John of God by which the latter took over the management and operations of the hospital. It appears that Louis XIV, in a letter to the town authorities on 22 August 1644, had asked that they "consent" to placing their institution in the hands of the brothers. The document concluded between Brother Bourtil, representing the vicar-general of the religious community, and the town representative committed the brothers "to administer, govern, and direct the ... chapel and hospital, its holdings and revenues forever and to admit, nourish, heal, and administer medicine to the poor sick from both inside and outside the town, but especially townspeople, as well as they can and even to shelter the poor vagabonds for one night only, unless they are sick."[54] Charged with the upkeep of the hospital and chapel, the brothers were to pay the traditional stipend of 200 livres a year to the prior and 100 livres to Notre-Dame church for a preacher. The contract forbade them to take up collections in the town to support the hospital, and it specified that the bourgeois from Pontorson were to retain their title of "patrons and founders of the hospital."

This takeover of the Pontorson hospital by the Brothers of Charity was but one local example of an important change in the direction of town and village hospitals throughout the kingdom. The new religious orders created during the Catholic Reformation directed their members towards involvement in the world. Besides evangelizing and conducting missions in the most remote areas of the kingdom, the orders addressed their activities to service and action in the fields of education, charity, and health. Their involvement in the latter two sectors fundamentally changed the organization and functioning of large and small hospitals everywhere. Reflecting the more professional approach of these orders, the brothers who took over Pontorson immediately reorganized the existing three rooms: the first, with four beds, was reserved for the sick, the second, with another four beds, for the traditional itinerants, and the third room for the brothers as a bedroom, kitchen, library, and pharmacy.[55]

If Caudebec and Pontorson give an idea of the newer tendencies in aid to the poor – in the first case, towards the consolidation of charitable institutions and in the second case, the involvement of newly founded religious orders in the management of hospitals – the small hospitals at Savenay and Malestroit in lower Brittany retained a profoundly traditional approach in their organization and functioning. Located at a crossroads linking routes between Blain, Nantes, St-Nazaire, and Pontchâteau, Savenay had become a traditional stopping-off point for travellers, and as early as the twelfth century, a hospice had been set up to lodge them. The first real hospital was established in the town around 1450, when Jean de Château-Giron, canon at the Nantes cathedral and recteur of the parish of Savenay, left the buildings and funds to finance what became the St-Armal hospital.[56]

In the act of foundation, Canon Château-Giron specified that the hospital was never to become an ecclesiastical living, but that the chaplain-administrator of the institution was to be a "worthy" man from the town and if not a priest, at least a member of a religious order. He was to be elected by the recteur and the parish wardens (*marguilliers*) and was to present a report on the hospital finances annually before the directors of the institution. As revenue, the chaplain-administrator was to receive a third of the annual contributions of the parishioners in the collection box of the St-Armal chapel and a long list of personal holdings left by Canon Château-Giron, to wit, a large house with garden located in the town between the two roads leading to St-Armal, twelve pasturelands, three fields, and revenues from a house and a field, along with a house in the village with two lots of grapevines. The revenues from these holdings were to finance six beds for the poor. Itinerants were to be received for one night going to and another night returning from their destination. If they were ill, they could stay until they were well enough to continue on their way, and in the meantime "they could beg from door to door for charity."[57]

A century after the establishment of this hospital, the accounts of Guillaume Morin for 1540 show revenues of 203 livres, indicating a relatively healthy management of the modest endowment left by Canon Château-Giron.[58] But for Léon Maître, historian of local hospitals in the Nantes region, this situation changed when the type of lay takeovers evoked at the beginning of this chapter upset the functioning of the hospice. The Hôtel-Dieu in Nantes tried to get control over Savenay in 1548 and 1555 using the powers granted to it by the royal edicts. However, the local administrators of the hospital successfully resisted these attempts.[59]

The foundation at Savenay seems to have been exactly the type of hospital that the crown viewed with dismay. It was seen as too small to be useful in combating poverty, and its permissiveness regarding vagabonds and passers-by conflicted with the new notions about "re-educating" the able poor. At the same time, the decrees and orders adopted by the crown to close or reorganize small institutions such as Savenay did not work. The administrators in Nantes were obviously too busy dealing with their own poor to spend time scrutinizing the modest 200 livres in the

Savenay accounts or overseeing the choice of small-town hospital administrators. Cities such as Nantes did not want to oversee these small institutions; instead they coveted the power to expropriate their modest resources.

Like so many other sixteenth-century institutions, the hospital in Malestroit had been founded by the seigneur of the town, but unlike the examples of seigneurial largesse in the southeast, the seigneur of Malestroit retained full control over the institution. According to the research of Louis Rosenzweig, a nineteenth-century specialist on local hospitals in the Morbihan, its foundation probably dated from the fourteenth century, and the first register of financial accounts was drawn up in 1441.[60] The hospital of Madame Ste-Anne was governed by a *gardien et administrateur* named by seigneurial officials. He had to approve all expenses and collect the revenues of the institution, which amounted to about 60 livres a year during the fifteenth century. In the following century, the administrator was helped in his work by a hospitaller, whose duty was to distribute food and care to the poor. Despite the municipalization movement that characterized the sixteenth-century approach to religious and seigneurial hospitals, the director, or provost, of the Ste-Anne hospital continued to be named by local officials of the seigneurial court (the judge and treasurer), before whom he presented his annual accounts.

This seigneurial control presented problems for the management of local charity; conflicts arose regularly between the town councillors and the seigneurial officials. As in Étoile and Grignan, the Malestroit town council appointed a recteur and two assistants (*économes*), who were responsible for establishing the list of local poor to receive alms. But the councillors had no control over the actual hospital or to what extent it respected their priorities in distributing aid. They argued that the men appointed to the hospital bureau often lacked the necessary legal and financial expertise to run the institution. After 1620 the community forced the seigneurial officials to enlarge their selection process for the provost and to name "nobles, bourgeois, notaries, lawyers, and solicitors" who possessed a certain knowledge of the law rather than limiting their selection to shopkeepers and merchants.[61] This action, together with the fact that after 1624, representatives from the town were permitted to assist and to criticize the presentation of the provost's accounts, set the stage for a long period of conflict between the representatives of the community and the seigneurial judges.[62]

As to the Malestroit hospital itself, at the beginning of the sixteenth century, it had consisted of a chapel, a lower hall (twenty-nine feet long by twenty feet wide), a small upper room, and a kitchen, added on to the back of the hall, where the staff were lodged. The large hall, which communicated with the chapel and the kitchen, was used to shelter itinerants. The patients who lived in the institution – men, women, and soldiers – were placed side by side in the windowless upper room without any distinction as to sex or communicable illness. Situated outside the town's walls in the lower section of the Ste-Anne district, these buildings were rebuilt and repaired from time to time, and they seem to have remained the basis of the hospital during its entire existence.[63]

One of the strengths of the Malestroit institution was its financing. The hospital buildings had been destroyed in three sieges of the town during the Wars of Religion, and in 1592 Henri IV gave the institution important royal taxation rights over twenty-five barrels of wine. These rights were linked to an annual competition, the *papegault*, in which the archer who hit the most clay targets during May Day festivities shared taxation rights with the hospital over the wine. The revenue from these taxes, together with invested annuities and income from houses, collections, and gifts provided the Madame Ste-Anne hospital with adequate finances to repair and rebuild the institution in 1625 and to continue functioning thereafter.[64]

The sixteenth century witnessed a series of marked contrasts in small-town poor relief.[65] Most communities in both the north and the south took an increasing interest in helping the needy; new institutions were founded in Caudebec and those in Étoile and Grignan revitalized. The problem of poverty was certainly most acute in the large cities, where it often led to violence and where city officials began to make charity more selective by trying to put the able poor to work while aiding the sick and handicapped. But at the same time, a second series of initiatives was directed at the problem of the poor outside the cities through the foundation of new hospitals or the reservation of the twenty-fourth part of the tithe for the poor as in Dauphiné. The problem for the non-urban institutions was that royal administrators remained convinced that the funds distributed as charity in the small towns and villages were being poorly managed or even squandered.

The resources available for the poor in the institutions under study varied enormously, ranging from an average of 130 livres distributed annually in Seyne to 827 in Étoile (see Table 1). The northern institutions

Table 1
Early seventeenth-century operating budgets of the eight hospitals discussed in the text

Hospital	Years	Average annual budget for the sick and poor (in livres)	Average budget for outside aid (in livres)	Average patients admitted	No. of beds
Caudebec	1612–30	671			3
Pontorson	1614[1]	635			8
Malestroit	1600–30	173			4–6
Savenay	1540	203			6
Grignan	1600–30	388	38	203	4
Étoile	1604–30	827	26	116	13
Seyne	1600–30	130			
St-Vallier	[2]				

[1] Hospital not yet under the direction of the Brothers of Charity.
[2] Hospital not yet created.
[3] Straw piled up in a room.

tended to be more independent of municipal governments. At Caudebec and Savenay, the director of the hospital was elected by a general assembly of hospital councillors, and in Malestroit he was named by seigneurial officials. On the other hand, the southeastern communities elected their recteur of the poor at the same municipal meeting at which the new town consuls were chosen. As a result, the recteurs in the south were responsible for the communities' global response to the problem of assistance. These larger powers explain the fact that the southern institutions allotted more resources to outside aid. This fact can be seen in Grignan, Étoile, and Seyne.

The example of Savenay and of Pontorson before its takeover by the Brothers of Charity illustrate the modest means and haphazard management of what probably represented the majority of the maladreries, hospices, and small hospitals in the kingdom. If Étoile, Grignan, Seyne, and Caudebec remained dynamic institutions, benefiting from the financial and moral support of seigneurs, consuls, and townspeople, most local hospitals seem to have been more marginal to community activities, neither as well endowed nor as well integrated into the functioning of town institutions. It was these latter hospitals that became the object of the crown's attempts to eliminate what it saw as redundant and poorly managed establishments.

By the reign of Henri III, the crown had become convinced that a centralized approach was necessary to root out graft and corruption in local charities. It was clear that the repeated royal edicts ordering local judicial officials to investigate the institutions in their districts had produced few results, and the crown remained convinced that the outdated leproseries and mismanaged hospitals possessed considerable revenues. Royal officials therefore conceived of a curious plan to divert what they saw as mismanaged local poor-relief funds towards the support of old and injured army officers. To do so the king's ministers planned to create a new military hospital in Paris with the power to expropriate the funds that abbeys were supposed to be distributing to elderly and disabled soldiers. The plan had been initially proposed in 1576 to reward service in the army while the crown was trying to bring an end to the conflicts that had marked the Wars of Religion. It was, however, never implemented at that time. Henri iv revived this project and added to its objectives. Besides establishing the Maison de la Charité Chrétienne for old soldiers in Paris, he sought to obtain the "mismanaged" funds of local abbeys and hospitals in order to pay pensions to former army officers. To do so, he set up a centralized royal commission – the Chamber of Christian Charity (Chambre de la Charité Chrétienne) – to investigate each foundation, maladrerie, and hospital.[66]

To understand the logic of this transfer, it is necessary to review the changing status of old soldiers and officers in a period between the end of the feudal confrontations that had characterized the Wars of Religion and the beginning of a the concept of a royal army as the backbone of the newly evolving "absolutist" policy. In looking at the status of old and physically handicapped soldiers prior to Henri iv's creation of a hospital for old soldiers (the Maison de la Charité Chrétienne), it must be emphasized that the royal actions in 1604, as well as those taken throughout the seventeenth century, continued to confuse notions of treatment according to age, social hierarchy, and physical handicaps resulting from wartime injuries. The 1604 edict applies to "gentlemen," "amputees," and "old and disabled soldiers." This lumping together of different categories of former soldiers was typical of the approach that preceded the 1604 reform.[67] From the thirteenth century on, aid had been granted to old soldiers, especially to those who had lost limbs.

The system of aid, called the *oblat*, made abbeys founded under royal charters responsible for taking in, feeding, and caring for a certain number of handicapped veterans.[68] Under François i, as the number of old and injured soldiers increased, the king tried to extend the oblat to all monasteries founded under royal charter that elected their head. But even this approach was not enough; the numbers of old and injured soldiers continued to rise as a result of increased hostilities during the Italian Wars and the confrontations with the Hapsburgs.[69] In these conflicts, the introduction of firearms and the large-scale use of cannons produced greater numbers of injuries and wartime amputees. The experiments of the late sixteenth-century surgeon Ambroise Paré in performing battlefield amputations and designing artificial limbs met a pressing need in face of the new realities of war. Providing care for these men after their amputation was one of the objects of the new legislation.[70]

The system of granting refuge to old or injured soldiers in French monasteries was neither unanimously accepted nor approved by the institutions in question. A problem of uneven distribution plagued the system, since the abbeys in the Paris area were overcrowded with veterans, while the more distant institutions took in fewer and fewer former soldiers. Arguing that the morals and habits of these men were incompatible with monastic life, most abbots tended to transform their obligations into monetary payments (pensions) that were granted to the soldiers in order to have them cared for at home. In addition, the places allocated to the oblats or lay religious (*religieux laïs*) in each abbey could by law also be occupied by servants or members of one of the monks' families, again reducing the number of places or pensions for soldiers who had the right to receive the oblat.[71]

Beyond these problems of adapting traditional responses to the new difficulties was the more wide-ranging challenge of reducing the royal army to 10,000 men and, of course, scaling down the numerous feudal armies. The French army during a few months in 1559 prior to the treaty of Cateau-Cambrésis had reached almost 50,000 men, and in 1562, on the eve of the Wars of Religion, there were still 28,000 on the rolls.[72] It is probable that the number of regular and irregular soldiers also increased dramatically during the civil and religious wars. To attain a lasting peace, it was necessary to reduce these forces and to stimulate economic recovery in order to provide for the soldiers who were to be demobilized. This was the issue discussed at the Assembly of Notables in 1596, when Chancellor Bellièvre presented the bleak financial situation of the kingdom: revenues came to 30,900,000 livres, but 24,000,000 of that amount had already been spent or was reserved to pay debts, and current expenses came to 24,900,000 livres, leaving a deficit of 18,000,000. In a desperate effort to balance his budget, Bellièvre proposed raising taxes and cutting expenses. In all, 5,400,000 livres were to be cut, and military expenses were to be rolled back to 4,500,000 livres.[73] As a member of the Conseil des Finances, which prepared the assembly,

Constable Montmorency appears to have succeeded in limiting the cuts in the military budget from the initial suggestion of 3,600,000 livres to the 4,500,000 eventually proposed.[74]

This assembly in 1596 has often been seen as a theatrical staging by royal officials, who presented the major problems facing the kingdom in order to force the represented notables to concede new fiscal revenues. Certainly, the problem posed by the large royal and feudal armies was accentuated and perhaps exaggerated, as was the necessity of pay-offs and compensation for those officers affected by the reductions. It was within this context that the crown tried to cut back its military without alienating the great nobles and army officers. Without creating too much disorder, it hoped to return regular soldiers, often old and injured, to their communities. At the same time that regiments were being disbanded, three different measures were taken to try to create the impression that Henri IV attributed great value to the services the soldiers had rendered.

Even as the 1596 assembly was taking place, the king had already begun looking into improving the treatment of elderly and disabled soldiers. In May that year an *arrêt* obtained from the king's council by Simon Le Musnier, the representative of the handicapped officers (*syndic des estropiés*), ordered that soldiers be housed, fed, and treated in the hospital that Henri III had turned over to their service by a 1577 edict.[75] The second step was taken in 1604, when this same hospital was the object of an edict officially designating it as La Maison de la Charité Chrétienne with the exclusive mandate of housing poor gentlemen and veteran amputees. The document went on to establish the structure of the institution, granting it revenues to be expropriated from the surpluses reported in the annual accounts of local and regional hospitals, from the sums paid by the monasteries for the oblat, and from fines imposed in the courts that were to be reserved to aid the poor.[76]

To preside over the institution and to supervise the collection of its revenues, the edict created a bureau composed of four officers or "personnes notables" and four gentlemen and old captains. They were to seek out revenues for the institution and to decide upon the admission of injured and amputated veterans and eventually to establish other houses and hospitals in the provinces.[77] Finally, the difficulties experienced by this bureau in carrying out the tasks specified in the edict, especially the expropriations, led to the third initiative, the creation in 1606 of the Chamber of Christian Charity, a veritable royal commission, which was far better structured to carry out the responsibilities of operating the Paris hospital and obtaining funds from local institutions for officers' pensions. As with the 1604 bureau, it was to expropriate all or portions of the funds held by the redundant leproseries or mismanaged hospitals and to centralize the management of the oblat, which had traditionally been handled by the abbeys.

From the beginning, this new commission was controlled by the authorities of the French army, and Constable Montmorency was appointed to draw up the list of poor gentlemen and handicapped soldiers who were to receive pensions. According to the text of the 1606 document, he was to study the gravity of the injury or amputation in each case and the date and place where the injury had occurred in order to be sure it had been received on the battlefield. On the basis of this inquiry, he was to recommend the amount of the annual pension to be given to each soldier. In drawing up this list, Montmorency was to be aided by the Duc d'Epérnon, colonel of the French infantry.[78]

The list of approved pensions was to be transmitted to the Chamber of Christian Charity, of which both Montmorency and Epérnon were members, along with Cardinal du Perron, the archbishop of Sens, who sat as *grand aumônier*, and the sieurs of Rochepot, Souvray, and Chateauvieux, representing the military orders. On behalf of the crown, there were to be one secretary of state and eight royal judicial officials; four of them were *maîtres de requêtes* (Louis Durant, Martin Langlois, Jean le Guay, and Jacques Merault), and four others were councillors from the Grand Conseil (Defriches, Bautru, Guynet, and de Bermont).[79] The possibility of certain replacements was also provided for in the 1606 text. The two oldest marshals could substitute for Montmorency or Epérnon, and an ecclesiastical representative could sit in for the archbishop of Sens. At least seven of the members were needed for a legal quorum, and they were to be convened under the direction of the *avocat de l'Hôtel du Roi*, Gilles de Champhnon.[80]

This chamber was to preside over the review and examination of the leproseries, poorly administrated hospitals, and monasteries that were not respecting the oblat. It was to send commissioners to inspect questionable institutions and order them to draw up a list of all such hospitals, leproseries, maladreries, and monasteries of the kingdom, along with their locations, and the amounts that they were ordered to pay in pensions. The 1606 edict noted that as a result of this review procedure, the chamber could condemn, without appeal, any institution to pay up to 500 livres.[81] This system was in operation from 1606 to 1610; both the appeals heard by the chamber and the decisions it rendered are preserved in the Archives Nationales. The appeals were numerous: for 1607 and 1609, the years for which the series are almost complete, 395 and 480 appeals respectively were lodged.[82]

The first register of minutes produced by the chamber illustrates the difficulties that the commissioners faced in trying to carry out their mandate. Between August 1606 and December 1607, the chamber met 117 times and rendered about 950 decisions concerning different issues. These were, however, primarily directed towards obtaining the documents necessary to decide the fate of the maladreries and hospitals under investigation, ordering the suppressions, and justifying the decisions they had taken. In the 950 decisions, the commissioners actually treated only 380 hospitals since the same cases returned over and over again as a result of legal obstacles, appeals, and delaying tactics; in the sixteen months for which the minutes have been studied, the hospital at Beauvais was treated 36 times, Montlhéry 34 times, Estampes 21 times, Oisemont 19 times, Francoville 18 times, and Lynois 18 times. Most of the hospitals that the chamber tried to suppress were within three hundred kilometres of Paris, although institutions in Angers, Loudun, Picardy, Beaune, and Moulins were also dealt with.[83] Officials in certain towns and cities, such as Beauvais or Mantes, appealed the suppressions of their hospitals almost every two months during the entire existence of the reform. This pattern indicates the resistance and the obstacles faced by the commission.

In the allocation of the pension payments, the grand aumonier received lists of the soldiers whom Montmorency and Epérnon had judged eligible to receive funds, and these men were accorded pensions from the amounts that the hospitals, leproseries, and abbeys were ordered to pay. The pensions seem to have varied, and although I could find none of the actual lists drawn up, appeal procedures indicate awards of between 60 and 80 livres.[84] The original oblat had been fixed at 60 livres. With the exception of the revenues needed to operate the Maison de la Charité Chrétienne, the amounts that local leproseries and hospitals were to pay were not to be transferred to Paris; they were to be paid directly in pensions to the eligible poor gentlemen and handicapped former soldiers who lived in the region of each hospital and who were given vouchers to be honoured by the institutions in question. For example, it was decided that Hiérosme Durant "from the town of Loriol in Dauphiné" was accorded a place as an oblat at the priory of St-Martin-Hazel in his native diocese of Valence.[85]

Although the chamber was not created to hear the complaints of individual veterans, a number did appear before the commissioners to testify that they had been given pension vouchers that had not been honoured by the local institutions. These hearings demonstrate difficulties in the functioning of this system. In a detailed study of the registers produced by the chamber between 1607 and 1611, André Corvisier has located 241 cases of "poor amputee gentlemen" or "poor amputee captains" who appeared to complain that their pensions or oblats were not, in fact, being paid. It is interesting to note that of the institutions ordered to pay these 241 retired soldiers, the overwhelming majority were abbeys, which had a traditional duty to pay the oblats: 176 abbeys were ordered to honour the chamber's vouchers compared to 4 priories, 8 hospitals, and 15 maladreries.[86] Certainly, the attempts to suppress the holdings of 380 hospitals and maladreries show that the chamber did try to go beyond the traditional obligation to enforce the oblats owed by the abbeys, but given the delaying tactics by the hospitals summoned before the chamber and the appeals registered by individual veterans who were not receiving their due, it is clear that the system did not work.

Such obstacles appear to have seriously compromised the efforts to fund military pensions, and almost immediately after the death of Henri IV, the whole experiment was ended. Funds were no longer to be transferred from lepers or the poor and sick to poor gentlemen, amputees, or old soldiers. A 1611 order by Louis XIII explained this decision, noting that "experience has taught us that the ordinary expenses and the destruction of [hospital] buildings during the recent wars [troubles] were so great that the revenues of their foundations were totally insufficient and the review of their accounts produced too little revenue to be of any aid to future soldiers."[87] The document goes on to make the totally false claim that the oblat was sufficient to maintain old and handicapped veterans. This order was completed by letters patent in 1612 that restated the necessity of continuing to review the accounts of local leproseries and hospitals, but it noted that the funds received from these inspections should be returned to their original purpose of aiding lepers as well as the sick and the poor.[88]

It is ironic that after noting the inability of the Chamber of Christian Charity to carry out its mandate properly, the letters patent of 1612 retained almost exactly the same form of commission with nearly identical composition and powers to continue the inspections and review. The new body, called the Chamber of the General Hospital Reform (Chambre de la Générale Reformation des Hôpitaux et Maladreries de France), eliminated the representatives of the army and the three major hospitaller orders. It also reinforced royal control over the commission; consultations with the bishops or ecclesiastical leaders were no longer mentioned in the document, and the grand aumônier, appointed by the king, became the director of the reform. But despite these changes in the objectives and composition of the commission, contemporaries do not seem to have seen it as fundamentally different from the Chamber of Christian Charity. This perception of continuity can be observed in the fact that as late as 1637, we find appeals to the commission still being addressed to the earlier body. It can also be seen in the integration of the registers of the Chamber of Christian Charity into the archives of the Chamber of the General Hospital Reform. It is clear that the royal-commission format continued under a new title and that the organizational structure does not appear to have been the fundamental reason for the change.

Why did Louis XIII abandon the policy of granting financial aid to old and handicapped veterans? The 1611 text argues that, besides the disappointing results of the attempts to expropriate hospital funds for the operation, there remained fundamental objections to the diverting of money earmarked for lepers and the poor in order to pay veterans' pensions. The document noted that lepers remained numerous in France and that the principal goal of the hospital foundations had been to aid them. The crown could not get around the fact that there were legal problems involved in using funds originally donated for one group in order to aid another. In addition, the legal right of the crown to order these transfers was questioned.

The objections to the work of the Chamber of Christian Charity certainly highlight the difficulties faced by the crown in trying to intervene in what were seen as essentially private abbeys, maladreries, and hospitals. The experience of the commission demonstrates this dilemma. During its first year of existence, it called over three hundred of these institutions before it, only to be confronted with appeals and delaying tactics. None of the eight hospitals examined in this study were among them, and most of the institutions called before the chamber never conformed to its orders to pay pensions to army veterans or turn over part of their revenues to the Maison de la Charité Chrétienne. However, the fact remains that with the hearings of the chamber, the movement to suppress and expropriate small institutions had been initiated.

This series of confrontations shows that municipal and royal officials believed that local hospitals were corrupt, redundant, and inefficient. Edict after edict spoke of the funds available in the increasingly deserted maladreries and in the poorly administered local hospitals. Even the church, accountable for most of the older foundations, came to admit that corruption was widespread. Certainly, when the pastoral visits of the period are consulted, the general weaknesses found in the distribution of local poor relief do confirm certain crown suspicions: in 1644 Charles-Jacques Leberon, bishop of Valence and Die, pointed out the cases of Rousset, where poor-relief funds were used to pay the schoolmaster; Barnave, Prébois, and La Croix-de-Cornillon, where they were employed to rebuild churches; St-Martin-de-Clelles, which used poor-relief funds to pay its bell-ringer; and Sinard, where members of the Confraternity of the St-Esprit appropriated revenues from their holdings to give themselves a banquet on Pentecost, with only the remaining funds going to the poor.[89] In the view of the crown, these corrupt local hospitals possessed considerable revenues and holdings, which if properly used, could care for all the poor of the kingdom.

2 Transferring Poor-Relief Funds to Old Soldiers: The Order of Mount Carmel and St-Lazare

On 4 July 1680 Maître Gaspard Cachod, agent of the general director of the Order of Notre-Dame of Mount Carmel and of St-Lazare, rode into Étoile to inspect the operations of the town hospital, which was located just outside the walls. He noted in his report that there was no caretaker and that he found only one inmate, a poor girl lying on a straw mattress in the rundown building. He concluded that the basic requirements for "hospitality" were not being respected.[1] Despite the protests of André Serret, recteur of the hospital, Judge Jean-Guy Basset of Grenoble upheld the negative aspects of the report and ordered the Étoile hospital to pay 100 livres a year to the order for pensions allocated to former army officers who were members of the order.[2]

The intervention of Gaspard Cachod in Étoile represented only one case of the first large-scale effort undertaken throughout the French kingdom to inspect the legal documents and the functioning of local welfare foundations. Attempts were subsequently made to close those that did not conform to the necessary criteria and to divert their funds towards the support of "gentlemen" who had served in the king's armies. After the relative failures of the Chamber of Christian Charity and the Chamber of General Hospital Reform, the king had learned valuable lessons about reforming or closing down local hospitals. The legal appeals and decisions showed that he could not intervene unilaterally, for these institutions were seen as an area where the church and the crown shared responsibility. It was also argued regularly that a founder's will had to be respected and that the crown could not simply decide that the revenues willed to an institution a century before for a specific purpose should now be turned over to another group. For these reasons the new inquiry was not carried out directly by royal officials. Responsibility for the investigations, hearings, and eventual interventions was turned over to a recently created military-religious order. In 1672 the Order of Notre-Dame of Mount Carmel and St-Lazare was given the right to investigate each hospice in the kingdom, with a mandate to close those that were judged redundant and to assume the management of any that were seen as not respecting the terms of their charter.[3] The revenues from all these totally or partially suppressed institutions were to be distributed annually to the members of the order.

This new reform tried to address the continuing legal problems confronted by the Chamber of the General Hospital Reform. It also had to face the fact that the abandoning of the military pensions created by Henri IV had been severely criticized by military leaders and the nobility. At the 1626 Assembly of Notables, the second estate asked that the crown look back to Henri IV's initiatives in order to find new means to support old and handicapped soldiers.[4] The nobility was one of the principal groups that the crown was trying to bring under its control in the course of the seventeenth century. This group's indiscipline and adamant defence of its decentralized, feudal power base made its objections particularly significant.[5] The Wars of Religion, the Huguenot Wars, and the Fronde all provided vehicles for greater and lesser nobles to oppose the increasing centralization of royal power; Louis XIV made it his absolute priority to obtain control over this group. The new approach relied on payments and patronage, including the re-establishing of pensions for army officers and members of the nobility, as a way of solidifying their loyalty and dependence upon crown largesse. William Beik has recently demonstrated how the nobility of Languedoc had been drawn into closer collaboration with the central government by being given increasing financial gains in both central and provincial government operations. The second attempt to use poor-relief funds to establish military pensions seems to have corresponded to this policy.[6]

In trying to address both the legal question of who had the right to intervene in local hospitals and the patronage issue of solidifying crown support within the military elite, Louis XIV's edict, issued in December 1672, astutely evaded the problem of legal rights by using a hospitaller order, and not royal officials, to carry out the expropriations. It repeated the claim that there was daily fraud and embezzlement of poor-relief revenues by the administrators of the maladreries, leproseries, hospices, and hospitals.[7] The document further empowered the nobles of the Order of Notre-Dame of Mount Carmel and St-Lazare to take possession of the holdings and funds of "all other military and hospitaller orders … that had been or were to be suppressed," as well as all hospices and maladreries that were not providing the services designated in their charters. They were to distribute the resulting revenues among their members.

The edict dwelt at length on the fact that the order, created in 1608, represented a fusion of St-Lazare, the oldest existing order of military and hospitaller origin, founded in the Holy Land during the fourth century and repatriated to France in 1137, and the Order of Notre-Dame of Mount Carmel, founded by Henri IV in 1608. The goal of the operation was to compensate army officers for their services.[8] From its very conception, the project sought to purchase the nobles' obedience, using the hospitaller order to reroute town and village poor-relief funds to the second estate. The new order thus became an ideal vehicle for carrying out the transfer of funds from the church-linked institutions of poor relief to the military. As a religious order, it could not be accused of laicizing ecclesiastical holdings, and since it was also a military order, the expropriated holdings could be turned over to army officers within its very structures.

The 1672 edict placed particular emphasis on the sweeping expropriation of other hospitaller or military orders, and it specifically noted that St-Lazare was empowered to take control of the holdings and funds of the orders of St-Esprit de Montpellier, the Holy Sepulchre, Ste-Catherine de Somport, of St-Louis de Boucheraumont, the Teutonic Knights, the Knights of St-Jacques de l'Épée, and all other orders that were to be declared "extinct, suppressed, and abolished."[9] This step in the expropriation movement gave the Order of St-Lazare blanket control over a large number of small hospitals or almshouses, particularly those of the Order of St-Esprit, which controlled most such houses in the south of France.[10] St-Lazare took immediate control of these institutions, and it did not need to become involved in long, drawn-out inspections and legal actions, as was the case when the order turned to the mismanaged local hospitals. Simultaneously, the expropriation measures taken against the hospitaller orders were challenged at a higher level and became a major bone of contention between the Vatican and the king of France.

The moving force behind the project to change the role of the Order of St-Lazare was François-Michel le Tellier, Marquis de Louvois,

Louis XIV's dynamic minister of war. This man had already demonstrated his interest in finding ways to compensate those who had served in the king's army. He had proposed the construction of a vast hospital to house injured and abandoned soldiers and officers. This project led the king to undertake the construction of the giant Invalides in 1670, a successor to the Maison de la Charité Chrétienne proposed, but never built, by Henri IV.[11] The directors of the Order of St-Lazare approached Louvois early in 1672 to ask for new measures to increase their funding.[12] In her study of the history of the order, Françoise Dissard argues that during these discussions the minister became convinced that St-Lazare would be an ideal means to investigate and suppress defunct or redundant foundations for poor relief and channel their funds to compensate French nobles for their service and obedience. The resulting edict of 1672 authorized the order to acquire two types of foundations: first, the hospices and maladreries that were not respecting their charters or where officials were engaged in graft and corruption and, second, the holdings of all other military and hospitaller orders whose rights to operate institutions had either expired or been revoked.[13] To accomplish these transfers and suppressions, the edict abolished the Chamber of the General Hospital Reform. According to the orders issued to establish a new chamber, the tribunal of the General Hospital Reform had received insufficient powers to carry out the desired suppressions, and most of its decisions had resulted in appeals and long judicial procedures. It was replaced by the Chamber of the Arsenal, which was accorded wide-ranging authority to receive all cases brought before it by the Order of St-Lazare, to give them first and last hearing, and to register declarations, edicts, and regulations concerning the "reform."[14]

While obviously aimed at buying and assuring the fidelity of the nobles, the project fell into the ambiguous notion of "charity" held by the seventeenth-century elite. Just as Kathryn Norberg has shown that charity in Grenoble extended to taking custody of the children of Huguenots and shutting them up in city institutions to educate them in the "true faith,"[15] so too the elite of the time praised the measures that compensated the king's commanders and soldiers. In the supporting documents submitted to the royal council at the time of the 1672 edict, it was argued that "it was the most just and glorious charity that the king could undertake to aid his officers of rank and merit, who spent their youth, were wounded, and used their own wealth in the service of the state." Another document noted that "they are the first and most illustrious poor of the state, and they are the most deserving of aid."[16]

Louis XIV also personally justified the rights given to the order, noting that with the aid of the military he had undertaken "great efforts" to ensure peace within the kingdom and to confront France's enemies, beating them back by the force of arms. The king further argued that it was perfectly reasonable to reward those who had been the principal instruments of this policy and that it would not be just to abandon the officers and soldiers of his army to "the misery that ordinarily accompanies those who have spent their lives and fortunes" serving in the armed forces. Finding themselves incapacitated by age or the injuries that they had received, these men were often driven to begging to earn their keep. Louis noted that to meet his obligations to these "valiant soldiers," he had established the Invalides, but he also felt that the officers should receive recognition and rewards in proportion to the merit of their actions. He had decided that the ideal means to do so would be to set aside the holdings and revenues of the oldest hospitaller order in the church and kingdom for the purpose of awarding pensions through its local branches, or *commanderies*, for the gentlemen and officers of his troops.[17]

To demonstrate his intention to direct and expedite this "reform" personally, Louvois had himself named vicar-general of the order. Among the thirteen members of the Council of St-Lazare, named in March 1673, seven came from the ranks of the judiciary. Through edicts registered in the provincial parlements, this group proceeded to oversee the confiscation of hospices and maladreries belonging to other hospitaller orders, such as the St-Esprit de Montpellier and the Teutonic Knights.[18] For the numerous charitable institutions independent of these orders, the councillors verified titles, contracts, and documents to determine their legal status. They sent commissioners to inspect their buildings, charters, and financial records to be certain that their responsibilities were being adequately fulfilled. The inquiries always concentrated upon discovering fraud, lack of conformity with charter provisions, absence of the type of disease for which the charity had been created, or forms of welfare that were no longer needed. Any of these reasons could motivate a request that the institution be "united" to the order and that all or part of its funds be transferred to that organization. The hearings on these demands were presented before the Chamber of the Arsenal.

The chamber was made up of five ordinary councillors and eight councillors and maîtres de requêtes, who were to carry out the necessary research for each request for suppression. Seven judges and at least one court councillor sat to hear the cases. During the first seven years of its existence, this group kept up a feverish pace as the council of the Order of Mount Carmel and St-Lazare presented hundreds of demands for the abolition of foundations and/or the transfer of their funds. In 1679 the number of judges was reduced to five, indicating that the suppression movement had peaked and that the number of cases to be heard had begun to decline. During the reform, the chamber heard over 1,700 often long, drawn-out cases involving suppressions in almost every diocese of the kingdom.

What was the actual effect of this "reform" on the structures of poor relief in France? It is clear that the Order of Mount Carmel and St-Lazare succeeded, first, in closing down or obtaining management rights over the holdings of thousands of small institutions and, secondly, in obtaining annual pension payments from thousands of other hospitals and institutions that continued to function. A register in the Archives Nationales drawn up in 1682 contains a list of institutions whose funds had been fully or partially transferred to the order, as well as the institutions over which it was still seeking control. The list includes 4,078 hospitals, maladreries, or bureaux of charity.[19]

Although the institutions suppressed or to be suppressed were located in virtually every diocese of the kingdom, the reform tended to concentrate on the more heavily populated areas surrounding Paris (see Map 3). Virtually all dioceses with more than 100 institutions either suppressed or to be suppressed were located in that zone: Sens, Bourges, Rouen, Chartres, Blois, Amiens, Tours, Poitiers, Soissons, Laon, Reims, Langres, and Dijon. In the smaller and poorer southern dioceses, such as Valence, Die, Uzès, or Tarbes, the order united or sought the right to "unite" between two and twenty institutions. The rare dioceses where hospice revenues were left untouched were clustered in the Comtat Venaissin and were under papal authority, or were situated along the French borders. The pensions that the Order of Mount Carmel and St-Lazare had distributed to its knights in 1672, before the expropriations, had totalled around 25,000 livres,[20] but this figure jumped to over 250,000 livres after the acquisition of local hospice funds. While this amount is considerable, Claire Guerin argues that Louvois had believed that the reform would enable the order to recuperate much more than 250,000 livres. A preliminary listing in 1675 of institutions to be united to the order in Normandy had included three times the number eventually taken over by it.

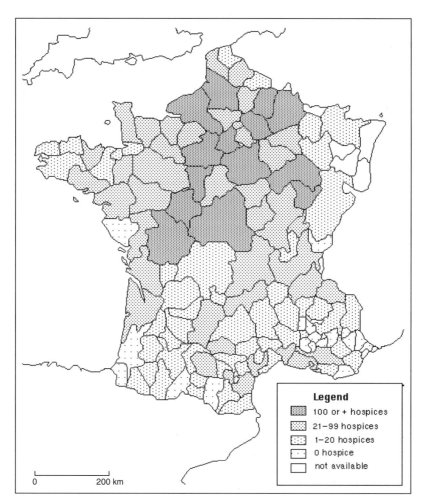

Map 3 Institutions of poor relief taken over or targeted for takeover by the Order of Mount Carmel and St-Lazare in each French diocese, 1672–82

These observations for Normandy seem to hold true for the whole of France. The uneven results of the regions contributing funds to the order can also be seen from the significant differences in the revenues that were paid to holders of the commanderies created by the Order of St-Lazare and listed in the 1682 register. The kingdom was divided up into five great priories, each of which contained twenty-nine command-eries that were distributed to members of the order. Each commanderie was funded from the hospitals, maladreries, and hospices united to the order within the dioceses of that region. Since the revenues collected in each commanderie were divided among the twenty-nine commanders, their payments depended on how much was collected. The differences were enormous: the revenues of 21,276 livres from the combined dioceses of Chartes and Blois, 18,305 from Rouen, 17,082 from Amiens, 13,929 from Paris, 13,156 from Sens, and 10,078 from Tournai dwarfed the other entries. With the exception of these dioceses, the results of the expropriations were often minimal.

The relation between demography, the hospitals, and the suppression movement is not particularly apparent since the heaviest populated dioceses of the kingdom did not necessarily produce the most revenues (see Map 4). Although the généralités of Paris, Rouen, Amiens, Arras, Caen, Rennes, and Alençon all contained over fifty inhabitants per square kilometre, only seven dioceses in that region actually procured more than 10,000 livres for the order.[21] The great priory of Brittany, among the most densely populated in France, contained only two dioceses (Chartes and Blois combined) in which the suppressions produced more than 10,000 livres, and the revenues from the other twelve dioceses listed in the register ranged from 123 livres for St-Malo to 7,601 for Orléans. Upon close examination of the sources of revenue of the four northern priories, it becomes obvious that absolutely no funds were received from most of the dioceses and that furthermore it was in the six dioceses surrounding Paris, where over 100 institutions of poor relief had been "united," that the contributions were the most substantial. The listing does not break down the aggregate figure for the great priory of Languedoc, and so it is impossible to calculate the funds actually provided by the southern dioceses.

These data dealing with the sources of financing for the commanderies created by the order demonstrate that the reform was very uneven. It did not follow demographic patterns, and it received the vast majority of its financing from a few dioceses close to the capital, where the Order of Mount Carmel and St-Lazare had been traditionally strong. The data also show that this reform, like the previous efforts at expropriating local hospitals, had seriously overestimated the wealth controlled by the supposedly prodigal local foundations and that it had also exaggerated the ability of the order to expropriate those revenues.[22] The funds received from the long, drawn-out procedures for suppression – the 250,000 livres – were only sufficient to fund about 145 pensions to "compensate" nobles for their military services.

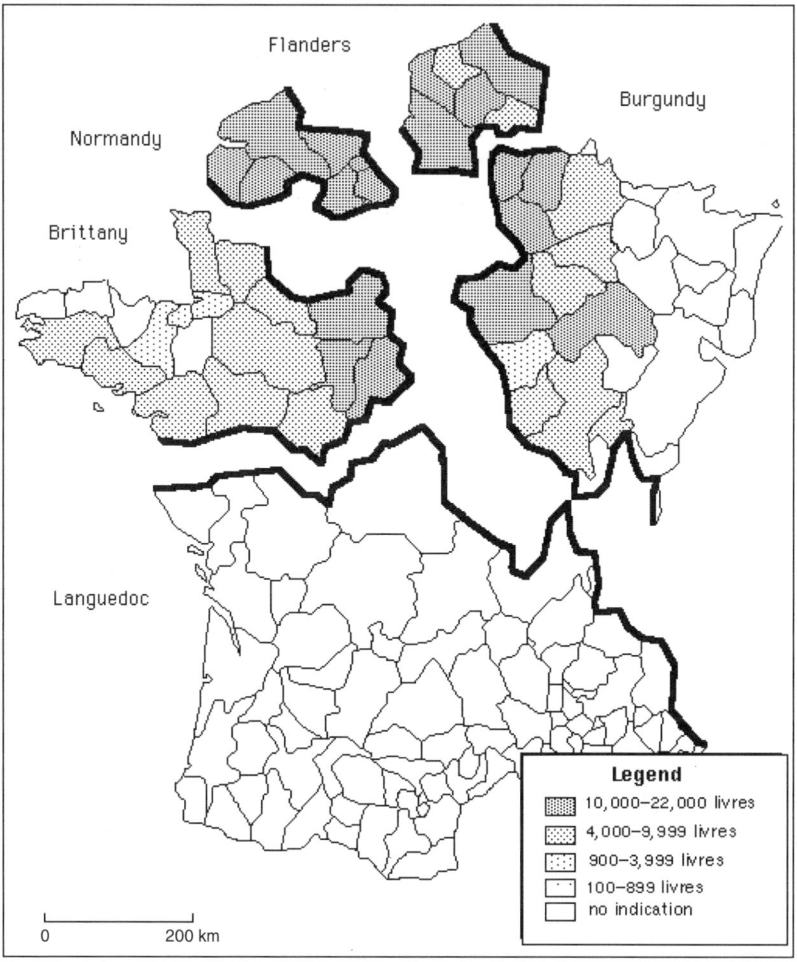

Map 4   Revenues obtained from the hospices "united" to the Order of Mount Carmel and St-Lazare in 1682, indicated by diocese, with total revenues for each great priory

Although the St-Lazare drive to suppress town and village poor-relief institutions failed to attain its projected goal of revenues, it did produce the first real, large-scale and effective intervention in a traditional field of town and village competence. Thousands of hospices and maladreries were in fact united on paper to the order, and the chamber ordered that their revenues be diverted to the former officers of the French armies. Yet the suppressions also necessitated the creation and maintenance of a large judicial bureaucracy, and the revenues obtained from the lengthy inquiries and proceedings did not at all reach expectations. In most cases, the orders that the hospitals and maladreries make annual payments to the commanderies of St-Lazare were never respected, and the order could not constantly send out collectors to obtain the minimal sums that the hospitals owed them. Louvois, like most royal officials before him, overestimated the revenues of the tumbledown and poorly financed institutions and underestimated the efficiency and local support structures of those poor-relief institutions that controlled substantial revenues. Furthermore, these institutions were generally successful resisting suppression, holding back the payments that had been accorded to St-Lazare.

Among other circumstances that contributed to the lower-than-expected revenues from the operation was the fact that this reform had to compete with a second, completely different movement that also had designs upon the "mismanaged" poor-relief funds. While Mount Carmel and St-Lazare was advancing Henri IV's goal of funding pensions for retired army officers, the second movement, born out of the urban humanist attempts to reform aid to the poor, was trying to distinguish between those who deserved aid and the phoney beggars who ought to be put to work. This movement aimed to establish hopitaux-généraux in the larger cities and towns to intern and reform the sturdy beggars.

From the end of the sixteenth century, the urban elite of the kingdom, stimulated by the dévot movement and the Company of the Holy Sacrament, had been working feverishly to construct this network of hôpitaux-généraux in which the poor, beggars, vagabonds, aged, and handicapped could be incarcerated and re-educated.[23] The members of this elite group inaugurated a powerful movement in favour of what Michel Foucault has seen as the "exclusion" from society of all who did not conform to an increasingly "bourgeois" social norm. Jean-Pierre Gutton has explained their initiatives as a reaction against the waves of rural poor who migrated to the larger centres seeking handouts. According to him, urban elites saw these demographic patterns as the causes of the increased violence and criminality, which became a menace to public order.[24] They sought therefore to confine the poor in specially created institutions, convincing the Lyon city council, for example, to build La Charité in 1622. This institution, a "hospital" that could lodge five to six hundred poor, had nothing to do with healing or caring for the sick; it was intended to clear the city streets of the poor. Behind its walls, these "marginal" elements of society were to be reformed; first, all were to receive lessons in moral and Christian doctrine, and secondly, the "able poor" were to be forced to acquire experience and work habits in the attached workshops or by being sent daily to labour for private manufacturers in the city.[25]

La Charité became a model for the hôpitaux-généraux to be set up across the kingdom. This type of institution was the basic component of the Europe-wide policy known in France as "the great confinement," a policy aimed at creating combination hospitals-workhouses-poorhouses in all major cities to contain the poor and thereby to rid the streets of undesirable elements. The premise behind this new approach, that assistance should be aimed at transforming the poor, had been widely criticized during the late sixteenth and early seventeenth centuries. The principal resistance came from the Catholic traditionalists, who defended individual alms giving as an act of charity that benefited the donor, eventually earning him or her the salvation promised in the Beatitudes.[26] The new humanist ideal favoured interventions directed at "saving" the poor and at recuperating and re-educating them, and by the 1650s, few voices were raised to defend traditional, indiscriminate charity or oppose the involvement of municipal governments and benevolent organizations in the reorganization of welfare. Even the major charitable orders of the Counter-Reformation church and leaders such as St Vincent de Paul eventually came to organize or serve in these institutions.[27]

In 1627 the residents of Grenoble contributed to the construction of a hospital along the same lines as La Charité. It was granted letters patent from the king setting out the rules for its administration and granting it the revenues of a new tax on meat cutters.[28] Similar initiatives to found hôpitaux-généraux were undertaken in Reims in 1632, Amiens in 1640, Marseille in 1641, Aix and Dijon in 1643, and finally Paris in 1656. These efforts by individual cities were encouraged by royal letters patent and by the contributions of individual donors, rural property and estates turned over or willed to the hospital by local notables, and duties on grain and cattle sold at the markets. The movement culminated in 1662, when by royal edict, all "cities and large towns" of the kingdom were ordered to establish hôpitaux-généraux to instruct the poor in "the piety and Christian religion and in the crafts of which they are capable."[29]

In the face of local resistance to this order, Colbert ordered the officials of all major cities and towns to convene their inhabitants in 1673 in order to convince them of the advantages (*commodité*) of establishing hôpitaux-généraux. Three years later the question of funding was addressed specifically when the king asked the bishops of the kingdom to promote the creation of these institutions and to turn over to them the revenues of all the small hospitals in their dioceses that were proven to be mismanaged and corrupt and were not already in the hands of the Order of Mount Carmel and St-Lazare.[30]

The suppressions of maladreries to create hôpitaux-généraux became the official solution to funding the new institutions; however, it was a solution that often conflicted directly with the expropriations by Mount Carmel and St-Lazare. In an edict issued on 24 March 1674, the king himself recognized the confusion that had been created by allowing both St-Lazare and the hôpitaux-généraux to target the same maladreries and local hospitals for expropriation. In effect, Louis XIV noted that in June 1672 he had given the hôpitaux-généraux the right to expropriate the holdings and the funds of the maladreries that were not respecting their obligations, and in a second edict in December that year, the same rights had been conceded to the Order of St-Lazare.[31] He therefore ordered that the institutions actually in the hands of the hôpitaux-généraux should be retained, but that the hospitals should pay the commanderies of St-Lazare an annual sum equivalent to the funds that they received from the maladreries in question.

The confusion resulting from this double grant was often complicated by successive individual grants, as was the case at Issoire in Auvergne. In 1671 the seigneur and town elite had asked the king for permission to found a hôpital général to which they could send the poor who were currently lodged in the Hôtel-Dieu, together with beggars and vaga-bonds from the region. One of the reasons for their request was the fact that, since the neighbouring cities and towns, Clermont, Riom, and Billom, had prohibited begging and set up hôpitaux-généraux to intern their poor, all the vagabonds of the province had become concentrated in Issoire. The king finally granted the letters patent for the new hospital in 1674, giving its administrators permission to expropriate the funds and holdings of the small hospitals and maladreries up to a distance of two *lieux* from the town. In 1676 he intervened again specifically to grant them rights over the small hospital of St-Bonnet-le-Chastel and the maladreries of Parredon, Groslier, and Durbize, all of which had been previously conceded to Mount Carmel and St-Lazare.[32]

At the same time that St-Lazare and the large hôpitaux-généraux were suppressing small, local hospitals and maladreries, a branch of the hôpital-général movement began working in small towns and villages to transform existing poor-relief structures through the creation of new or reformed local hospitals and bureaux of the poor. This movement grew out of the municipal reforms of charity carried out during the sixteenth and early seventeenth centuries; it was stimulated by the royal edict of

1662 ordering the large cities of the kingdom to create hôpitaux-généraux, and it was actively promoted by missionaries and by the local assemblies of the Company of the Holy Sacrament working to extend the values of the Catholic Reformation. The difference between the great confinement movement created by these groups in the cities and the extension of its values into the towns and bourgs of the kingdom was that the new movement promoted more simple and spontaneous measures for creating smaller hôpitaux-généraux: the Franciscan method, which consisted of simply taking up a collection in the parish or town to set up what were often makeshift facilities to house and aid the poor and at the same time give them lessons in Christian doctrine.

During the 1670s several members of the groups promoting this movement had begun writing pamphlets encouraging the crown to create a "central direction" to oversee the establishment of these new institutions for poor relief outside the large cities. Around 1680 the king replied to this pressure by naming a minor nobleman from Brittany, Sieur Gabriel Calloët-Querbrat, as "avocat général des pauvres" and secretary of the Assemblée Charitable de Paris.[33] The new avocat was closely connected with a Jesuit priest, Father Honoré Chaurand, who together with his assistant, Father Pierre-Joseph Dunod, began criss-crossing the kingdom on a preaching mission, advising city and town councils on how to set up the new institutions.[34] Joined later by a third Jesuit, André Guevarre, the two priests advocated new initiatives in the field of poor relief in Provence, Languedoc, Dauphiné, Normandy, Brittany, and Poitou, the same peripheral provinces where Mount Carmel had had great difficulty attaining its expropriation goals. The three Jesuits are credited with establishing over 126 so-called hôpitaux-généraux.[35] Although inspired by the urban model, these institutions were conceived to meet the needs of the local poor and not for internment along the lines of the great confinement. They were generally located in smaller cities and large towns, and in their smallest versions, they consisted of little more than one or two rented houses to receive the poor.

Honoré Chaurand was the first of the Jesuits to preach in favour of these institutions. Trained as a missionary to convert Huguenots, he had begun his efforts to convince municipal governments to create hôpitaux-généraux during a series of missions in Normandy in 1657.[36] According to the description of Abbé Laffetay, Chaurand started at Vire in Lower Normandy on 10 March 1657. "Ringing the church bells, he described in pathetic terms, before the assembled bourgeois, the misery that he had witnessed in the cities, the lack of revenues to aid [the poor]."[37] Chaurand then asked his audience to take up a collection in their town to found a hospital for the poor. His proposal was accepted, and on 5 April a wing in the town hospital was temporarily set aside for this purpose.

Chaurand and his assistant, Father Dunod, continued the same type of mission, holding meetings with the towns people in the rural Cotentin region of Normandy. They also travelled to Valognes, Cherbourg, Coutances, St-Sauveur, Granville, Carentan, and Thorigny, re-establishing the St-Lô hospital and promoting spontaneous public collections – "the Franciscan approach" – to obtain revenues for these institutions.[38] Between 1677 and 1685 Chaurand extended his activities and missions to Brittany, where he persuaded the elite of Tréguier to set up a hospital in November 1677.[39] In his proposals for Tréguier, which were later printed and distributed by Calloët-Querbrat, Chaurand suggested renting a few existing houses to form the hospital. The buildings would be furnished with donations from local residents, and the poor nourished from the collections taken up by the local women's confraternities. He put great emphasis upon this approach, by which a community could see the concrete results of its donations, since the hospital would be opened almost immediately after the initial collections. He contrasted this approach with the more traditional "Benedictine method," in which donations and legacies were collected for years before buildings could be constructed and letters patent obtained that would enable the institution actually to open its doors.[40] Chaurand's preaching in Brittany resulted in over thirty-eight communities deciding either to set up new hospitals for the poor or to revise the statutes of existing institutions to correspond to the objectives of the hôpitaux-généraux.[41]

Since it was oriented towards community-created and supported hospitals or houses for the poor, one of the principal challenges of this campaign was to convince members of the town elite to create such institutions and to solicit the financial contributions of the local population in order to assure their support. The missions of Chaurand and his assistants were directed especially towards changing popular attitudes in the face of indiscriminate alms giving by encouraging the French to concentrate on organized attempts to provide solutions to the problem of poverty.

Proposing reduced versions of the larger hôpitaux-généraux, the campaign was directed not only towards smaller cities, but also to small towns and villages. In this context, a 1681 document, certainly inspired by Father Chaurand during his work in Brittany, goes well beyond the

structures recommended by St Vincent de Paul and the earlier missionaries and provides a key to the new forms of organized charity that were
proposed for small communities. The document, published in Paris,
probably by the Assemblée Charitable de Paris under Calloët-Querbrat,
asks for the creation of charitable assemblies (*assemblées politiques de
charité des paroisses*) in all the parishes of Brittany. The introduction to
the text claims, as did the sixteenth-century *aumône générale* movement,
that in the parishes of Brittany where assemblies had been created to
manage poor relief, traditional aid had been sufficient to nourish the
poor, and their numbers had declined by two-thirds since the lazy and
the sturdy beggars had been cut off the poor rolls and had left the
villages.[42] Repeating the urban rhetoric that direct handouts to the poor
encouraged laziness and multiplied the number of beggars, the Brittany
document argued that in each parish, the curé, *vicaire*, judge, or noble
should convene an assembly where the people could choose officials to
preside over local charitable initiatives during the coming year: a director,
secretary, treasurer (*receveur*), and assistant (*distributeur*) were to distribute the aid received.

These officials were to fix the eligibility rules for receiving aid and set
limits on the distribution of charity to itinerants and vagabonds, but
their first and foremost goal was to maintain services to the real poor,
overseeing collections in the parish church and from house to house.
Where possible, they were to acquire a house or other building where
the sick could be received and ensure that a woman whose morals were
above reproach was assigned to treat them and that a doctor or surgeon
would visit them.[43] The document concluded by envisaging a number of
hypothetical objections or problems presented by the new policy and
furnishing solutions, such as practical tips on how to increase the revenues of the poor-relief fund (fines for drinking in taverns during mass,
requests for donations at the time of weddings and baptisms, and the
placement of collection boxes with merchants and tavern keepers). It
also suggested cheaper treatments and remedies for the poor and in
particular demonstrated the way to put together a list of the poor eligible
for relief by weeding out the undeserving or phoney poor.[44]

By 1686 Chaurand was back in the south, working in the Comtat
Venaissin, in Nîmes, Aix, and Marseille. In the course of this organizational work in Provence, Chaurand and Dunod were joined by their
younger Jesuit colleague, André Guevarre, who went beyond the individual missionary rhetoric and promoted hospital organization by producing a pamphlet in 1687 for the campaign in Aix, a document that

became a model for the hospital movement. Much as in the earlier Chaurand–Calloët-Querbrat approach, this publication used a question-and-answer format to discuss how and why cities and towns should adopt the hôpital-général model for their poor-relief facilities. Entitled *La mendicité abolie dans la diocèse d'Aix par l'établissement d'un hôpital général ou … par un bureau de charité en chaque lieu ou l'on ne pouvait pas enfermer les pauvres*, it was originally composed in Latin for Pope Innocent XII, and the text was thereafter adapted to numerous cities or regions.[45] After Aix, an edition was tailored to Montauban north of Toulouse in 1693 and to Grenoble in 1712. The document was essentially a plea for smaller cities and towns to follow the lead of Paris and Lyon in establishing hôpitaux-généraux, but through its replies to preconceived objections, it tried to orient individuals away from the traditional patterns of charitable donations. Treating such hypothetical objections as "aiding the poor is not an obligation," "it is the clergy who should come to their aid," "doing good works is just as rewarding as aiding the poor," or "before the great confinement, it cost less to nourish the poor," Father Guevarre constantly tried to foresee objections that might arise from the creation of the new hôpitaux-généraux to intern the poor.

In one of his longest replies (twelve pages), he denounced in no uncertain terms those who continued to give indiscriminate handouts directly to the poor after the establishment of an hôpital-général or house of charity.[46] It is obvious that the manual was directed not just at creating the new hospitals, but also at changing the charitable habits of the French by inducing them to contribute generously to the new institutions and stop giving directly to the poor. In its work in Normandy, Brittany, Dauphiné, and Provence, this movement renewed the objectives and methods for financing small hôpitaux-généraux at the same time as it campaigned for new financing and extensions of large institutions located in the major towns and cities. Both these initiatives reduced the number of mismanaged, redundant local hospitals and entered into direct conflict with the suppressions of the St-Lazare movement.

Certainly, the hôpital-général movement was one of the reasons that the suppression of small hospitals and maladreries by Mount Carmel and St-Lazare fell short of its expected revenues; this outcome was particularly evident in Brittany. However, the long, drawn-out procedures for expropriating smaller institutions also help to explain the shortfalls of the St-Lazare operation. As in the case of the Chamber of Christian Charity and the Chamber of the General Hospital Reform, appeals, complicated legal procedures, resistance to the Chamber of the

Arsenal, and refusal to comply with its decisions all limited the results of the efforts at suppression. From 1672 to 1679 the Chamber of the Arsenal had actively sought to expropriate the capital and landholdings of the foundations that fell within its mandate – maladreries that had been abandoned or where foundation revenues had been diverted to other purposes – and the holdings of regular and hospitaller orders whose rights to operate hospitals had expired or had been abolished. But the revenues realized from these operations were limited, and in order to increase its funding, the order eventually went beyond these two types of institutions and sought to acquire funds from all maladreries where hospitality was not maintained.[47] Using these three criteria, but placing special emphasis upon the maintenance of hospitality, the chamber sent commissioners to every questionable institution to observe its functioning.

The Mount Carmel and St-Lazare suppressions affected three of the eight local hospitals retained for analysis in this book. One of them, Étoile, was located in the province of Dauphiné, and the other two, Savenay and Malestroit, were in Brittany. In Dauphiné, twenty-six maladreries and hospitals were "united" to the order in the diocese of Grenoble, twelve in Die, and fourteen in Valence.[48] As mentioned at the beginning of this chapter, the Étoile hospital was visited in July 1680 by an inspector who recommended that it be united to the Order of St-Lazare. Most of the neighbouring hospitals – Beaumont, Loriol, Montélier, Montélimar – had their funds expropriated and services partially or totally suppressed. Typical of what seems to have been the haphazard method of the reform, the Grignan hospital never figured in the register, nor did Seyne, which was situated in a relatively inaccessible border diocese where no maladrerie was annexed.[49]

What were the reasons evoked by the officials of Mount Carmel and St-Lazare to unite Étoile into their Valence priory? The basic accusations against La Charité in Étoile can be found in the correspondence of André Serret, recteur of the hospital for 1681. He protested against the decision to annex Étoile taken by Judge Jean-Guy Basset of Grenoble, a member of the royal chamber. The initial protest from Serret, written on 7 January 1681, noted that the Basset decision was based on a visit on 4 July 1680, when, as we have noted, an inspector, M. Cachod, had observed that no caretaker was present at the hospital and that the institution contained only one poor girl lying on a straw mattress on the floor.[50] The inability of Étoile to provide the care called for by the hospital's 1531 charter, specifically the absence of a caretaker and the lack of care for the hospital's only inmate, became the essential points in the St-Lazare case that hospitality was not being maintained at the institution.

The reply for Étoile was argued in detail in June 1681, when Serret advanced three major points. First, he stated that it was unacceptable to judge the hospital on the basis of the regulations promulgated in 1531 by Guillaume de Poitiers since, legally speaking, they did not constitute a charter. Secondly, on the point concerning the lack of hospitality, Serret produced the minutes and accounts of the bureau of the poor to prove that there had always been a caretaker, that the buildings were kept up, and that a daily mass was said in the chapel according to Guillaume de Poitiers's regulations. Thirdly, he presented annual hospital accounts to demonstrate that neither foundation funds nor revenues destined for the poor had been tampered with. Furthermore, he specifically denied that the accounts from 1672–78 had been readjusted to produce a more favourable image of the institution.[51] However, the judgment against Étoile was upheld in hearings in 1683, 1685, and 1686, and the administrators of the hospital were ordered to pay 100 livres from their annual revenues of 1,500 livres to the commanderie of the Order of St-Lazare in Valence.[52] Nevertheless, in the accounts of the hospital, no entry indicates that the annual payment was ever made to the order, and it is unlikely that the administrators ever conformed to the court order.[53]

In Brittany too, St-Lazare sought to appropriate revenues or holdings from institutions in every diocese; its inspectors visited fourteen maladreries and fifteen hospitals in the diocese of Rennes, eleven maladreries and nine hospitals in Vannes, eighteen maladreries and thirty-three hospitals in Nantes, thirteen maladreries and four hospitals in St-Paul-de-Léon, eight maladreries and hospitals in St-Malo, eleven maladreries and ten hospitals in St-Brieuc, twelve maladreries and four hospitals in Dol, and ten maladreries and five hospitals in Tréguier.[54] In the end, despite systematic inspections of all the targeted institutions and long, drawn-out legal proceedings, the order succeeded in appropriating revenues or holdings from only twenty-nine institutions.[55]

Savenay and Malestroit were two of the hospitals that the order singled out for suppression in Brittany, and each illustrates different experiences with the legal procedures of the operation. Concerning Savenay, the Chamber of the Arsenal issued a judgment in 1674 ordering Pierre Bezard, chaplain of the St-Armal hospital, to give up his rights to the institution, to repair the buildings, and to locate the titles to hospital property and the accounts of its revenues over the last twenty-nine years. Furthermore, he was instructed to turn all these documents over to the Order of St-Lazare, which was to lease out the holdings for 200 livres a year.[56] This judgment was probably appealed because a second ruling, issued in 1677, confirmed and further justified the initial decision. According to this document, the Savenay hospital had been in complete ruin in 1674, without doors, roofless, and its chapel bare. Since the takeover, however, the leaseholder for St-Lazare had placed two wooden beds with straw mattresses in the dormitory of the hospital.[57] In the end, the institution seems to have been put into the hands of the representatives of St-Lazare.

The process of suppression in Malestroit was totally different. The institution was listed as one of those to be "reformed" in the diocese of Vannes, and Julien Garson, Sieur de la Guichardaire, the provost of the hospital, was convoked by the *grand vicaire* and commander of the Order of St-Lazare to appear before the Chamber of the Arsenal on 28 June 1675. At the hearing, he was condemned to turn over to the Order of St-Lazare all the revenues and holdings that the institution had acquired over the previous twenty-nine years.[58] The general assembly of the community met several times during the summer of 1675 and named a special commission of five bourgeois to defend their hospital. The procedures, hearings, and appeals concerning the affair lasted until 1681, and in the end Malestroit succeeded in defeating the St-Lazare attempts to appropriate either a part of the hospital revenues or its holdings.[59]

The uneven results of the expropriation process in Étoile, Savenay, and Malestroit, as well as the 1,700 other cases brought before the Chamber of the Arsenal, seem to account for the failure of Mount Carmel and St-Lazare to receive the revenues that it had anticipated from the suppressions. Of the three hospitals, the order succeeded in expropriating only the holdings of Savenay – an institution in ruins. In Étoile and Malestroit, as elsewhere, the town and village institutions with the highest revenues were precisely those best able to resist expropriation or to limit the payments that they were ordered to make to the commanderies of the order. The problem was that the hospitals that were truly corrupt or had ceased to maintain hospitality generally had no funds. In order to secure financing for their commanderies, the commissioners for the order had to turn to hospitals such as Étoile or Malestroit and try to prove that their holdings, too, should be wholly or partially expropriated.

Local resistance to the expropriation of well-run hospitals slowed the movement overall, but ultimately the Mount Carmel and St-Lazare reforms were stopped, not so much by the protests of the small communities as by two influential groups: the disgruntled hospitaller orders that had been dispossessed of their holdings by St-Lazare and the dévots who had worked since the 1620s to reorganize new urban charitable structures and to spearhead the creation of the hôpital-général network to incarcerate and reform the able poor. These opposition groups concentrated on two aspects of the St-Lazare reform. First, they attacked what they portrayed as the scandal of the diversion of poor-relief funds to compensate former army officers and soldiers rather than the poor for whom the foundations had been created. Secondly, they cited the absence of prior papal consent to the confiscations of holdings that had belonged to the Teutonic Knights, the Order of the St-Esprit de Montpellier, the Knights of St-Jacques, and the Order of the Holy Sepulchre.[60] The objections of the hospitaller orders to the reform won concrete results in the 1690s because of continuing disputes with the pope over Louis XIV's attempts in the 1670s and 1680s to encourage French bishops to support the Gallican concept of the church, in which the king disposed of widespread patronage and political rights. With the king trying to settle his differences with Rome, the pope insisted that no general agreement could be obtained without a resolution of the problem of expropriation of the traditional hospitaller orders.[61]

The death of Louvois on 16 July 1691 deprived the Order of St-Lazare of its principal protector at the royal court just as the combined group resistance to the St-Lazare reform became critical. By December that year the seriousness of the opposition to the order led the king to appoint twelve commissioners to examine all objections to the 1672 edict.[62] During the resulting inquiry, the commissioners studied the statutes of the order and pointed out the legal problems inherent in applying the edict. They began by noting that the 1672 resignation of M. de Nerestang from the position of grand vicaire of the order to make way for the nomination of Louvois had been totally illegal. The king, in the absence of papal consent, did not have the authority either to receive the resignation or to name a new Grand Vicaire. Furthermore, given the rights of the church over the different holdings that had been incorporated into the Order of St-Lazare, the crown alone did not have the right to permit it to proceed with expropriations. The document produced by the commission noted that the process of seizure had totally ignored the rights of the founders of the hospitals and maladreries in question, although the commissioners did not make any specific recommendations concerning this point. Instead, they turned to the legal basis and precedents evoked by Louvois to justify the crown initiatives, and they claimed to have found only specious arguments and unconvincing precedents. For them, the basic problem with the whole process was the absence of papal bulls confirming the king's rights to intervene.[63]

The Louvois project did not go undefended, however, and the Marquis de Chamlay, secretary of state for war, who had been closely associated with the creation and functioning of the order, presented four different reports concerning the project. Two of them were submitted directly to Louis XIV, and one contained notes written in the margins by the king. The increasingly critical approach to the St-Lazare project by both the commission and the king is evident in the change in tone of Chamlay's reports. In his first intervention, he strongly defended the project, while his later submissions made distinctions between the positive and negative aspects of the experience. He noted that the commanderies established in 1680 had been greatly appreciated by the king's officers, that the initiative had not intentionally violated canon law, and that the problems could be resolved if the king requested papal bulls to ratify the actions taken. In the later texts, the marquis tried to overcome the criticism that funds donated for the poor had been diverted to pensions for army officers by suggesting a change in funding for the two major military institutions: he argued that the money currently spent to run the recently created Invalides could be used instead to fund army pensions and that the revenues from the expropriated hospitals and maladreries could be directed to the care of the poor and handicapped soldiers treated in the Invalides, this approach being more in conformity with the original intentions of the donors.

In his final report, however, Chamlay seems to have realized that the revenues of St-Lazare were too modest to finance the Invalides. He modified his previous position, arguing that to function adequately, the Invalides required all the revenues presently in the hands of the Order of St-Lazare, a part of its current funding from the military budget (the *extraordinaire des guerres*), and the revenues that Louis XIV had ordered the abbeys of the kingdom to furnish for the replacement of the oblats. In this final submission, Chamlay contended that the commanderies of St-Lazare should be paid out of a part of the extraordinaire des guerres, but at a much lower level. The number of commanderies should be reduced and the criteria for admission to the order tightened. Members should merit admission by serving in the army for a certain period of time, nobility should no longer be one of the criteria, naval officers should be allowed to join, and members should no longer have to pay for their admission.[64]

Despite the attempts of Chamlay to defend the St-Lazare project, even he had to admit that the king did not have the right either to name Louvois to the position of grand vicaire of the Order of St-Lazare or to authorize the transfer of the holdings of other hospitaller orders to the order without papal consent. The commission named by Louis XIV had been specifically preoccupied with the legal precedents of the 1672 edict, and Chamlay presented no arguments to contradict their essentially negative conclusions. The results of the inquiry led to an edict in March 1693 repealing the 1672 legislation that had permitted the order to take control of small, local institutions and expropriate all or part of their funds.[65] The king therefore ordered that all the holdings seized over the previous twenty years be returned to their original owners, and he appointed twelve commissioners to carry out this restitution.

In a declaration the following August, however, Louis revealed the new direction of charitable reform: he ordered that in cases where the revenues of local institutions were insufficient to maintain hospitality and provide efficient aid to the poor, they should not be re-established, and their funds should be turned over to what he considered the more efficient regional hospitals.[66] This directive confirms the activity of the dévots and the great confinement movement in opposing the St-Lazare reform. The dévots sought to take over the funds of small institutions for themselves in order to continue their vast projects of urban reform, specifically the extension of the hôpital-général system.[67]

Like most attempts by the state or its agents to intervene in local areas of jurisdiction in early modern times, the various reforms were handi-capped by several factors: the meagre resources of the suppressed hos-pitals, the determined resistance of community leaders, and the continual judicial challenges by the affected villages. Royal authorities had seriously overestimated the wealth of the small foundations that they had charged with graft and corruption. Like Savenay, most of the suppressed insti-tutions possessed few or no funds, and most of those that did have significant capital or landholdings were not at all corrupt or redundant. Like Grignan, Caudebec, Pontorson, and Malestroit, they were managed efficiently following the model of most urban charities, and the St-Lazare agents had great difficulty finding excuses to expropriate their resources. The uneven results obtained by the ambitious St-Lazare reform, together with the earlier failures of the Chamber of Christian Charity and the Chamber of the General Hospital Reform to reappro-priate the funds and holdings of the supposedly mismanaged local hos-pitals, demonstrate the limits to the crown's power to interve directly or indirectly in a new field of jurisdiction. The large number of hearings, judicial procedures, appeals, and judgments making up the records of the three semi-royal commissions all testify to the difficulty of establishing royal rights to intervene. They also show the modest or total lack of revenues of the institutions where corruption could be proved. As in Étoile, Savenay, and Malestroit – even in cases where the hospital was in total ruin, such as Savenay – local officials still appealed the commission decisions, and in cases where the hospital was clearly active, administrators either ignored court orders, as in Étoile, or obtained their annulment, as in Malestroit.

The St-Lazare experiment was actually directed towards providing pay-offs to the military elite. Using the funds of the "mismanaged" hospitals and maladreries, it provided pensions to former officers and attempted to get around the legal obstacle to direct crown intervention by leaving the suppression and expropriation to a military-hospitaller order created by papal bull. This reform was hastily abandoned in the face of vigorous opposition from groups purporting to defend what they called the rights of the sick and the poor. From the beginning, it had competed against the well-organized movement for the creation of urban hôpitaux-généraux to incarcerate and reform the able-bodied poor and with the more marginal and more spontaneous effort by Calloet-Quebrat and Chaurand to revise the mandate and functioning of small, local hospitals in order to "save the souls" of the poor outside the cities. Both of these movements benefited from the grass-roots support of the dévots and the increasingly organized missionary initiatives. The creation of hôpitaux-généraux in the cities was designed to incarcerate the poor, re-educate them, and teach them work skills in order to eliminate beggary. While never the object of a centralized reform attempt, large numbers of small hospitals and maladreries were turned over to hôpitaux-généraux in the individual letters patent signed by the king. Furthermore, in provinces such as Brittany, hôpitaux-généraux even became part of the small-town and rural infrastructure, in many cases extending and reinforcing the network of small, local institutions at the same time as the St-Lazare movement was trying to suppress them.

Although there was much resistance to these different solutions and attempts at suppression, it is evident that they did achieve some results. They destabilized the local hospital network and sent inspectors to thousands of small institutions seeking arguments to invoke their suppression. The hearings of the Chamber of the Arsenal show that the majority of these small institutions did receive orders of closure or judgments demanding that their revenues and holdings be partially or totally incorporated into the domains of larger city hospitals or into the commanderies of the Order of St-Lazare. These incursions were constantly challenged and the suppression process slowed down, but as Colin Jones has noted, it appears that the reform effort destabilized and compromised numerous institutions of assistance, leaving a mountain of paperwork, without ever really achieving their suppression or expropriation. Most of the commanderies of the Order of St-Lazare were never able to trace the holdings that had supposedly belonged to the local hospitals, and many of the suppressed institutions continued to function.[68] In the aftermath of the St-Lazare experiment, the network of hospitals had to be re-examined, and control by the city hospitals over local institutions of poor relief was even accelerated as the rationalization continued to consolidate the urban infrastructures.

3 The Aftermath of Notre-Dame of Mount Carmel and St-Lazare: The Closures Continue

On 4 May 1697 the administrators of the hôtel-Dieu and hôpital-général of Le Havre asked that an inquiry be held into the new expropriations of seven maladreries in and around the town of Fécamp.[1] After the 1693 decree had ended their "union" with the Order of Mount Carmel and St-Lazare, these institutions had been taken away from the Seigneur de Refuge of the commanderie of Fécamp. The Conseil d'État had ordered that since they were too small to function normally, they should be closed down and their revenues used to found an hôpital-général in Fécamp. However, in a series of meetings in May and October 1697, the administrators of Le Havre opposed this decision, arguing that the resources of these seven hospices should not be used to establish an hôpital-général, but should instead be turned over to the existing hospital in Le Havre. All of the hospitals of the region were consulted on this question, and the administrators of the Caudebec hospital met with François de Romé, Seigneur de Fresquiennes, a *conseiller* in the Parlement of Rouen, along with representatives from the hospitals at Fécamp, St-Romain-de-Colbosc, and Montivilliers. Before this group, the Le Havre administrators argued that besides the sick and poor of the region, their hospital was committed to care for sailors from the royal navy and impoverished seamen. The revenues from the expropriated institutions would allow Le Havre to improve services to all these groups. After much debate among the representatives and within the Counseil d'État, the revenues of the seven institutions were finally turned over to Le Havre by a royal edict issued on 7 May 1700.[2]

This type of dispute between small towns and villages became common after the 1692 decision to revoke the right of the Order of St-Lazare to dispose of the revenues of maladreries, hospices, and hospitals. Since their initial expropriations, the order had, in fact, initiated procedures to close down many of these institutions, and for others they had expropriated buildings, revenues, and archives. It was almost impossible for most of the hospitals simply to resume their operations. Nor was it the intention of the crown to allow the reopening of what it had always seen as small, ineffective institutions. Capitalizing upon the destabilization of these hospitals and maladreries during the St-Lazare experiment, the crown itself undertook a massive series of suppressions, mergers, and expropriations that actually executed many of the rationalizations that St-Lazare had been unable to carry through. This new reform took place in two different phases. The first series of mergers was carried out between 1693 and 1705, when regional hospitals were created with the revenues of the thousands of small maladreries and hospices that were not re-established after having been closed down for almost twenty years. The second phase occurred after 1724, when a new series of decisions was made in which Louis xv took the unprecedented step of designating a limited number of these regional hospitals to receive crown subsidies to incarcerate the poor, the beggars, the sick, and the handicapped of the great confinement.

The royal edict ordering the restitution of the hospices and maladreries taken over by the Order of St-Lazare was dated December 1692, and it was issued at Versailles the following March. The details of the restitution were published on 15 April; they specified that the founders or owners of the expropriated institutions were to be given two months to present legal titles or charters proving their ownership of the maladreries, hospices, or hospitals. These documents were to be submitted to the commissioners named to execute the restitutions.[3] But four months later, in a second edict, it became clear that the crown's objective was not to reopen the thousands of small charitable institutions whose operations it had denounced for over a century. The new edict on 24 August ruled on cases where the revenues of the maladrerie or hospice to be restored were considered "not sufficient" for it to function adequately. The document openly promoted the merging of such small charitable institutions, specifying that in the cases where village maladreries or hospices were closed in order to transfer their revenues to larger regional institutions, the seigneurs of the villages affected retained certain rights over the new hospitals. They were to be consulted on the nomination of administrators and any changes in the hospital statutes and were to be given quotas for the poor of their villages in the new regional institutions. The edict clearly retained the principle of the 1561 declaration that each village was responsible for its own poor, but it provided the opportunity for such communities to meet these obligations by uniting their resources to create regional hospitals.[4]

This modification was explained in detail in a 1693 report to the archbishops, bishops, and intendants, who were asked to aid the royal commissioners in implementing the new policy. The letters patent issued in April 1693 named twelve commissioners to examine the cases where ownership of a maladrerie, hospice, or hospital could not be established. Among them, the Sieurs de la Reynie, de Marillac, d'Aguesseau, de Ribeyre, de Harlay, and de Fourcy were councillors in the Conseil d'État, and the Sieurs le Blanc, Quentin de Richebourg, Pelletier de la Houssaye, Ferrand, de Fieubet, and Camus de Pontcarré were maîtres de requêtes. The procedure to be followed in the resulting inquiries was set out in the document. First, for each of these institutions, the commissioners were to establish whether or not the knights of the Order of Mount Carmel and St-Lazare had improperly exploited the lands and buildings that had been transferred to them by cutting trees, selling off furnishings, or permitting buildings to deteriorate. Secondly, they were to examine the revenues received from the hospital holdings in order to decide what to do with the institution. The document presented them with three options. If the revenues of the hospice were sufficient to support the services required by an institution's charter without any new capital investment, it could reopen its doors. If not, a second possibility might be to group the revenues of several maladreries and hospices to form one regional hospital to which the sick and poor of surrounding villages could be sent. The third option suggested that regional authorities might prefer to transfer the revenues from all the small maladreries and hospices to an existing hôpital-général in a nearby city.[5] The application of these criteria set the tone for a decade of disputes between towns and villages, which fought to get their hands on the poor-relief facilities of others and to prevent their own institutions from being shut down.

Using these royal directives, the commissioners examined the revenues and holdings that had been expropriated by the Order of Mount Carmel and St-Lazare in 106 dioceses. The results of their work, published in

1705, contain their recommendations for each of the suppressed institutions; the maladreries and hospitals to be restored were to be merged with larger existing hospitals or have their funds and holdings used to create new hospitals. These recommendations are presented in Map 5.[6] The commissioners examined 1,768 cases of hospitals, maladreries, or foundations that Mount Carmel and St-Lazare had expropriated. They recommended that 608 of the institutions should be re-established using the revenues and holdings that had been taken from them in the 1670s and 1680s. But in the great majority of the cases treated (1,632 hospitals, hospices, and maladreries), the commissioners opposed restitution, frequently recommending instead that the expropriated revenues and holdings of defunct institutions be transferred to the most active of the local hospitals or that the funds of a number of suppressed hospitals be used to found a new and more important local or regional institution.

These transfers were very uneven, and the number of small poor-relief institutions that were turned over to larger urban hospitals was far greater than those merged with other rural institutions: no less than 24 local hospitals were suppressed to fund the Hôpital pour les Pauvres Malades de Perpignan, 21 went to the Hôpital de Beziers, 16 to the Hôpital St-Jean-d'Arras, 14 to the Hôpital de Lisieux, and 16 to the Hôpital-Général de Vienne. However, the vast majority of the institutions benefiting from the suppressions received the holdings of only one or two local hospitals.

A second element that can be discerned from the 1705 list is the fact that most of the institutions treated by the commissioners had, in fact, continued operating despite the Mount Carmel and St-Lazare "suppressions." Frequently, it was noted that an institution should no longer have to pay the allocations that had been awarded to the knights of Mount Carmel, thus indicating that the hospital had remained open. It is also clear that the 1,632 suppressions in the 1690s represent only a little more than a third of the 4,078 that the order had tried to carry out. The more limited scope of the redistributions ordered by the royal commission between 1693 and 1695 may have been due to the crown's desire to avoid the legal protests that had marked the earlier suppressions. More probably, it may have been because the weakest of the hospitals and maladreries had already disappeared in the earlier round of expropriations.

If the suppressions recommended by the commissioners in the 1690s were far fewer than in the earlier period, the geographic distribution of the hospital shutdowns was very similar. Just as the large northern dioceses around Paris had been the primary targets for the Mount

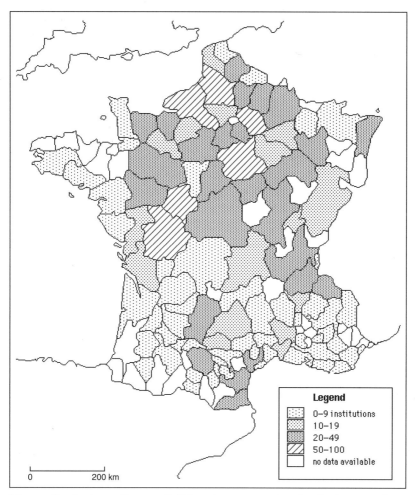

Map 5   Institutions of poor relief that the crown ordered to be integrated into larger hospitals after their restitution following expropriation by the Order of Mount Carmel and St-Lazare, 1693–95

Carmel and St-Lazare expropriations, so they once again became the focus for the re-examinations launched in 1693. Of the six dioceses in which the holdings and revenues of 50 to 100 hospitals were to be redistributed (Sens, Soissons, Rouen, Amiens, Tours, and Poitiers), all but Poitiers had been in the category of 100 or more expropriations carried out by the Order of Mount Carmel (see Map 5). Just as in the expropriations of 1672–93, most of the small southern dioceses, as well

Table 2

Distribution of revenues of 145 maladreries, hospices, and hospitals in Dauphiné in February 1692 (in livres)

10 or less	11–50	51–100	101–400	401–1,000	1,001 or more
6	71	32	29	6	1

as those of Brittany, either were not touched or fell into the categories of 0 to 9 or 10 to 19 redistributions. The 1705 document illustrates the exceptional importance of the holdings of the Confraternity of the St-Esprit in Provence. In the diocese of Aix, 9 of the 18 confirmed or re-established hospitals belonged to the confraternity; in Fréjus it held 9 out of the 18 that were returned; in Grasse it owned 2 out of 4, in Marseilles 7 out of 11, and in Riez 1 out of 4. Only in Sisteron and Toulon was the confraternity absent from the lists of re-established hospitals.[7]

In two of the four provinces examined in this book, the archives on the restitution process allow us to go beyond the official listing of suppressions and restitutions and to gain further insight into the way that church and crown authorities limited the number of institutions to be reopened by distributing the revenues of many of the suppressed hospices to the better financed and usually larger hospitals. For Dauphiné, Guy Allard, a nineteenth-century historian, reconstituted a list of 150 maladreries, hospices, and hospitals either belonging to Mount Carmel and St-Lazare or being claimed by the order in February 1692. The revenues for 145 foundations are indicated in the lists drawn up by Allard, and they amounted to 20,955 livres 13 sous. But as Table 2 indicates, the distribution of these revenues was very uneven. Seven of the hospitals possessing between 401 and 1,000+ livres accounted for a quarter of the total revenues. Hospitals such as Étoile supposedly contributed 100 livres a year to the order, but, in fact, the Valence commanderie never received any payment from Étoile. Others, such as Renel or Bellegarde, contributed 10 livres, and Alixan, near Valence, produced an annual revenue of only 13 sous.[8]

The local bishops in Dauphiné apparently went even further than the royal commissioners in convincing local officials that it was in the best interest of communities with impoverished charitable institutions not to reopen their hospices, but to transfer the revenues to fund the activities of a nearby hospital properly. The essential debates over the operation of these suppressions took place in the king's council and in the Grenoble Parlement. Royal commissioners such as the Sieurs Quentin

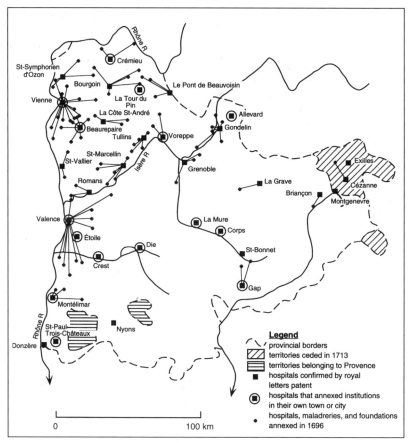

Map 6   Local hospitals, maladreries, and foundations annexed to hospitals in the province of Dauphiné in 1696

de Richebourg, le Blanc, le Casmier, Fievbre de Reuvillon, Ribeyre, and Guillaume de Vieville, all maîtres de requêtes, and the Sieurs de Fourcy and de Marillac, counseillers d'État, were sent into the province. They examined the closings and transfers that could be carried out for the institutions "detached" from the Order of St-Lazare, and the council subsequently approved their recommendations.[9]

René Favier has shown that the Parlement of Grenoble discussed and approved the transfers, which sought to establish or reinforce the 33 recommended regional hospitals financed by the appropriation of funds from 17 almshouses, 40 hospices, and 52 maladreries (see Map 6).[10] In some cases, it was necessary to re-establish hospitals in regional centres before they could receive the revenues from surrounding institutions. Nyons was one of these special cases where hospitality was reinstituted. Since it was a Protestant town, its hospital had been suppressed after the revocation of the Edict of Nantes, and the buildings and property of the institution had been transferred to the Grenoble hôpital-général. The Nyons hospital was re-established in 1696, and the commissioners authorized its directors to recover the institution's former holdings to pay for building repairs and future operating expenses. However, unlike the majority of the restored hospitals, Nyons received no new funds transferred from hospital closings in the surrounding villages.[11] In the region, the major beneficiary from the transfer of funds controlled by rural hospitals was the hôpital-général of Valence; it received the revenues of the hospitals at Allex, Alixan, Chabeuil, Montélier, Chabrillan, Beaumont, Grâne, Loriol, and Mirmande.[12] Even the Étoile hôtel-Dieu received the revenues of a disbanded town maladrerie in addition to 45 livres from the hospice at La Vache.[13] The results of these expropriations and transfers are not always clear: the Nyons hospital could never function adequately since it received no new funding, and both Valence and Étoile complained that they had not been able to take possession of many of the holdings accorded to them. The hospitals that they acquired had lost all their archives and land registers. None of the villagers would admit to having appropriated former hospital lands, so that Valence and Étoile were never able to get control of the holdings that they had supposedly received.

In Normandy the same type of local hospital expropriations were carried out. Crown and church authorities singled out small-town and village hospices, which they saw as underfunded, recommending that their revenues be used for the creation of regional institutions. As in Dauphiné, maîtres de requêtes such as Sieur Lefevre d'Ormesson and conseillers d'état such as the Sieur de Marillac were sent in to review the status of the "re-established" hospitals and maladreries.[14] Here too it was the Parlement of Rouen that discussed the number of transfers, giving its stamp of approval to the operation. Between 22 October 1694 and 7 May 1700, the Parlement approved the creation of 32 regional hospitals in Normandy funded by the transfer of revenues from 89 suppressed maladreries and small hospices, 4 hospitals, and 2 monastic foundations. In Normandy as in Dauphiné, it becomes obvious that the policy of mergers was aimed at building up regional hospitals and that in the criteria for retained or re-established institutions, geographical location was very important. An example of this policy was that a new hospital was ordered to be built in Vaudreuil "on the most convenient

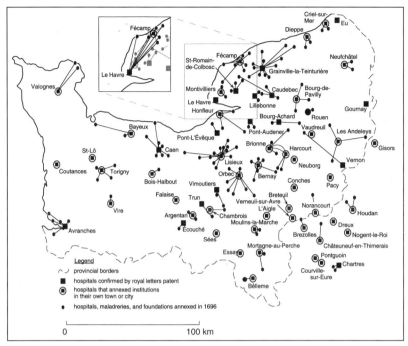

Map 7   Local hospitals, maladreries, and foundations annexed to hospitals
in the province of Normandy in 1696

site for distributing aid to the poor."[15] The 32 regional hospitals were
distributed around the province to try to reduce conflicts between institutions and avoid redundancy in their services (see Map 7).[16]

The presence of a hospital played an integral part in assuring the
regional pre-eminence of an urban centre: besides opening up patronage
opportunities for the local elite, the existence of one of the new hospitals
ensured that the community had access to a doctor or surgeon and an
apothecary and that it possessed a relatively imposing building to house
the facility. Since potential regional centres struggled among one
another to acquire the best of the disbanded rural institutions, the policy
produced important conflicts when it came to designating hospital
towns. It was for this reason that the hôpital-général of Le Havre
opposed the designation of Fécamp for a regional institution. A decision
of the Rouen Parlement on 22 October 1694 had turned over seven
maladreries to the Fécamp hospital in order to provide for the founding
of a new regional institution. However, the administrators of Le Havre
claimed that a previous royal decision in 1669 had granted them rights
over all the former leproseries in the region, and they argued that the

seven maladreries were all former leproseries. They went on to assert that since they were responsible for lodging and treating the men of the royal navy and other seamen, they should be compensated for their services. This disagreement led to regional meetings in May and October 1697, as Fécamp sought support from the surrounding towns.[17] Le Havre eventually won out, however, receiving the seven contested institutions, including the maladreries of Fécamp, which alone produced annual revenues of over 800 livres.

A similar dispute between Caudebec and Le Havre broke out over the distribution of the maladreries of St-Amator-d'Auberville, St-Léonard near Lillebonne, and St-Julien-de-Lugan, a parish of Lillebonne. The Parlement had initially granted these institutions to Caudebec in 1695, but the administrators of Le Havre claimed rights over the three maladreries on the same grounds that they had used to dispute the transfers to Fécamp. In a meeting at Caudebec in 1697, this new dispute was discussed between the administrators of the hospital and François de Romé de Fresquiennes, councillor in the Parlement of Rouen, the judge who had also dealt with the Fécamp case. This time Caudebec turned the tables on Le Havre, agreeing to give up its claim to the maladreries and support their transfer to Lillebonne, a town in which two of the three institutions were located. It was more difficult for Le Havre to deprive a town of its own institutions, and in 1705 the Parlement officially accorded the three maladreries to Lillebonne.[18]

Along the same lines, a dispute broke out in lower Normandy between the administrators of the hospitals of Orbec and Bernay. In 1708 conseilleur d'état Marillac accorded to Orbec the maladreries of Ferté-Fresnel, la Barre, Lire, Notre-Dame-du-Valet, du Buzot, St-Martin and St-Denis-d'Echauffour, St-Nicolas and Ste-Marguerite in the forest of St-Evroult, La Ferrière, and the hospital of St-Jean in Chambrois. Some of these institutions had been awarded to the Bernay hospital in 1698, and its administrators accused Orbec of soliciting letters from the bishop of Lisieux to support their claims. Furthermore, it was shown that the subdelegate of Intendant d'Alençon had mistakenly confirmed Orbec's rights over all of the institutions in question. The final decision by the Conseil d'État in 1710 restored to Bernay the maladreries that Orbec had tried to expropriate.[19]

The approaches employed in Dauphiné and Normandy to "restore" the institutions expropriated by the Order of Mount Carmel and St-Lazare seem to have been typical of the process of revising the welfare system throughout France. Crown administrators wanted to avoid the previous haphazard dispersal of rural poor-relief services, and yet they were anxious to ensure a certain presence of local welfare institutions. They walked a tightrope between the complaints and appeals of small towns, such as Caudebec and Fécamp or Orbec and Bernay, that dreamed of becoming regional centres and the demands of the even larger urban centres, such as Le Havre or Valence, with their insatiable appetites for absorbing the institutions that were to be "restored." The process of "restitution" permanently eliminated a large proportion of the maladreries, hospices, and hospitals that had previously been expropriated by the Order of Mont Carmel and St-Lazare.

The new crown policy was carried out by royal councillors and maîtres de requêtes, who recommended the suppressions and mergers that were subsequently approved by the parlements in both Dauphiné and Normandy. These bodies discussed and executed the recommendations of the commissioners and frequently had to hear appeals and reconsider their initial decisions. The process caused the crown and the provincial governments to be inconsistent in implementing their new welfare policy. Starting out with the goal of creating a new "urban" welfare landscape in their respective provinces, they revised their plans and retreated on their intentions whenever the opposition of the towns and villages became too strong. Colin Jones considers that, despite its drawbacks, this exercise in the realignment of the hospital system produced a lasting and potentially more efficient structure for local poor relief.[20]

The second stage in the creation of larger, more centralized, and more urbanized charitable institutions came with the designation in 1724 of 156 hôpitaux-généraux to carry out the new official policy of "eliminating beggary forever." Under this policy, all those who could not support themselves were either to go voluntarily to be interned in one of the designated hospitals or, if they were caught begging in the streets or loitering on the highways, the newly reinforced maréchaussée, or constabulary, would compel them to be confined. Within these "hospitals," they were to be put to work on the textile looms, in woodworking shops, or in the adjacent manufacturing centres. The 156 designated institutions were to be partially subsidized by grants from the crown, but part of the funding for these grants was, once again, to be found in the suppression of local charities and town and village alms distributions.[21]

The new policy constituted a radical departure from the 1566 Edict of Moulins, which had specified that each village was accountable for its own poor and that rural immigrants who were found begging in cities should be returned to their native villages. The royal declaration of 1724 allowed fifteen days after the publication of the edict for the poor to return to their places of birth in order to find work or report to the nearest hospital for internment (article 1). Thereafter, if they were caught begging or loitering, they were to be arrested by either the police, the archers in the towns, or the newly reorganized constabulary in the countryside. They were then to be led to the nearest hôpital-général, where they were to be interned for a period to be fixed by the institution's administrators.

A double standard of internment was established that corresponded to earlier distinctions between able-bodied beggars (*valides*) and the physically and mentally handicapped (*invalides*). The able-bodied were to be interned on bread and water for no less than two months for their first offence and for no less than three months for their second arrest, with the additional penalty of having an *M* (*mendiant*) branded into the flesh of their upper arm. Thus identified, men who were arrested for the third time were to be sent to the galleys for no less than five years, and women were to be confined in the hospital for no less a period of time (article 3). Begging by invalides was regarded as a less serious offence; the duration of their confinement depended upon their condition, although upon a second arrest they were to be punished by confinement for the rest of their lives. Children were to be held until they were old enough to earn a living (article 1). The edict also encouraged those who could not find work to report to the hospital as *éngagés*; they would be lodged and nourished by the institution, which would organize them into groups of twenty under the command of a sergeant in order to provide the manpower for public works projects. The profits realized from this work were to be used to supplement the revenues of the hospital (article 2).[22]

In the decision to arrest, intern, and enforce work habits upon the vagrant population, the 1724 edict laid down two important innovations: first, that the principal police force responsible for enforcing the law was to be the newly reorganized royal constabulary (articles 7, 8, and 9) and, secondly, that the crown promised to subsidize the hôpitaux-généraux that were to be responsible for incarcerating the beggars and vagabonds turned over to them (articles 3, 4, and 5). In the preamble to the new law, the crown recognized that past attempts to control and eradicate beggars and vagabonds had been hampered by the lack of effective enforcement. The reorganized constabulary was to change all that. Initially created by François 1 and Henri 11 to punish minor offences committed by the military, the constabulary was at the same time a police force commanded by the *prévôt général*, under the orders of the *maréchaux de France*, and a legal body with the right to judge vagabonds, highwaymen, deserters, counterfeiters, and rebels.[23] Understaffed and underpaid, constables had played a minor role in maintaining social order up to 1720, when a new royal edict totally reorganized the force. It disbanded the old venial companies and replaced them with a new organization and an improved pay scale so that every generalité in the kingdom would have a company divided into brigades and commanded by a prévôt général.[24] The généralité of Caen in Normandy was divided into twelve brigades, each stationed at a strategic location. In 1726 there were two brigades in Caen, one at the seat of each subdelegate, and two others in smaller towns (Pontfarcy and Aunay) situated along major highways.[25]

Recent historians have shown that a reorganized constabulary was a prerequisite for the implementation of the 1724 edict. Jean-Pierre Gutton was the first to have clearly established the link between policing and the new attitudes toward the poor that developed in the late sixteenth and seventeenth centuries. His work on the coming of the great confinement concentrated upon the repressive aspect of the new hôpitaux-généraux begun in the early seventeenth century, and in his discussion of the 1724 edict, he argued that the reorganization of the royal constabulary was a necessary element in taking social control a step further.[26] Gutton never actually measured the ability of the reorganized police force to carry out the heavy task assigned to it, but in his conclusion to *La société et les pauvres*, he recognized that such a "demography of poverty" would be a useful complement to existing research.[27]

A recent volume by Robert Schwartz has provided just such a complement. Concentrating upon lower Normandy, it links improvements in the organization of the constabulary to the ability of the hôpitaux-généraux effectively to incarcerate the poor and undesirables. It measures the efficiency of the constabulary after the 1724 decree in terms of its ability to round up beggars, vagabonds, aged, and infirm in each of the nine designated hospitals of lower Normandy. Schwartz has shown that the reorganized force generally carried out its mission. During the initial period after the decree, there was popular opposition to the arrests made by the constabulary and community solidarity with the "persecuted" poor. However, by the 1780s the police were much better accepted, even in rural communities, and, in a complete reversal of attitudes, it became the idle poor, the beggars, and the vagabonds whom the population saw as the bigger social danger.[28] Of course, Schwartz's conclusions must be tempered by the work of Iain Cameron, who argues that the efficiency of the constabulary differed considerably from one province to another,[29] but it remains clear that the new effectiveness of the reorganized constabulary was one of the keys to the carrying out of the provisions of the 1724 edict.

In analysing past problems, the preamble to the 1724 edict considered insufficient funding of the hôpitaux-généraux to have compromised previous efforts to eliminate vagrancy. The text indicates that some hospitals had been so short of funds that they had simply opened their doors and emptied the institution rather than organizing work projects for the able-bodied beggars and subsistence for the aged and handicapped. The crown ordered its administrators to support the hospitals and, wherever institutional revenues were insufficient, to supplement them from the king's own resources. Asking the people to contribute as well through charity to the upkeep of their hospitals, the text continued the traditional crown attacks on indiscriminate charity, arguing that if each subject gave half the money to the hospitals that he or she distributed in handouts to the poor, it would be enough to finance all the institutions of the kingdom.

The administrators of the hôpitaux-généraux were given wide-ranging responsibilities in the direction of the confinement. They were to be in charge of deciding the terms of incarceration for those arrested (article 3), issuing passports to avoid arrest for those vagabonds who wanted to return to their native villages (article 4), maintaining a register of those arrested so as to account for repeat offenders (article 3), and transmitting data on all those interned to the hôpital-général in Paris, which was to maintain a central registry for all those arrested in the kingdom (article 5).

The text of the edict never defined exactly which hôpitaux-généraux were to be subsidized and become responsible for enforcing the new law. Apparently, the crown itself had not yet made this decision at the time the edict was issued. Jean-Pierre Gutton has shown that between 1720, when initial drafts of the proposal for interning the poor were sent to the intendants, and the publication of the 1724 edict, crown authorities were torn between creating totally new institutions under their control to incarcerate the poor and using the existing hospital network.

At the same time that they requested information on existing hospital facilities, royal officials seem to have preferred the solution that would have given the state complete control over the instrument of repression.[30] On 31 January 1724 the controller general, Dodun, wrote to each of the intendants concerning the availability of unused chateaux, crown properties, or buildings in each généralité that could contain the poor. However, the replies seem to have been less than enthusiastic. The intendant of Auvergne answered that the king possessed nothing in his province and that the purchase of a sufficiently large building would cost at least 2,000 livres.[31] On 7 July 1724 Dodun wrote back to the intendants that, having studied their replies, the king had decided that it would be too costly to create a new network of institutions and that the existing hospital structures would be used. Furthermore, the selected institutions were to be repaired and enlarged. His letter then asked the intendants to comment upon the condition of those hospitals that they felt could be employed.[32]

The replies to Dodun's letter varied considerably from intendant to intendant. In Dauphiné, Intendant Fontanieu had a list of possible institutions prepared, and on 18 July 1724 he wrote suggesting that internment centres could be organized in the hospitals of Grenoble, Gap, Embrun, Vienne, Romans, Valence, and Montélimar, the principal cities in each region. It was important that centres be on major travel routes. Vienne, Romans, Valence, and Montélimar were situated along the heavily frequented Rhône valley, and Gap and Embrun were on the well-travelled route from northern Italy leading from the Montgenèvre pass near Briançon down the Durance valley through the mountains of Dauphiné and Provence. Fontanieu calculated that 21,500 livres would be needed to prepare the buildings of these institutions to receive the poor and beggars of the province and that 9,820 livres in new furnishings would have to be procured. Such investments would enable the seven selected institutions to admit 1,068 inmates compared to their present capacity of 552. Fontanieu also noted that a certain number of the poor, especially the invalides who were arrested or had reported to the hôpitaux-généraux of Dauphiné, could be transferred to the smaller, non-subsidized hospitals in towns of the province. He further indicated that at least 60 handicapped inmates could be sent to those institutions to create more room for the able-bodied poor, who were to be forcibly employed in the different workshops to be attached to each of the hôpitaux-généraux.[33]

René-François Richer, intendant of Caen, undertook much more wide-ranging consultations than Fontanieu. He immediately asked the officials of his généralité for their evaluations of sixteen hospitals under consideration as possible internment centres: Caen, St-Lô, Vire, Coutances, Bayeux, Avranches, Carentan, Pontorson, St-James, Mortain,

Valognes, St-Sauveur-le-Vicomte, Cherbourg, Montebourg, Thorigny, and Granville, as well as Periers and Villedieu.[34] The resulting study chose the first eleven of these institutions, but the intendant concluded that the modifications required to prepare the buildings of Pontorson, St-James, and Mortain would be too costly.[35] As a result, he reduced his list to ten hospitals, adding Valognes and St-Sauveur to the first seven.[36] The ten institutions retained in lower Normandy were considerably more than in most of the généralités of the kingdom, and this outcome was probably due to Richer's ability to justify his choices by arguing that the widespread dispersal of the poor in his region made it necessary to provide space in each area to incarcerate those arrested. It was also to stop Normans from emigrating to Paris, where increased vagabondage constituted one of the crown's principal urban problems. Richer estimated the space available in the ten institutions at about 1,400, of which Caen alone accounted for 500. The distribution of the remaining places around the généralité provided eight of the nine subdélégations with at least one hospital, the exceptions being Mortain, where no institution was retained, and St-Sauveur, which was the second hospital in the subdélégation of Valognes on the Cotentin peninsula, a region of extreme poverty. The other selected institutions were located in the principal cities of each region of the province, in the seats of subdélégations or élections that were generally the headquarters for a brigade of the constabulary.

The same criteria – the cost of undertaking repairs to existing hospitals, the distribution of institutions among the principal cities of each region, and their concentration along the major highways – were applied differently in each généralité. As can be seen in the case of Caen, certain intendants obtained larger quotas of the 156 hospitals than did others. It is clear from the exchange of correspondence between Dodun and Intendant de la Granville in the généralité of Auvergne that the controller general was often exasperated in his attempts to limit the number of hospitals proposed by intendants. A month after his letter of 7 July 1724 asking de la Granville for a list of the selected hospitals in his généralité, no less than 22 were proposed.[37] The intendant explained that Auvergne contained a large number of beggars and vagabonds who posed a major problem, and he noted that the 22 hospitals were to be divided into two categories: permanent institutions for internment were to be retained for Riom, Thiers, Clermont, Issoire, Brioude, St-Flour, Aurillac, Mauriac, and Salers, while thirteen other smaller hospitals were to be used in the initial period of enforcement of the 1724 edict so that the threat of internment would be clearly felt by vagabonds in every part of the province.

Dodun initially replied that two or three hospitals would suffice for Auvergne, and when de la Granville eventually proposed to reduce his list to the seven or eight principal establishments, Dodun replied that that number was more than adequate.[38] The controller general remained convinced that de la Granville had exaggerated his needs, and in October 1724, when the official list of hôpitaux-généraux was released, Auvergne was granted only five: Riom, Montferrand, Clermont, Thiers, and St-Flour. The negotiation continued, for de la Granville would not accept this selection. Refusing to recognize fewer than seven hôpitaux-généraux, he eliminated Montferrand from Dodun's list and added Issoire, Brioude, and Aurillac, institutions that received official subsidies until 1734.[39]

As the selection of St-Sauveur and Valognes in the généralité of Caen, Embrun in Dauphiné, and the 22 hospitals that de la Granville wanted to retain indicates, it was not always the largest cities whose hospitals were chosen to enforce the 1724 edict. There seems to have been some indecision among the intendants as to whether the new measures were to be directed at preventing migration to the larger towns and setting up preventive detention centres in smaller towns and along the routes to the urban areas or simply at interning the vagabonds and beggars once they arrived in the cities. With seven institutions selected, Rouen, the second généralité of Normandy, combined both policies and even selected the small hospital of Caudebec to become a hôpital-général. Again, the migration of the poor from Normandy towards Paris probably influenced the choice of Caudebec since along with Le Havre, Rouen, and Vernon, it was on the direct route up the Seine valley to Paris.

In the 1724 edict, the king had declared that he was ready to subsidize the selected hôpitaux-généraux, and in subsequent years, the crown experimented with method after method to try to live up to its promise. Initially, the *Instruction* issued to the intendants on 24 July 1724 proposed that every fortnight they should compensate the hospitals for the deficit they had run up. The funds for these subsidies were to be taken from the *régie des droits*, an indirect tax levied on minor offices, such as inspectors of weights and measures, slaughterhouses, and breweries.[40] A second edict, issued during the same month, eliminated a series of municipal offices and positions of governor, lieutenant, and major that had been restored and put up for sale two years earlier. Half the revenues previously set aside to pay the salaries of these officers was to be turned over to the hospitals.[41]

The problem with the latter tax was that the offices had already been sold and, in order to turn over half of their revenues to the hospitals, they had to be bought back. This operation was not popular at the grass-roots level, as can be seen in the town of Grignan. The Comte de Grignan had paid the 27,500 livres imposed upon his county as part of the national policy to buy back the offices sold under the August 1722 edict. At their meeting of 18 April 1724, the town consuls adopted a proposal from him for a tax of 15 sous per florin of assessment to repay him for the funds that he had turned over to the crown.[42] This assessment came on the heels of a very high royal levy (*taille*), and the town consulate was obviously uneasy. The new officials selected at the 27 December 1724 meeting did not even show up for their official installation, and the minutes of the meeting mention that "murmurs" from those assembled led the bailiff to cancel the meeting.[43] At the one held over a year later, on 3 February 1726, the affair had not yet been concluded; the consulate sent a delegate to the intendant asking him to reduce the town's annual payment because of the poor harvest, and at the same time it sent archers to collect back payments from those who had not yet contributed to the new tax. By 23 August the consuls themselves supported a proposal that town residents "delay" payment of their taxes because of the poor harvest and the resulting inability of Grignan to meet the payments.[44]

In addition to these two sources of revenues, which it seems to have had great difficulty collecting, the crown also counted heavily upon funding the hôpitaux-généraux by closing more town and village charities and expropriating their income. The specific target of this new reform was the alms distribution by certain monasteries and convents. These alms consisted of money or of bread bought with revenues left in wills. Often begun far back in the Middle Ages, the distributions were carried out at the doors of the institutions in question at certain times of the year: Easter, Holy Week, or during the winter months. This type of aid, indiscriminate in nature and given without distinguishing between the able-bodied poor and the physically or mentally handicapped, did not at all correspond to the new work-oriented criteria established by the crown for poor relief. Royal authorities recommended that the foundations for financing such aid be turned over to the hôpitaux-généraux, since the July 1724 edict had assured shelter and nourishment for all invalides and the possibility of work for all able-bodied poor.[45] A first step in trying to obtain control over these funds can be seen in the questionnaire sent out by Controller Dodun on 6 October 1724. Besides asking the intendants to evaluate the ability of the hospitals in their généralité to receive beggars and vagabonds, it requested a list of the alms that could be taken over to finance the expansion of the hospitals.[46]

In the face of crown preoccupation with finding new sources of revenue for its policy of ridding the kingdom of beggars and vagabonds, the replies of the intendants varied. In Dauphiné, Fontanieu listed no sources of alms, but he did propose that the twenty-fourth of the dîme that each parish was supposed to reserve for its poor could be turned over to the hospitals, noting that "the king's intention being to ban begging from his kingdom forever and to obtain for the hospitals responsible for the upkeep of and for supplying nourishment to the beggars, additional revenues to aid them in meeting these expenses, it is normal to seek out these revenues in the twenty-fourth, which will produce considerable financial returns."[47]

Fontanieu argued that since the dîme in many parishes was in the hands of laymen or members of outside ecclesiastical orders, the twenty-fourth frequently went unpaid or consisted of only a token payment. Yet he held that the *feux* evaluations carried out by Intendant Bouchu between 1698 and 1706 had estimated the twenty-fourth to be worth about 20,000 livres in the province of Dauphiné. Fontanieu believed that he could obtain 23,000–24,000 livres from this tax, amounting to about half the cost of interning the poor in the new hôpitaux-généraux of the province.[48]

In response to this proposal, the intendant received an ordinance from the king's council authorizing him to turn the revenues of this tax over to the hospitals of the province.[49] To set up the new collection system, he ordered each hospital chosen to intern beggars and vagabonds to establish a *receveur des pauvres* responsible for ensuring payment of the twenty-fourth and the use of those payments to subsidize their internees.[50] These receveurs were not to collect the traditional twenty-fourth of the dîme in crops harvested, but were to tax those who held the rights to the dîme at 20 per cent of their lease price. They were also to return a quarter of the resulting revenues to parish priests to support the "honourable poor." To further simplify the collection process, the villages that owed less than 300 livres for the twenty-fourth would be exempted from payment.

This elaborate system to evaluate and collect the twenty-fourth never worked. As early as 1728, Fontanieu wrote that his attempt to appropriate the revenues for the hospitals had been unsuccessful. As a result, the whole project for interning the poor in Dauphiné was now in jeopardy, and he made an urgent request to the king to supply new revenues to compensate for the loss of the twenty-fourth. While the exact reasons for the failure of Fontanieu's project were not explained, René Favier believes that they lay in the opposition of church officials to the intendant's plan. As early as 1681, Le Camus, bishop of Grenoble, had insisted that the bishops of the diocese bore the ultimate responsibility and right to levy the twenty-fourth on church property and to distribute it to the poor.[51]

In Brittany, Intendant Feydeau de Brou sent out a questionnaire in 1724 asking his officials to suggest new sources of revenue for the hôpitaux-généraux, and he received at least one reply recommending an approach similar to the Dauphiné project. Like Fontanieu, the sub-délégué from Quimperlé suggested that a portion of the dîme be set aside for the hospitals, noting that since "some curés, in a normal year, receive more than 2,000 livres, there will be enough left over for [the hospitals'] usual needs."[52] Most of the replies to Feydeau de Brou, however, merely obeyed the official request and transmitted lists of traditional alms and foundations that could be expropriated. Proceeding by diocese, the intendant's synthesis of the replies noted that the monasteries of Léon, Dol, Tréguier, and Quimper distributed no significant alms, and even for the dioceses where he recommended the transfer of alms to the hôpitaux-généraux, the amounts to be obtained were very modest. In the diocese of Rennes only the priories of St-Nicolas-de-Montfort and St-Pierre-de-Breteil were cited, and they distributed a mere 20 minées of rye (worth about 260 livres) to the vagabonds and poor of the neighbouring parishes. For Nantes, eight institutions were mentioned, including the Convent of Villeveuve, which distributed 2 septièmes of rye to the poor every week on Mondays and Thursdays and offered dinner and a silver coin to fifteen poor every Holy Thursday. Moreover, at the death of each nun, a poor beggar was given bread, wine, and a monetary allocation for a period of thirty days.

Most of the others followed the same model, distributing grain two or three times a week at the door of the monastery, while the Aumône Doudon also lodged the poor travelling to and from the pilgrimage of St-Méen. The total quantity of rye distributed in the alms recommended for suppression in the diocese of Nantes amounted to 261 septièmes, 18 boisseaux (worth 34 livres), 1 tonneau, 5 minées (65 livres) of rye, and 1,306 livres. In the remaining dioceses of Vannes, St-Brieuc, and St-Malo the alms that could be recuperated were worth roughly 1,650 livres, plus 104 boisseaux of grain (worth 250 livres), 12 tonneaux of grain, and 10 minées of rye (130 livres).[53] The whole operation of taking over the annual revenues reserved for alms distributions would not have produced even 4,000 livres for the hospitals.

As for the foundations that could be expropriated outright in Brittany, the sums involved were more enticing. The intendant's list indicated two foundations in the diocese of Rennes that would produce 2,954 livres, three in Nantes worth 1,306 livres, three in Quimper evaluated at 8,040 livres, and four in Vannes that distributed various unidentified quantities of grain, including the Chartreuse d'Auray, which had received 10,000 livres left by the Sieur de Rochefort for its hospital.[54] For Dol and St-Brieuc, he noted that he had received no reply, and for St-Malo he mentioned the abbey of St-Jacques, which had formerly distributed grain to the poor. The total income of the foundations that the intendant thought could be taken over amounted to a respectable 22,300 livres, presuming he was able to get his hands on the Rochefort legacy.

While at first glance, the 22,300 livres to be recovered seems to have constituted a profitable operation, the other side of Feydeau de Brou's document evaluated the cost in Brittany of implementing the 1724 edict "to abolish begging." In the seven institutions selected as hôpitaux-généraux, additional annual revenues of 24,388 livres had to be found to cover the 1,523 vagabonds who were incarcerated in 1727. Even if the 22,300 livres from the foundations covered the operational costs of the hospitals for one year, this figure represented a one-time contribution, and the basic challenge was to find long-term revenue. To subsidize the upkeep of seventeen hospitals in the province, including five hôpitaux-généraux, Intendant de Brou had already allocated 31,398 livres in 1727, and he sought another 25,970 livres to increase the sums accorded to twenty-three other institutions.[55] As is clear from the remarks of Fontanieu for Dauphiné, reserving a certain number of functioning institutions for beggars and vagabonds had obvious ramifications for all the other hospitals of the province. A certain number of old and sick patients had to be transferred to smaller, non-subsidized establishments to make room for the new inmates of the great confinement. The physical structures of the selected hospitals had to be altered to accommodate the new type of inmate, and the other hospitals were forced to receive additional patients for whom the 1724 royal edict had not made any financial provision.

In Brittany, just as in Dauphiné, it was very difficult for the crown actually to obtain the other sources of revenue earmarked for the great confinement. Such was notably the case for the funds that were to be transferred to the hospitals after the elimination of the series of minor offices that had been created in 1722. In Grignan the problem had been to find the money to buy back the offices that had already been sold, while in Brittany there was great difficulty in recovering the back pay that had supposedly been set aside.[56] The revenue from the *octrois* in Brittany, created to support new municipal offices, amounted to 51,723 livres a year in addition to the 142,202 livres of back pay.[57] But as Christine Chapalain-Nougaret has noted, the back pay was not often available because, despite crown directives, most municipalities had not set aside funds to pay the unnamed officials, and even Intendant de Brou judged that most municipalities in his généralité needed their revenues just as much as did the hospitals.[58]

Twelve to fourteen months after the creation of the hôpitaux-généraux, it had become clear that in order to carry out the desired internment policy, these institutions needed far more than the revenues generated from half the *octrois* and from the funds recovered from the town and village alms and charitable foundations. In Dauphiné, Brittany, and Normandy, all the intendants noted that the projected revenues from the two principal sources of financing had fallen below expectations, while the costs of maintaining the new hospital system were steadily rising. They therefore requested further revenues to meet the new hospital objectives.

Small hospitals constituted one of the principal difficulties for crown administrators in carrying out the new policy. As previously mentioned, a number of the institutions retained as hôpitaux-généraux were relatively small and had been chosen because of their geographical location along a major migration artery or in a particularly poor region of the country where beggars and vagabonds were numerous. However, these institutions tended to cost far more for the crown to operate. In the diocese of Rennes, Christine Chapalain-Nougaret has shown that the crown revenues necessary to operate the hospital in the town of Vitré were proportionately much higher than those needed for the hospital in Rennes (see Table 3).

Rennes, with a potential capacity of one hundred inmates, possessed both capital and operating revenues equivalent to around 50 per cent of the annual costs of the institution, while Vitré, with a capacity of twenty, covered only about 30 per cent of its operating expenses. In both hospitals, income from the inmates' production in the textile workshops or woodworking centres fell far below initial projections. Proponents for the great confinement and crown administrators had even hoped to cover

Table 3
Hospital revenues for Rennes and Vitré, 1729–30 (expressed in livres with percentage of revenues in parentheses)

	Capital revenues	Operating revenues	Alms	Income from inmates' work	Crown grants
RENNES					
1728	5,098 (15.2)	16,800 (50.1)	100 (0.3)	2,500 (7.5)	9,000 (26.9)
1729	5,098 (13.4)	17,520 (46.3)	720 (2.0)	2,500 (6.6)	12,000 (31.7)
1730	5,098 (10.5)	17,520 (36.2)	240 (0.5)	2,500 (5.2)	23,000 (47.7)
VITRÉ					
1728	2,000 (25.3)	469 (6.0)	21 (0.3)	400 (5.0)	5,000 (63.4)
1729	2,000 (23.5)	585 (7.0)	21 (0.2)	400 (4.7)	5,500 (64.6)
1730	2,000 (14.0)	1,314 (9.1)	530 (3.7)	400 (2.8)	10,093 (70.4)

the full costs of the hôpitaux-généraux through the revenues from inmates' work. In Brittany, as elsewhere in the kingdom, the marginal revenues from the workshops were a major disappointment. The soaring costs of the internment in Brittany made it necessary for the crown to increase its grants continually, and yet Vitré and Rennes, as with all the other hospitals in Brittany, ran deficits for almost every year of operation from 1724 to 1730.[59]

What was the experience of the great confinement like for the small-town hospitals that became hôpitaux-généraux? Certainly, their selection and the financial aid they received from the crown placed them in an enviable position among other smaller regional institutions. When Vitré received its first 300 livres on 16 March 1725, it proceeded to purchase cloth for the inmates' shirts, 150 boisseaux of rye and 50 of blé noir, straw mattresses, and looms for the children's workshop. The administrators also began to enlarge their buildings and to purchase new furnishings. Presented with the costs of these renovations and the increases in grain prices, Intendant de Brou increased his 1726 grant to Vitré to 12,000 livres.[60] In 1728 and 1729 the hospital received 5,000 and 5,500 livres respectively, and its grant hit a maximum of 10,093 in 1730 in order to carry out important repairs. However, from 1726 on, the authorities warned the hospital every year that it had to reduce its expenses. On 28 February 1631 the intendant notified the Vitré administrators that their grant would be reduced, and by June it was rumoured that the aid would even be cut in half. In February 1732 the cut was announced; Vitré was to be authorized 2 sous 9 deniers a day for each inmate, compared to the 8 sous it had previously received. By 1733, with the outbreak of the

Polish War, the new municipal offices were finally sold, and the tax credits that had been rerouted to the hospitals had to be returned to pay the salaries of the new officials.

In Normandy the choice of Caudebec as an hôpital-général produced a similar expansion of a small-town institution. New buildings on the rue des Capucins had been acquired and renovated in 1685, and the hospital had been installed there in October 1693.[61] Up to the 1724 edict, the Caudebec institution functioned like most other early modern hospitals, combining poor relief and aid to the sick and dying. An admissions register begun in 1705 indicates that the institution had started the year with thirty-five to fifty-five residents and served another thirty-five to sixty in the course of the year. In 1705 there had been thirty-five admissions between September and December; for the twelve months of 1710 that number jumped to fifty-eight before falling back to thirty-three for the twelve months of 1711. The women and children admitted far outnumbered the men: in 1710 there were only five men listed among the patients, compared to twenty-seven boys and twenty-six girls and women.[62] An analysis of the admission registers of the hospital shows the same trend for the first six months of 1724: five men were among the thirty-one admissions, although two of them, Jacques Consant and George le Bateur, *dit* "le gazelle," were discharged after three and five months respectively, the first as a "drunkard and blasphemer" and the second for his "insolence." During the same period, seven women, nine boys, and ten girls were admitted.[63]

These registers show that patients were taken in almost every month of every year, although the admission rate during the winter period was always higher. Among those entered in the register, the majority were not ill, most were old, or invalids, and a good number of the children were orphans, illegitimate, or abandoned. This group constituted the "permanent residents" of the hospital; an example is Catherine Gavin, seven years old and an orphan from the parish of Hautot le Tattoes, "to be nourished and cared for until she was old enough to earn her living."[64] Nearly all shorter-term patients were sick or injured, such as Martin Mauger, who had been crushed in a limestone furnace when he was admitted on 28 April 1717. He died the next day.[65]

The mortality rate for the patients at Caudebec prior to the 1724 law was generally low, although it soared in periods of widespread disease: two of the thirty-five short-term patients admitted in 1705 died in the hospital, compared to five of the fifty-eight admitted in 1710 and to fifteen of the thirty-three taken in in 1711. The year 1718 was particularly disastrous since there were sixteen fatalities among the thirty-two longer-term patients and four among the twenty admitted in the course of the year.[66] In contrast, in 1721 there were no deaths either among the twenty-five residents or among the seven who had recently entered the institution. From 1724, even before Caudebec was selected as a hôpital-général, the register begins to list the ages of the patients living in the institution. From this information, it becomes clear that they were grouped around two poles: the aged and the young. Among the residents of the hospital at the beginning of the year, there were four men whose average age was sixty-seven and nine boys who averaged eleven years, that figure being increased by a twenty-two-year-old classed as an idiot. The average age of the seven women listed was sixty-one, and there were eight girls whose average age was eight. None of these patients died that year, and five were sent back to their homes. Among the forty-three new admissions, André Dragon, a soldier, died in February, and Marie Gaulere and her daughter both died of a "flux de sang" in April.[67]

This portrait, typical of the activities of most small-town hospitals, changed radically after the designation of Caudebec as an hôpital-général during the summer of 1724. The new regime began in the hospital registers on the first of September, when the institution began to admit those who "asked for admission" or who "were led to the hospital of Caudebec according to the terms of the royal declaration of 18 July." From the beginning of September to the end of December, the registers show that seven women, five from outside the town, were voluntary admissions, and nine women, eight of whom were from outside the town, were escorted to the institution after being arrested by the *brigadiers* and charged with vagrancy. The most significant difference after 1724 is the fact that men came to constitute a majority of the internees: from September to December, seven men, all from outside Caudebec, presented themselves voluntarily to the hospital for admission, one was brought to the institution by his mother for internment and eighteen, almost all from outside the town, were led to the institution by the brigades of Caudebec and Goderville.

At the same time the number of children in the hospital dropped dramatically. Five of the women interned were accompanied by their children, and two boys from Caudebec also were admitted.[68] The number interned in the institution jumped to forty-nine for the first six months of the new regime, and men constituted more than half of the total, of whom almost 60 per cent were involuntarily interned. The *raison d'être* of the Caudebec hospital was transformed from its more neutral role of providing shelter and food for a relatively docile group of poor, marginal, sick, and elderly people to an institution participating actively in a movement aimed at incarcerating and detaining on an involuntary basis a younger, increasingly male, and more aggressive and hostile segment of the population.

The budget of the Caudebec hospital underwent fundamental changes as well. Prior to its selection as an hôpital-général, the annual income of the institution had averaged 3,214 livres from 1700 to 1708, dropping to 1,593 between 1709 and 1720 and levelling off at 1,658 livres from 1721 to 1723.[69] After 1724 it jumped to 8,543 livres between that year and 1727; by 1728 the institution received 12,410 livres; this figure dropped to 7,136 in 1729 and rose again to 13,717 in 1730.[70] The increase in revenues came from two sources. First, direct payments were made by the intendant to the hospital administrators for the upkeep of the inmates. Amounts of 1,553 livres were turned over to the hospital between 22 November and 22 December 1724, 8,410 in 1725, and 8,059 in 1726.[71] A breakdown of the Caudebec budget does not reveal the same type of financing as was used at Rennes or Vitré in Brittany. The grant of 8 sous per day per inmate never seems to have been applied at Caudebec, where it is noted that the hospital generally received a lump sum of around 4,000 livres derived from royal taxes.

This figure was far below the level of financing in Brittany: at 8 sous per day per inmate, Caudebec would have been paid 1,968 livres in 1724 instead of the 1,553 it received; in 1728 it would have received 19,710 rather than 4,000 livres and in 1730, 9,928 livres in the place of 4,000.[72] After 1732, when the level of financing at Rennes and Vitré dropped to 2 sous 9 deniers per day per inmate, the more informal Caudebec financing system produced superior returns, and for that year the hospital received 3,000 livres, compared to the 2,058 it would have been granted under the Brittany formula.[73] The comparison between the treatment of these three institutions – Rennes, Vitré, and Caudebec – illustrates the disparate and local nature of both the management and the financing of the hôpitaux-généraux. At the same time that Brittany created a province-wide formula, which it was not able to maintain beyond 1732, Normandy turned rapidly to lump-sum grants three or four times a year to the institutions that made up the system. The level of financing throughout Normandy was consistently lower than in Brittany, and the hospitals in Avranches and Carentan, with 144 and 102 inmates respectively, received grants roughly similar to those received by Caudebec.[74]

The other source of revenue for Caudebec, just as for Rennes and Vitré, was the work carried out by the inmates. Between 1728 and 1732 the registers of the hospital noted that 5,499 livres 10 sous had been received from the sale of cotton spun in the workshops of the hospital.[75] On 1 September 1725 a stove had been purchased for the refectory, which was also the hospital workshop, and a basin installed in the garden to wash the cotton and the hospital linens.[76] As elsewhere, crown administrators counted heavily on the income from inmates' work to pay the expenses of each hospital, but as in the other cases examined, the income from cotton sales at Caudebec never came close to meeting expenses: between 1728 and 1732 sales amounted to barely 18 per cent of the total hospital expenses, although by 1733, when the crown had begun reducing its grants, cotton sales had risen to make up 21 per cent of the total budget.[77]

The population of the Caudebec hospital hit a peak of 135 internees in 1728, before the fiscal pressures of the internment forced a reduction in the scale of the movement. The Caudebec budget reached a high point in 1732 with receipts of 8,589 livres, including the return of surpluses from the previous year. But by the 1740s, income had returned to the 5,000 to 6,000 range, and by the 1750s, it rarely amounted to more than 8,000 livres, with cotton sales becoming ever more important (in 1750 they produced 2,685 livres, or almost half of the institution's budget). These amounts were a vast improvement over the 1,000 to 3,000 livres that had made up the hospital's income prior to the 1724 experiment. The great confinement left Caudebec with a reinforced infrastructure, personnel, and workshops, which continued to be in operation long after the crown had abandoned the attempt to "eliminate beggary forever."

The Caudebec hospital made some gains out of its designation as an hôpital-général, just as a number of other small institutions came out of the 1724 experiment with higher profiles. The crown's attempt to control and eliminate beggary accelerated the tendency toward hospital centralization begun by the work of the royal commissioners after 1693. The selection of certain local hospitals to take over the holdings of institutions that were to remain closed obviously represented a further step towards the organization of a network of poor-relief centres and hospitals throughout the kingdom. After the failure of the Mount Carmel and St-Lazare movement, royal commissioners meticulously examined all the hospices, leproseries, and hospitals that had been taken over by the order. Following royal directives, they tried to set up a rational system of small hospitals in regional centres and larger cities. To that end, they generally sacrificed the small, poorly financed foundations for poor relief in out-of-the-way villages and rural regions. They made their choices according to the financial health and physical location of each institution. It was, in fact, the hospitals comprising this system that became the basis for aid to the sick and poor during the rest of the Ancien Régime. These institutions remained the essential French hospital network well into the nineteenth century.

The 1724 edict went even further than the previous efforts by designating and granting special privileges to the 156 institutions selected as hôpitaux-généraux. Many historians of eighteenth-century France have seen such interventions as playing an essential role in the constitution of an evolving urban network.[78] This network was made up of large cities and towns along major highways that assumed a regional vocation. Having hospitals made these towns more important as centres for the population of their surrounding area. Those with hôpitaux-généraux, besides their hospital facilities, usually possessed a brigade of the constabulary to bring in the arrested vagabonds and local seats of justice to condemn them. Even on a smaller scale, it was important to possess hospital facilities. Towns competed with one another for the right to one of the new regional hospitals that the crown had ordered to be set up using the revenues and holdings of the smaller charitable establishments that had been taken away from the Order of Mount Carmel and St-Lazare in 1693. Fécamp, Caudebec, and Le Havre wanted their hospitals to get control over the revenues of neighbouring institutions that were to be closed. They realized that if they were not in a position to strengthen themselves by expropriating other small institutions, they could be the victims of any future reform.

PART TWO

Consolidating and Reinforcing Local Hospitals

The attempts to reform local assistance to the poor and the sick brought numerous investigations of and litigation against the hospitals and hospices that had distributed such aid. Two major movements emerged to argue in favour of reforming charity. The first was a practical approach in reaction to what was seen as the corruption and inefficiency of local hospitals. Beginning in 1543, royal edicts had started to ask crown officials to investigate the way that local hospitals were being managed. They were perceived as squandering the grants and legacies that had been given to them to aid the sick and poor. Attempts were made to "reform" these institutions – in many cases, by closing them, expropriating their holdings, and redirecting their revenues toward other royal priorities such as old and handicapped army officers, who benefited from newly instituted crown relief in 1604 and 1672.

A second offensive against poor-relief institutions began at the same time as these new royal initiatives. More theoretical, it originated with the proponents of new humanist values, who sought to reform assistance to the poor and called for a distinction between the real poor (orphans, disabled, insane, sick, and dying) and what was seen as the phoney poor: those able to work and actually earn their living. These reformers, mainly members of the urban elites, argued that hospitals should help only the first group and not encourage the laziness

of the second by indiscriminate charity. Their arguments were integrated into the approaches towards charity proposed by certain agents
of the Catholic Reformation. Experiments along these lines were
undertaken by the dévots in Lyon, Rouen, and Grenoble in the 1530s
and 1540s. They were also linked to the hôpital-général movement of
the seventeenth century, which attempted to cut back on small, local
institutions in order to build up urban facilities.

   In the course of the seventeenth century, at the same time as these
two movements were producing attacks upon local hospitals, another
approach was developing. It placed far more emphasis upon reinforcing the infrastructure and staffing of local hospitals and making them
more adequate to serve the needs of the poor and the sick. The
Christian charity movement, also inherent in the ideology of the
Catholic Reformation, re-emphasized the importance of assisting marginal members of the community. The initiatives of this movement,
which was spearheaded by St Vincent de Paul, resulted in increased
donations to charitable organizations and, most important, in the
foundation of numerous new women's religious orders. Organized to
work "in the world," most of these new orders were created towards
the last half of the century only after a long dispute with Rome over
the moral acceptability of nuns leaving the cloister to serve in schools
and hospitals. In the course of the late seventeenth and early eighteenth centuries, these orders took over the direction of the majority
of hospitals that survived the reform movement, whether they were in
villages, towns, or cities. Their place in these hospitals gave women a
new visibility in society and opened new doors to them outside the
traditional areas of the household or domestic service.

   These practical changes had profound effects upon the organization of local charitable institutions. The attack on local hospitals had
been led by the crown or its agents, who described the institutions as
redundant and inefficient. However, just as their reforms were
launched, many of these local institutions, influenced by agents of
the Counter-Reformation, were engaged in reinforcing their finances
and organization. Town and village elites collaborated with them in
resisting the centralized attempts to close down local poor-relief
agencies. They contributed generously of their time and money to
maintain local hospitals and supported legal proceedings to block
the recommended closures and expropriations of these community
facilities.

It is ironic that just as royal agents and members of the urban elite undertook serious efforts to eliminate local charitable foundations and rationalize the hospital system, towns and villages received the long-needed ideological and practical support to reinforce their poor-relief structures and resist centralized attempts to continue cutbacks and rationalization.

4 The Hospital, the Church, and the Local Community: Control, Support, and Involvement

In late October 1736 the members of the Grignan bureau of the poor met to carry out a surprise inspection of the local hospital. Having prayed together at the St-Roch chapel, the group proceeded to the institution, where they found Jeanne-Marie Peyronnette, the servant and caretaker, and the inmates: Bonpenase Viellet, who was handicapped, Jeanne Burque from Messire and Isabeau Roux from Courdeille, both slightly deranged, the six- or seven-year-old illegitimate son of Jean Andiol's wife, a three-year-old illigimate son of Jeanne Buffete, the wife of Bartholomé Luschuges, the widow Malquroin, and Marie Casandrine. The members of the bureau found that the last three "could earn their own living and as a result, they were to withdraw from the institution and to return to their homes." The others could remain in the hospital, but under more stringent conditions. Finding that the institution bought them bread at the bakery, the bureau ordered that in the future they were to be supplied rye to make their own bread. It also decided to negotiate to buy rye and wheat at the best possible price.[1] This inspection and crackdown on hospital practices came five months after the visit of Daniel Joseph de Cosiac, bishop of Die, who had met with the town council to find ways of reinforcing and ensuring the application of the regulations for aid to the poor and the functioning of the hospital.[2]

On a superficial level, the impromptu inspection of the Grignan hospital seems to confirm the long-term crown conviction that small institutions mismanaged poor relief. Despite the presence of the caretaker, the bureau decided that virtually half the inmates should not have been admitted to the hospital, and they criticized the extravagence of the institution for buying bread instead of baking it. In fact, the beneficiaries of Grignan relief came from the ranks of the traditional poor, and on a smaller scale they were not very different from the clientele of city hospitals such as Grenoble. Kathryn Norberg's research concerning the much larger Grenoble hospital shows that, except for the period of internment in the 1720s and 1730s, the majority of the inmates were the elderly, the handicapped, the sick, and the insane, who were joined by orphans, bastards, unwanted children, rejected women, and widows,[3] virtually the same groups found in Grignan. Certainly the Grignan visit appears to confirm the arguments of Olwen Hufton, who judged that poor relief in eighteenth-century France was haphazard and fundamentally insufficient. She argued that the numerous radically new solutions (hôpitaux-généraux, internment, and the subsequent dépôts de mendicité, or workhouses) involved continual restructuring of relief approaches and that they never had the funds or the long-term support that characterized the more traditional and stable English responses to poverty.[4] In England the system remained virtually the same from the late sixteenth century to the 1800s; it was locally based, with intervention from neither the central government nor the church.

It is certainly true that the 1736 inspection demonstrates the weaknesses of local poor relief, which French law saw as the jurisdiction of the community and which had traditionally been administered with the participation of the church. There had always been some ambiguity in this arrangement as was clear from the Edict of St-Germain-en-Laye in 1545, which had sought to eliminate religious communities from the control of poor-relief institutions. Going even further, the Edict of Moulins in 1566 had clearly dictated that the communities where the poor were born were to be held responsible for their upkeep. Despite the temporary interruption of this principle after 1662 with the widespread establishment of the hôpitaux-généraux and after 1724 with the systematic attempt at internment for beggars and vagabonds, towns and villages continued to be seen as responsible for their own poor. But to what extent did the church remain involved in the direction of poor relief, and to what degree were the communities really capable of providing food, shelter, and aid to their weaker members? To answer these questions, this chapter treats the community response to changing orientations in relief to the poor and sick. It initially concentrates upon the respective duties of local religious and civil leaders in encouraging support for the poor and for the hospitals founded to serve them. Secondly, it looks at the new initiatives taken to extend the types of aid and financial resources furnished to the different institutions by their respective towns. Finally, it discusses the ways in which local notables reinforced their own social dominance using the hospital structures and the relations that these institutions maintained with the poor.

Traditionally, the community and the church had shared the obligation for aiding the local sick and poor.[5] This shared responsibility is illustrated in the meeting between Bishop de Cosiac of Die and the Grignan town council several months before the inspection of the local hospital. It set forth new rules for the hospital and led to the 1736 inspection, showing how church and town officials often got together to introduce new rules before carrying out inspections and then collaborated in implementing their decisions. This joint action was particularly evident during the seventeenth century, when the missionaries of the Catholic Reformation in France became the instruments used by both religious and crown officials to intervene at the community level. The Jesuits, Lazarists, Eudists, and other missionary groups tried to persuade local notables of the need to reform poor-relief practices, such as the traditional forms of indiscriminate alms giving. They suggested instead that communities set up local assistance agencies and bureaux of the poor and induce perspective donors to direct their aid towards the new institutions, which could organize more rational forms of welfare.

The division between church and community responsibility for poor relief had never been clear-cut; Jean Imbert has demonstrated that the early modern church, like that of the Middle Ages, claimed primary and exclusive jurisdiction over hospitals and assistance to the poor. During its fourteenth session, the Council of Trent reiterated the long-standing church contention that the bishops were the "executors" of all pious bequests, whether they were in the form of wills or donations, and that these same bishops should receive hospital accounts annually and visit and inspect all the institutions in their jurisdictions.[6] Earlier sessions of the council had gone even further in restating church pretensions, holding that only a bishop had the right to alter the goals of an institution, close it down, or transfer its funds to another foundation or hospital.[7]

Obviously, these claims to exclusive rights over the hospitals conflicted with the attempts by the French crown to "put order" into the poor-relief system by extending community efforts and rights in the field with the goal of limiting church involvement. Imbert notes the existence of this conflict, arguing that it was one of the reasons that the integral text of the canons of the council were never adopted in France. The sixteenth-century jurist Charles du Moulin had pointed out that the claims of the church as expressed in the council documents contradicted the royal edicts and ordinances of 1543, 1544, 1546, and 1561 concerning hospitals.[8] When the General Assembly of the French clergy met at Melun in 1579, it did not try to appropriate all the power over poor relief claimed at Trent. The assembly merely specified that the holdings of the hospitals should henceforth be consecrated to the needs of the poor, and it asked bishops to intervene: first, to verify that the acts of foundation of the institutions were being respected, with local administrators being named and carrying out their mandates according to the will of the founders, and secondly, to ensure that discipline in the institutions was continually observed.[9]

At the same time, it is obvious from the directives of the council that the church realized it must improve its record as overseer and frequently also as manager of poor relief. The bishops grappled with complaints of corruption levelled against religious hospitals and foundations. In their later sessions, the fathers of the council implicitly recognized the weaknesses in the system of poor relief, and in 1563 they called for all who possessed church livings, especially those who had been named to hospitals, to carry out their responsibilities properly. Henceforth, they were to submit separate accounts for their hospitals, failing which they could be stripped of their livings. Those who had embezzled or misappropriated hospital funds were to be dismissed and obliged to pay back all missing revenues.[10]

These different attempts to put order into local hospital management have often been seen as the basis of the subsequent reform of French poor relief. However, the bold declarations of the fathers of the council concerning church involvement in charity, specifically in the managing of hospitals, had only vague repercussions upon the eventual development of French poor relief. The traditional thesis of Abbé Bremond argued that the Catholic Reformation had a profound effect upon French society through the spreading of the new doctrines by the pastoral visits of bishops, the founding of new seminaries and colleges, and the interventions of the Jesuits and the other "shock troops" of the Catholic Reformation.[11] However, a number of more recent historians have shown that a large gap existed between initial transmission of the new church message about charity and its eventual reception by the population. In fact, the work of Jean Delumeau, Louis Pérouas, and Alain Croix has pointed out that the initial preaching of the new message frequently met with hostility from the peasants of small towns and villages.[12] Croix goes on to explain that the early Jesuit missionaries in Brittany, Le Nobletz, and Maunoir, in the years 1608–83 were often led to transform the new doctrinal positions in order to make them comprehensible and acceptable to their listeners; they resorted to imagery, scare tactics, and an intermixing of the new church message with traditional beliefs and Breton cultural values.[13]

Charity and assistance to the poor had always been an integral part of the traditional religious culture. The new attitudes and initiatives in the field of hospital reform and poor relief were based upon the premise that both the clergy and the laity must improve the treatment of the poor and that each should undertake a number of new charitable initiatives. To what extent was this message carried to the people, and how was it received? Research on this question has shown that the peasants and rural communities often resisted the suggested reforms, seeing them as strange urban initiatives imposed upon them. The proposals for action relating to poor relief and the reception of these initiatives in the eight communities examined in this book reveal a great deal about the respective roles of religious and lay leaders in bringing about changes in the administration of community welfare measures.

One of the earliest of the new initiatives coming out of the Catholic Reformation was the charitable confraternity (*confrérie de la charité*), or bureau of charity. The church had always preached the obligation of individual Christians to aid their needy brothers and sisters in order to attain their own salvation, but the approach emphasized by the new theology showed the necessity for collective, organized aid. Drawing upon the examples of Charles Borromeo, archbishop of Milan, Vincent de Paul introduced confraternities – lay brotherhoods or sisterhoods – in France, and they became a model for the new church. In 1625 he directed his priests "to establish confraternities everywhere you go as missionaries."[14] In their initial conception these charitable organizations were to extend the material and spiritual aspects of religious missions, but in face of the hardships and devastation of the Thirty Years War, they often became the principal goal of the missions. The same was true of Vincent de Paul's successors, the Lazarists, who in the diocese of Montauban during the crisis of 1693, replaced all their preaching and spiritual exercises with organized distributions of bread and soup to the poor.[15]

The confraternity recommended by Vincent de Paul became a bureau of charity for many of the other missionaries. These bureaux resembled the community institutions that had traditionally taken care of poor relief, except that in the conception of Monsieur Vincent the local clergy were to play a far more active role, serving on the new bureaux and ensuring that they were oriented towards action rather than being distant, bureaucratic institutions. In Brittany, the missionary, Jean Leuduger attached a lawyer who had since become a priest to the bureau created at St-Brieuc, and this priest-lawyer "took care to settle lawsuits and civil proceedings" that affected the poor.[16] In his *Direction pour les missions* (1646), Father Bourgoing, an Oratorian, recommended the creation of a "compagnie de charité" to assist the "sick poor," the handicapped, and the mentally retarded, as well as the "pauvres honteux." He wanted these institutions to be headed by "ladies of quality," who were to serve as an example for others. They should be assisted by helpers and by several women from each neighbourhood, who would visit the sick poor and attend to them according to their needs, even to aid them to receive the Holy Sacraments.[17]

The process of creating these institutions of local intervention can be examined in detail at St-Vallier, where they eventually led to a renewal and reconstruction of the town hospital. The St-Vallier confraternity was founded on 8 November 1637 by Father Gernus, a priest from St-Vincent de Paul's Lazarist missionary society in Paris. He had been brought into the town to preach a mission at the request of the archbishop of Vienne, Pierre de Villars, and following his talks and services, the Lazarist convened the ladies of the parish to set up a confraternity. Over forty women from the ranks of community notables joined the new movement, electing four officials, two of whom were widows. Among other tasks, the members of the group were to take up two separate collections on Sundays and holy days, the first to assist the poor of the town and the second to aid the indisposed who had been taken to the hospital.[18] The results of these collections seem to have been very uneven. The financial accounts of the hospital prior to 1689 have been lost, as have most of the registers of the group. We know that in 1684–85, three cardinals passed through the town and were solicited for donations and that the funds received from the women's collections in the 1680s and 1690s varied from about 100 to 200 livres annually, before dropping back to around 55 livres in the early 1700s.[19] Even during the early years, however, the amounts received were probably not very substantial, because in 1656 the women considered consolidating their two collections.

A more detailed examination of the workings of this type of collection is available for the hospital at Caudebec in Normandy. There, throughout the seventeenth century, the "bourgeois" men and women of the parish took turns soliciting their fellow parishioners, but they do not seem to have been members of an organized confraternity. From 1611 to the 1680s they took up two collections. Just as in St-Vallier, the *plat des pauvres* was collected to help the poor of the town and the *plat de l'Hôtel-Dieu* to assist the town hospital. Different residents were designated every three months to collect donations in front of Notre-Dame church, and four different entries were listed for each of the two collections each year.[20] The revenue obtained from these collections is illustrated in Figure 1; it is expressed in grain equivalents to compensate for currency devaluations. The graph indicates that after initially starting off well between 1611 and 1614, revenues remained relatively marginal throughout the seventeenth century. At times, as in 1632, it was noted that the bourgeois had even been unable to find collectors.

Collections became more lucrative in the 1690s when the structure was changed; a ladies confraternity, the Dames de la Miséricorde, took up one of the collections and the parish priests the other. The specific uses of the revenues were no longer designated, but in 1694 it was noted that the plat de l'Hôtel-Dieu had been reinstituted, possibly to ensure that certain revenues were turned over to the hospital. These three collections continued well into the eighteenth century, although they rarely produced more than 10 to 15 per cent of the hospital revenues. At Pontorson a collection box placed in the St-Antoine chapel rarely yielded more than 10 livres a year for the hospital, and the contract signed in 1644 between the Brothers of Charity and the community was inter-preted in 1662 as excluding them from the right to solicit donations in the community. Nevertheless, the brothers did continue to receive grants, especially from local notables and the wealthier houses of their order. In 1749, perhaps an exceptional year, the hospital obtained gifts and legacies totalling over 4,000 livres out of total revenues of almost 17,000.[21] Certainly, the bureaux of charity installed in numerous parishes and hospitals by the Lazarists and the new missionary groups brought fresh life and initiatives to a number of local poor-relief activities. However, to judge from the attempts to establish local collections to supplement poor-relief funding, the revenues were erratic and the initi-atives difficult to sustain.

A second and frequent clerical initiative in poor relief was the *mont de piété* and *grenier d'abondance*. The monts de piété were a type of community lending agency. In the cities they were to act as popular pawnbrokers from which cash-strapped workers could borrow money on objects left as security. Churchmen and missionaries considered usury

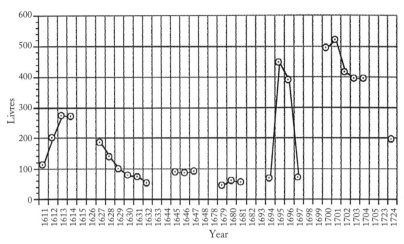

Figure 1   Revenues from the collections for the poor at Notre-Dame church, Caudebec, 1611–1724 (in *livres tournois*)

one of the principal reasons for the indebtedness and misery of the people, and through these agencies they sought to control such interest rates.[22] In Avignon the mont de piété was to lend money at rates not exceeding 2 to 2.5 per cent, and the initial rate in Paris was 2.5 per cent as well.[23] A similar type of institution to provide alternatives to peasant indebtedness was the grenier d'abondance, or *mont de grain*. These agencies were spread out in rural areas of southern France. They consisted of banks of seed grain to be distributed to hard-pressed peasants at planting time; the banks were to be repaid with interest at the harvest. Both institutions were originally Italian initiatives, and they seem to have spread into southern France through the papal possessions in the Avignon area. Marc Venard notes that the proposal to establish a mont de piété in Avignon had been made as early as 1541, two years after the creation of a similar institution in Rome. But it was only seventy-one years later, in 1612, that the Avignon institution began operating under the auspices of the confraternity of Notre-Dame de Lorette.[24] The monts de piété in general were frequently run by local confraternities, and one was opened in Nice in 1590; however, the real wave of such creations occurred much later in the seventeenth century: Paris in 1638, Angers and Montpellier in 1684, and Grenoble in 1692.[25]

The smaller towns and villages of the south were more affected by the seed-grain banks. These monts de grain were set up in virtually all the towns and villages of the southeast in the course of the eighteenth century. In Grignan the bureau of the poor, meeting on 5 March 1709, noted that famine was rampant, and together with the town consuls its members worked throughout the spring to gather grain to allow peasants both to plant their crops and to nourish their families until the next harvest. The canons of St-Sauveur gave them a six-month interest-free loan of 300 livres to meet the needs of the community, and from this fund grain was purchased and loaned out to the peasants.[26] There are no other indications of the functioning of the mont until August 1761, when the directors of the hospital again approached the townspeople for donations. The solicitation produced a bank of 35 *saumées* 5 *eyminées* of grain (125 kilolitres), which was to be stocked in the hospital for eventual distribution. This is the only evidence of a large-scale collection being directed by the bureau.[27] It was noted on 14 April 1770 that the members of the bureau had decided to "recreate" the institution. The renewed interest probably stemmed from the town's request that the hospital produce a better organization for the bank, which was then made up of the grain collected and revenues from a sum of 500 livres left in 1752 to the poor of the town by the late André-Joseph de Peron, former dean of the canons. His will had specified that the money was to be used to found a mont de piété.

The mont in Grignan seems to have remained a rather informal institution, for the 1770 meeting brought together consuls and former recteurs of the poor, apparently to reply to criticism from the community concerning the management of the seed bank.[28] The structures set up in the neighbouring villages reflected the same irregular interest in seed banks. At nearby Rousset there were discussions in 1714 concerning the "reconstitution" of the granary, indicating that some sort of structure had existed earlier.[29] At Remuzat in 1737 it was noted that the community owed 300 livres to the mont.[30] At both Marsanne in 1727 and Vinsobres in 1782, the communities considered proposals to use poor-relief funds to buy grain for the seed banks.[31]

The mechanics of these seed banks are most evident at Vinsobres, where the bishop of Vaison created the institution on 16 June 1721, setting forth its rules and regulations. According to this document, the administrators of the institution were to be the curé, the châtelain, the consuls, and the village elite. The grain was to be stored in a granary under double lock with one key held by the curé and the other by the châtelain. It was to be distributed between Christmas and May; each of the borrowers was to be sponsored by three solvent townspeople. They could receive 2 eyminées (.5 hectolitres) each and were to pay back the grain in September at an interest of 5 per cent, or 1 *cosse* (litre) for each eyminée borrowed. To maintain the stocks of the seed bank, two townspeople were to solicit grain from their neighbours at harvest time.[32] Of course, despite the high hopes of their founders, most of these monts de grain were sporadic affairs, founded and refounded according to the needs of the times. By emphasizing seed grain and the idea of keeping the peasants from abandoning their land, the new institutions placed the same accent on the work ethic that was evident in other innovations of the Catholic Reformation, but they do not seem to have spread much beyond the southeast. Moreover, with their limited stocks of grain, the monts were rarely able to meet the needs of the poor in years of true famine.

A third kind of new charitable initiative taken by the missionaries of the Catholic Reformation was the action of Father Chaurand and his associates to try to convince large and small towns to open local versions of the hôpital-général. Just as in the larger cities, these institutions were to take in the local poor and encourage them to turn from drifting and begging to a search for work. As mentioned in chapter 2, Chaurand's activities gave birth to a large-scale propaganda movement coordinated by Breton nobleman Gabriel Calloët-Querbrat. By sending out copies of Chaurand's letters describing the need for the new hôpitaux-généraux and the ways to create them, the movement tried to convince communities as well as bishops and parish priests to follow his advice and create the new institutions everywhere. Just like the early Breton missionaries, leaders of this movement employed scare tactics; among the documents distributed was an "histoire horrible" in which Chaurand or Calloët-Querbrat related the story of a poor widower in the diocese of Mans who, in the midst of a great famine in May 1678, slashed the throats of his three starving young children and hanged himself in despair after his brother, influenced by his wife, had refused to loan the widower some seed grain to plant his crops. Considering himself responsible for the tragedy, the brother strangled his wife and in turn tried to hang himself. The villagers intervened, preventing the suicide, imprisoning the brother, and attacking the parish priest, whom they considered responsible for the deaths. The moral drawn from this "histoire horrible" was that if the parish had created a confraternity of charity as its bishop had ordered in a 1675 pastoral letter, the peasant would have had recourse to the food and grain normally distributed, and all the lives would have been spared.[33]

To avoid such catastrophes, the documents sent out by Chaurand and Calloët-Querbrat tried to convince all communities, urban and rural, to set up confraternities. These associations were to grow out of parish assemblies and be headed by the local pastor. In cities and large towns they were to take steps, particularly the collection of money, to create hospitals that would then coordinate aid to the poor. In small towns and rural parishes, Chaurand recognized the limited means of the population, and he asked that confraternities create bureaux of charity instead in order to coordinate aid to the poor, who were to remain in their homes. Among the documents distributed was a 1677 ordinance by Bishop Lescar noting that local priests should emphasize the obligation of the rich and ordinary townspeople to contribute to the needy and that the men and women taking up these collections should not hesitate to go into taverns (*cabarets*) to solicit funds.[34] For their part, Chaurand and Calloët-Querbrat emphasized that the poor who received aid should be rigorously selected to eliminate the lazy and undeserving and to demonstrate to donors that their aid was being well spent. To that end, they sent out a sample list of criteria for evaluating the need of each applicant for aid.[35]

The recommendations that the aid given be justified and well spent take on particular significance in the documents circulated by Calloët-Querbrat. It appears from these ordinances, letters, and recommendations that the movement met considerable resistance from the local population, and all the documents suggested ways to meet objections. In a pamphlet prepared to explain to the local elite how to establish charitable institutions, Chaurand bluntly confronted what he saw as the principal obstacles to the creation of the confraternities, the first step to establishing local hospitals and bureaux of charity. First and foremost, he argued, it was necessary to convince the local notables that it was in their interest to create these institutions. To do so, he noted that he regularly read from the pulpit the king's edicts and ordinances on the subject, as well as decisions of the parlements. In addition, he frequently cited the texts of St John Chrysostom proclaiming the responsibility of the rich to feed and house the poor, and he described the example of the Lyon Aumône Générale to show all the good that such initiatives could do. He went on to flatter the elite, arguing that they were "the most qualified" to initiate such a project and adding that it would be up to them to name commissioners to visit the homes of the poor and draw up the lists of those to receive aid.[36]

The second major obstacle to which Chaurand alluded was the cost of establishing the hospitals. From the inception of the movement, the potential expense of new hospitals seems to have caused the local elite to resist and even oppose his proposals. One of the major documents sent out by Calloët-Querbrat was organized in a question-and-answer format; it dealt at great length with preoccupations concerning the cost of the initiatives. The replies argued that in addition to collecting money to set up the hospitals, women's confraternities should be established and made responsible for soliciting food and furniture. Women should be named to care for the sick in the institution and others selected to visit the poor in their homes and organize the distribution of bread and grain to the needy. All these measures were to be carried out through donations, and Chaurand never hesitated to return to St John Chrysostom or to St Matthew, who had argued that such donations would save the rich from damnation.

In face of the objection that it cost less to maintain the poor in their homes than in the hôpitaux-généraux, Chaurand replied that experience showed that the number of poor was cut in half when they were interned, that the lazy and the beggars saw hospitals as prisons where they would be forced to work. To the objection that alms distributed indiscriminately in the streets, in front of the churches, and at the city gates constituted a small burden compared to the onerous levels of support necessary for a hospital, he answered that if every ordinary inhabitant contributed as little as 5 sous a month, it would be sufficient to finance a hospital that would rid the community of beggars, with their thieving and contageous diseases. To the argument that the creation of hospitals and the internment of the poor would deprive the faithful of an opportunity to practise charity, Chaurand replied that the collections by the directors of the hospital would replace alms giving to beggars and that the directors would solicit donations every month in the homes of the community. He even argued that donations would increase since the dying rarely left considerable sums to beggars, but experience proved that they were far more generous to hospitals.[37]

It is evident that the propaganda movement coordinated by Chaurand and Calloët-Querbrat was essentially directed at convincing the local notables that they would be well served by the proposed confraternities and hospitals, but the results of their efforts generally reinforce the notion that the introduction of major elements of the Catholic Reformation into smaller towns and villages was often met with indifference, if not open resistance. It is true that the propaganda sent out by the movement in 1680 claimed that in the previous two years Chaurand and his associates had founded, or brought about alterations in the statutes of, twenty-five institutions in Brittany in order to create hôpitaux-généraux with the mandate to intern and reform the poor. During the same period, fifteen other hôpitaux-généraux in Normandy and the southeast had been set up.[38] In recent research, it has been estimated that Chaurand, during his stay in Brittany, succeeded in creating thirty-eight hôpitaux-généraux.[39] But even these institutions had limited success in combating poverty and vagabondage, which a 1705 report from the intendant of Brittany noted had reached alarming proportions.[40] At the same time, the documents published by the movement indicate a continuing hostility, especially among the smaller communities, to Chaurand's initiatives. In effect, all the hôpitaux-généraux were set up in cities or large towns, and there was little sign of the bureaux of charity that he had advocated for the smaller towns and villages; only in Guerche and Pornic were lasting bureaux established.

While spectacular, most of the clerical attempts to change poor-relief structures and create new institutions of assistance had limited effects both in scope and in time. One of the problems in applying these new solutions was the lack of collaboration between the missionaries and the crown officials on the one hand and the local community leaders and elites on the other. It was not that local leaders were necessarily opposed to the new measures, but they often resisted because they felt that they had not been sufficiently consulted or involved in the attempts to apply the new reforms or because they saw their leadership challenged by the newcomers. Certainly, Father Chaurand realized the implications of this problem, and in the documents distributed by Calloët-Querbrat, he alluded to "natural leadership," arguing that the local notables should always be consulted before attempts were made to set up the new structures. At the same time, however, he did not hesitate to impose a clerical vision on the initiatives, proposing that the parish priest be head of the confraternity and that he distribute the aid collected by the notables, both suggestions that left much ambiguity concerning the leadership role of the lay elite. Alain Croix has noted that in Brittany the earliest missionaries were also well aware of the necessity of ensuring the cooperation of the lay elite and that as the conversion movement became more organized in the eighteenth century, one of the principal directives given to local missionaries was to meet with the local notables prior to carrying out their mission and involve them in the efforts to "convert" the community. But in these cases too, the essential leadership in the reforms was to be clerical.[41]

It cannot be assumed, however, that there was a natural antagonism between the local lay elite and the Catholic renewal. Recent studies by

Table 4
Presence of the priest at the distribution of the twenty-fourth in Dauphiné

	Parish majority	
	Catholic	Huguenot
Priest present at distribution	14	4
Priest absent for distribution	17	15

Philip Hoffman and Keith Luria have both noted that, on the contrary, the initial application of religious renewal frequently came through the laity, local governments, or community leaders.[42] An interesting example of lay initiatives in applying the principles of the Catholic revival to poor relief can be found in the previously mentioned law adopted by the Parlement of Grenoble in 1564, ordering that a twenty-fourth of the tithe be turned over by parish priests to community poor relief. Maurice Basque has studied the application of the order eighty years after its creation through the records of the pastoral visit of Charles-Jacques de Léberon in 1644. Léberon was bishop of Die, a small Dauphiné diocese extending from the Rhône valley on the west to the Prealps on the east and from the Vercors mountain range on the north to the Comtat Venaissin on the south.

Basque found that information about aid to the poor or the distribution of the twenty-fourth was present in 75 of the 150 parishes visited. Sixty-four of them gave specific information on the twenty-fourth: in 13 the aid was not distributed at all, while in the remaining 51 parishes some form of the twenty-fourth was present. These documents again provide evidence of the respective roles of priest and laity in the towns and villages that distributed the twenty-fourth. A 1620 directive had ordered that the priest, the consuls, and the seigneur should preside over the distribution, but it was rarely respected. In the same sense that large towns and cities in the sixteenth century had tried to take control over religious hospitals, in the diocese of Die, lay authorities tended to monopolize the distribution of aid to the poor and to exclude parish priests. Certainly, the Huguenot influence in the region may have been partially responsible for this tendency, but as Table 4 shows, even in non-Huguenot parishes the priest was more often absent than present for the distribution of the twenty-fourth.[43]

Bishop Léberon was very critical of this progressive elimination of his priests from village assistance, and in the text of his pastoral report he noted that every priest should "support the charities and other obligations to which he is committed." In several parishes, such as Sinard, he even called upon the curé to maintain the traditional charities inherited from the Middle Ages.[44] Certainly, evidence from the twenty-fourth tends to reinforce the thesis that the role of the laity in both religious and charitable change has been underestimated. The application of the new doctrine and institutions of the Catholic Reformation was far more linked to the lay leadership than has been previously thought.

The role of the priest or curé in the towns and villages was often ambiguous. Was he a member of the local elite or not? Certainly, the reforms of the Council of Trent were directed at reinforcing the privileged status of the local priest. He was to be better educated, to be descended from the social elites, to establish a certain distance between himself and his flock, and to play a more active role in defending the position and holdings of the church in the community.[45] In some cases these "new" priests originated from the communities or regions that they served, and in others they were outsiders, brought in because a lack of local-born priests. Obviously, this factor played an important role vis-à-vis the local notables, who were often related to the priests.[46] However, it was the responsibility of defending the church position with regard to the community that most often put the curés at odds with local notables. Long-running disputes arose over tithes, the fencing off of cemeteries, precedence of the elite families in church pews or processions, and, of course, the role that the church claimed in the distribution of poor relief.[47] In the case of an aggressive curé, his stand on all these issues often set him apart and in opposition to the community elite.[48] In cases of the restruction of local charity, he was often seen as having a vested interest in the reforms proposed by the missionaries and church officials.

It becomes clear that many of the clerically dominated attempts at restructuring charity were only marginally successful. At best, the missionaries and bishops created a climate and a doctrine that were favourable to the extensions of the new religious message as well as to the charity and welfare reforms that were eventually carried out by local notables. There is, of course, a persistent notion that in the northwestern provinces, such as Brittany and Normandy, poor relief was more concentrated in the hands of the clergy as compared to the more municipally oriented hospitals of Provence and Dauphiné. Certainly, the type of hospital run by the Brothers of Charity in Pontorson and initiatives such as those of Chaurand in Brittany were more frequent in the northern provinces. The role of priests in distributing community aid, as in Caudebec, also varied from the southeast, where hospitals carried out weekly distributions of bread and grain and controlled the sums of money allotted to the honourable poor. The confraternities and bureaux of the poor established by missionaries such as St Vincent de Paul or Chaurand were dominated to a greater extent by members of the clergy than were the more traditional bureaux in the south. Religious institutions, monasteries, convents, and mother houses of religious orders were more concentrated in the north, where dioceses were larger, wealthier, and more powerful.

But this northern clerical thesis has often been exaggerated; emphasizing the handouts and alms giving by the convents and monasteries in the north often overlooks the southern charitable network of groups such as the Order of St-Esprit de Montpellier, whose activities and houses had been temporarily expropriated by St-Lazare. It is also clear that the popular, Italian-inspired clerical reforms – pawnbrokers, seed banks, and confraternities – eminating from the Comtat Venaissin strongly influenced charity in the southeast. Despite the apparently greater involvement of religion in northern efforts at poor relief, the structures and functioning of local assistance were not very different in the two regions; the local notables played an increasing role in hospital contributions and administration in both northern and southern areas of the kingdom.

The importance of local elites in reforming assistance to the poor can be demonstrated from their contributions to charitable initiatives in their towns and villages. They were generally at the forefront of the structures established to distribute aid as heads of the confraternities, members of the bureaux of the poor, recteurs of the bureaux, and directors of the hospitals. From these positions they generally collaborated with representatives of the urban elite, bishops, missionaries, and crown officials to tighten up the criteria applied to the poor in the attempt to reduce the number of able-bodied receiving assistance and to promote a work ethic among the poor.

All indications are that the contributions of many town notables to local charitable institutions increased throughout the period and that the increase was often totally independant of clerical initiatives. Although there was never adequate funding to carry out the multiple obligations required of local poor relief, charitable donations rose throughout the seventeenth century in six of the eight communities that I have studied. Such increases do not represent isolated examples, for Kathryn Norberg, Cissie Fairchilds, Michel Vovelle, and Pierre Chaunu have all demonstrated through their studies of wills that there was an important increase in charitable donations everywhere in France, even if the same social groups were not always responsible.[49] Patrice Berger has demonstrated the involvement of nobles, in particular the Pontchartrain family, in promoting new forms of charitable aid on their rural estates in the late seventeenth century.[50] At the same time, Vovelle and Norberg have shown that by the mid-seventeenth century, bourgeois families had begun imitating the example of noble donations.

Like the Pontchartrain family, nobles and members of the community elite in the southeast were very generous to charity organizations. Michel Vovelle had demonstrated this new outpouring of aid in his study of eighteenth-century wills in Provence. Donors consciously or unconsciously imitated urban patterns and gave generously to found new rural and small-town hospitals or to supplement the revenues of existing institutions. In 1720 Monsieur de Castellane-Pontèves left a grant producing 100 livres a year to set up a four-bed hospital at St-Laurent. In 1735 Mme de Lombard, Baronne de Chateauneuf, left 200 livres to the town of Grasse to found a hospital, specifying that if it did not open, her money should be transformed into four alms distributions of 50 livres each, to be given to the poor by the consuls.[51]

Almost half of the towns and villages in Provence possessed hospitals (83 of the 190 recognized communities), although the equipment, number of beds, and capacities of these establishments were often very limited. They were not well distributed either, for in the central part of the province, the sénéchaussée of Aix, the number of hospitals per community was far greater (over 40 per cent) than in the west around Arles or in lower Provence. The donations to hospitals were just as important as the individual gifts in the wills studied by Vovelle – 15 to 20 per cent – but they were more concentrated in towns, while alms distributions tended to be favoured by donors in villages and rural areas.[52] This pattern generally confirms the work of Maurice Basque on the distribution of the twenty-fourth portion of the dîme in the Dauphiné diocese of Die, where larger communities were generally more capable of aiding the poorer members of their community.[53]

The support of local noble families was often a critical factor in maintaining poor relief. As previously mentioned, the Adhémar family was particularly active in supporting and directing the Grignan hospital; it did so over several generations. Three major grants to the institution were left in family wills during the seventeenth century: one in 1660 by the Comtesse Marguerite d'Ornano bequeathed 1,400 livres; the second, by Louis d'Adhémar eight years later, left 600 livres; and the third by Charles-Philippe d'Adhémar donated 800 livres in 1672. These grants seem to have established a model imitated by other members of the community. The collegiate chapter of St-Sauveur church made an annual grant of 4 charges of rye to the hospital amounting to an average gift of about 30 livres, or about 3,000 livres during the century. Individuals, too – canons, notaries, county administrators, and wealthy residents – gave to the hospital. In the accounts from 1656 to 1700, twenty-one different donations can be identified, ranging from 3 to 204 livres and adding some 1,482 livres to the hospital funds.[54]

The social and religious importance attached to such legacies often led people on their deathbeds to will substantial holdings or sums of money to hospitals or the church. Their heirs, often surprised by such "generosity," did not hesitate to contest such grants, and the hospitals were frequently before the courts defending their rights to these gifts. In some cases, such as a 1723 grant of 300 livres made to the Grignan hospital by Mlle Janine Serre, the issue came before the town council, which ordered the hospital directors to dispute the refusal of the late Mlle Serre's brother-in-law, Claude Gourjon, to turn over the money.[55] In other instances, the councillors opted to leave the grant with the heirs when the terms of the will were unclear; such was the case in March 1723, when holdings worth 150 livres were returned to Claude Heraud, heir of Sieur Denanes, since it appeared that the lands were already mortgaged.[56] In situations where the holdings left to the institutions were of value, heirs often tried to discredit the will so as to retain the property of the deceased. They did not do so in the case of the Adhémar legacies, which were duly entered into the accounts of the Grignan hospital, but uncertainty as to whether many of the other legacies were actually paid is an argument raised against the reliability of conclusions drawn from the global studies of early modern wills.[57] For this reason, I have not retained them as indicators of the grants made to hospitals; instead I have concentrated directly upon the financial accounts of the institutions under study.

Partly because of social attitudes developed by Counter-Reformation Catholicism,[58] interest in charity accounted for a spectacular increase in the revenues of small-town, as well as city, institutions. For the eight hospitals studied here, with the notable exception of Malestroit and the limited data on Savenay and St-Vallier, annual revenues grew more than tenfold during the seventeenth century. Even when the revenues in livres are translated into quartals of wheat to compensate for the effects of devaluations and inflation, the increases in hospital revenues remain just as impressive. For five of the eight institutions, they go from the levels

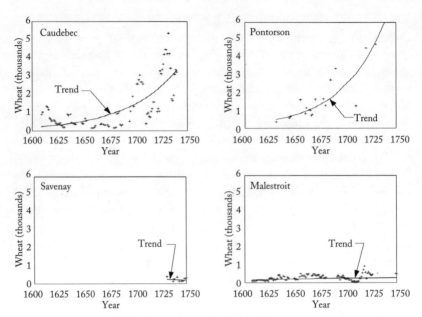

Figure 2   Income of the hospitals in Caudebec, Pontorson, Savenay, and Malestroit, expressed in quartals of wheat, for the period 1600–1750

of 100 to 200 quartals at the beginning of the seventeenth century to averages of 1,000 to 3,000 by the 1750s (see Figures 2 and 3).[59]

Of course, these revenues do not reflect real annual donations to the institutions. Gifts of land or capital were generally noted once as a total value in the revenue section, and thereafter their incomes were integrated into the hospital holdings and rented or loaned out by the recteur. Their interest produced several of the entries listed as revenue in the annual hospital accounts. The revenue curve is influenced by these sporadic donations, as can be seen from the deviations in the Étoile graph between 1675 and 1700 and in the regular ups and downs in that for Seyne. Additional explanations for disparities in the graphs come from the fact that each recteur upon balancing the accounts of his term in office usually included a certain number of late lease or interest payments; sometimes these accounts were not closed up until two or three years after his term of office expired, so that late payments were constantly being entered into the revenue section. The erratic comportment of Caudebec revenues between 1724 and 1732 is due to injections of funding for the beggars and vagabonds who had been incarcerated as a result of the 1724 royal edict. Other revenues included long-term investments; most hospitals

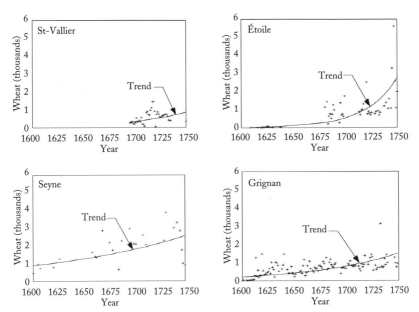

Figure 3   Income from the hospitals of St-Vallier, Étoile, Seyne, and
Grignan, expressed in quartals of wheat, for the period 1600–1750

possessed fields and houses that they leased out. For example, Malestroit
owned and rented houses in the centre of the town, and the Caudebec
hospital even held a house in Rouen, which it rented out.

Camille Bloch studied the financial condition of the larger hospitals
of the kingdom using replies to a 1764 inquiry launched by the controller
general, and he found most of them to be deeply in debt.[60] In contrast
to his findings, the eight hospitals studied in this book generally balanced
their budgets and rarely spent more than they took in for any extended
period of time. The revenues illustrated in these graphs are therefore
relatively good reflections of general hospital expenses (payments to
doctors, surgeons, apothecaries, caretakers, and nuns, repairs to the
buildings, the cost of beds, sheets, and food, sums loaned out, and
amounts paid in interest on borrowed money). However, it should not
be assumed that because their revenues increased, these hospitals were
better able to meet the needs of the sick and the poor. On the contrary,
one after another, they complained that they did not have sufficient
funds to care properly for their patients and their community.[61]

A key to the apparent contradiction between increasing revenues and
complaints that they had difficulty meeting the needs of their inmates

lies in the hospitals' inability to expand their physical facilities or their services. Even with increasing revenues, the institutions studied ran into difficulty whenever they undertook any new construction. This fact can be seen at Pontorson and Caudebec, both of which launched expansion projects during the eighteenth century. In 1715 the Brothers of Charity built a new building eighty by twenty-one feet to house a new chapel, apothecary shop, and rooms for the brothers. Even with revenues increasing, the expenses of this construction and the repairs on the existing buildings made it more and more difficult for them to balance their budget, and they had to call upon other houses of their order to help them meet current expenses. In 1757 they undertook the construction of another new building presented to the father provincial as a *maison de force*, a centre for those sent for internment by their families. Since the families compensated the hospital to have their kin locked up, it was argued that this building would pay for itself and produce surpluses, enabling the community to balance its increasingly strained budget.[62]

In the case of Caudebec, the deficits incurred by construction projects were even clearer. At its meetings of September and December 1765, the hospital board decided to build a new extension, the cost being estimated at 4,000 livres.[63] By the meeting of 2 April 1766, it had brought in contractors, who calculated that the planned building would cost "much more than double the sum" anticipated.[64] By 1769, when the extension was finished, an examination of the accounts of Sr LeDuc, the administrator, showed that the building had cost 11,381 livres.[65] Such expenses and the loans needed to carry out these construction projects obviously had a major impact upon the capacity of hospitals to continue normal operations. It took several years for the new Caudebec facility to be furnished and become operational, and relief to the poor was actually reduced during this period.

Although the increases in revenue registered by most of the hospitals under study were not really enough to transform or improve assistance, they extended well into the eighteenth century and contradict current notions that charitable donations tended to decline after the 1700s. Michel Vovelle for Provence, Kathryn Norberg for Grenoble, and Pierre Chaunu have all traced a contraction in the revenues contributed directly or bequeathed to charitable institutions as a result of the "dechristianization" movement – the decline in religious fervour and practice that began towards the end of the seventeenth century.[66] Does this mean that the elites of small towns were slower to react to the changes in the *mentalité* governing poor relief? Were they more influenced by the church message in favour of charity? Or were the charitable institutions in question simply more fully assimilated into the social fabric of the towns in which they were situated?

One of the reasons for the increases in local hospital revenues was the determined actions of the directors, recteurs, and town councillors, who actively sought new sources of funding for their institutions. Over and above the revenues and holdings donated to the hospitals by local residents, the directors pursued new types of patients and inmates for whom they would receive reimbursement – soldiers, orphans, and abandoned children, as well as the mentally ill. Caudebec concentrated upon soldiers, and after receiving from 1 to 8 sick or injured men per year from the nearby garrisons during the period from 1739 to 1749, the directors took in 14 soldiers the following year and 31 in 1751; their numbers skyrocketed to 89 in 1756 before returning to around 60 by 1757 and 1759.[67] According to the 1759 deliberations, the board of directors seems to have negotiated with each battalion to set a daily rate for their men. It was noted that the Touraine battalion had agreed to increase its daily payments from 10 to 14 sous per soldier, and it was hoped that the Montreuil regiment would also honour the increase since "for the last few years the hospital is considerably burdened by sick soldiers for whom it has received only 10 sol a day, of which half comes from the soldier's pay and the other half from crown subsidies that are currently a year overdue."[68] The average hospitalization for the 89 soldiers treated in 1756, even before the increase, had amounted to twelve days, resulting in payments of 534 livres, or about 8 per cent of the total revenues of slightly over 7,000.[69]

The administrators of other small hospitals were just as aggressive as Caudebec in seeking out new paying clients. At Pontorson, when the Brothers of Charity attached the maison de force to the hospital, it began by receiving 6 inmates interned by their families in 1702 and increased that number to 22 by 1725, 28 by 1750, 50 five years later, 42 by 1765, and 59 by 1779.[70] As the brothers had argued at the time of its construction in 1757, the revenues from the maison de force by the 1760s and 1770s came to constitute over half the annual income of the institution.[71]

At Seyne and Étoile the hospital administrations sought to increase their revenues by taking in orphans or abandoned children. The deliberations for the Seyne hospital from 1753 to 1780 indicate that the administrators of the small institution regularly admitted such cases: an average of three orphans a year were presented to the bureau.[72] For Étoile the deliberations available between 1768 and 1787 show a similar interest in abandoned children, and there as well, three or four cases a year seem to have been added to the hospital register. The institutions were able to request compensation for these children, as others had for soldiers. The Seyne deliberations indicate that the subdelegate paid 1 or 2 sous a day for their care, and in 1763 the Assembly of Procureurs of Provence voted to pay hospitals 120 livres for each child that they agreed to take in and raise.[73]

As Kathryn Norberg has pointed out, the organization of the bureaux of the poor and the hospital boards were clear reflections of a patronizing, hierarchical conception of society. It is clear, as she has also indicated, that the individuals who made up these boards consistently worked to increase the revenues distributed to the poor and the needy. The new paying inmates enabled the hospitals to stabilize their financial situation and offer better services to the poor members of the community. In many cases, the notables of the town actively sought out additional financing. The women's confraternities took up collections at the church doors, and the men who served as directors of the hospitals and hospices regularly sought new means to increase institutional services and extend aid to the poor who remained in their homes. The notables of the different towns were profoundly interested in maintaining their control over local hospitals and over the lands and revenues that they possessed. This fact can be clearly seen in the case of Pontorson, where the town lost control over its hospital. A 1644 letter from the king had asked the community to transfer the revenues and holdings of the hospital to the Brothers of Charity. The inhabitants of the town, particularly the elite, acceded to the royal request, but never really reconciled themselves to giving up their rights over the institution. They took legal action in 1654, arguing that the brothers were not respecting their obligation to pay 200 livres a year to the chaplain of the hospital.[74] A 1656 decision of the Parlement of Rouen on the case tried to strike a compromise by reducing the payment owed to the hospital chaplain.

However, the decision marked only a truce, and hostilities broke out again in 1721 when the Pontorson consuls sent a letter of complaint to the bishop of Avranches. They noted that they had been "obliged" to give up their hospital in 1644 and that the brothers were making considerable sums of money from the institution and were not respecting its charter. It was noted that despite promises to serve all the town residents, the brothers refused to admit or treat the women and girls of the community. All these grievances were repeated again in 1738–39 when

Louis xv asked for the official registering of the letters patent confirming the 1644 acquisition of the hospital by the brothers. The town hired a solicitor and sent a report to the Parlement. The document denounced the brothers for not respecting the terms of the original grants to the institution and for squandering its revenues on food, new buildings, and "large gardens, with elegant pathways on all sides, to beautify their house."[75] These charges and countercharges continued up to 1747, and they indicate the deep resentment felt by the notables of Pontorson, who saw traditional town resources being disposed of by the brothers.

Why were town notables so insistent upon managing the poor-relief institutions? Why did they become so involved in seeking and soliciting new revenues for the local hospitals? Their efforts were obviously linked in part to the rhetoric of the dévot movement, which underlined the responsibilities of the elite towards their needy brethren, but this activity also consolidated their position as members of the community elite.[76] They supported the hospitals not only because of their Christian responsibilities, but also because they enjoyed the social control that they derived from managing institutions for the poor and the sick.[77] Contributions to the hospital and service on the board constituted one of the marks of membership in the local elite. Donors not only helped to bring about the well-being of the poorer members of their town, gained prestige, and ensured their Christian salvation by aiding the members of their community poorer, but they also assured themselves a certain patronage role in distributing aid.[78]

With the exception of Pontorson, where the Brothers of Charity had taken over the management of the hospital, all the other bureaux of charity examined were managed by the community, especially by the elite. The recteur of the poor was generally named at the same town assembly as the consuls, the political leaders for the upcoming year, and he was chosen from the same group of individuals who eventually became consuls or councillors. This pattern is evident from a comparison of the persons named to different community institutions in Grignan and Seyne (see the appendices). An analysis of the position of recteur at Grignan between 1661 and 1722 shows that the count himself was recteur for seven years, five other notables served two terms, Jean Dumas, a notary, three times, and forty-six other members of the local elite held the position at least once. Only ten of the forty-six had not or did not accede to the position of first or second consul. Among the remaining thirty-six were eight notaries, one lieutenant de baillage, two merchants, one doctor, one surgeon, and five blacksmiths. Thirty-two of them can be retraced on the 1681 taille roll, where they were assessed an average of 16.11 sous on a roll where the average payment was only 4.75 sous.

In Seyne the same type of portrait can be drawn. When the available data on first consuls there is compared with the list of recteurs for the period from 1713 to 1751, it becomes apparent that the retiring first consul was generally named to head the hospital. The resulting recteurs were an integral part of the community elite. Merchants, notaries, lawyers, doctors, and "bourgeois" succeeded each other in the position, and some such as Jacques Arnaud, a doctor, were returned three times to the direction of the institution. François-André Laugier, notary, held the position four times, as did Louis-André Savournin, "bourgeois."

This participation by the elite in the management of poor-relief structures legitimized the privileged position that they held in the community. In no other area was this hierarchical approach more evident than in the distribution of aid to the poor. In all the towns studied, the recteur presided over various types of aid: the supervision of the caretaker who worked in the hospital buildings to care for the sick poor, the making up of the list of "outside" poor who lived at home and received weekly distributions of bread or grain to nourish their families, and the determination of the honourable poor, the formerly well-to-do who had fallen on hard times and been obliged to seek charity. The members of the community elite were the clear arbiters of both the latter categories, judging who should be aided and who refused. In order to be placed on the role for the weekly distribution of bread or grain at Étoile, the individual in question had to provide the recteur with a slip of paper signed by a town notable attesting to his or her need. The hospital archives at Étoile contain a certain quantity of these slips, generally preserved with the annual accounts.[79] The number of recipients of these weekly grain distributions was considerable both at Étoile and in most of the other hospital towns.

However, the types of distribution varied, and while Étoile gave out considerably more grain in the winter and spring months, the records at Grignan show that similar distributions continued twelve months a year there. In the northwestern towns, the municipal structures were less involved in "outside" poor relief. At Pontorson the Brothers of Charity maintained a certain distribution of alms, and at Caudebec it was the pastor of Notre-Dame church who administered the fund to aid the outside poor, although there too, recipients had to be recommended by town notables. The signature of a notable on each request for aid demonstrates the role played by the local elite in deciding who should benefit and what criteria should be applied to candidates for relief. This control was even more evident in the cases of the honourable poor, for there as well it was the recognized elite who decided that a certain person could be considered as a former member of their ranks, deserved a higher level of aid than most poor, and have his or her name concealed from the community.

In addition to having their patronage role reinforced through their power to decide who should receive aid, the elite's control over hospital structures made them arbiters of important sources of community wealth. The recteur received the revenues and lands of the hospital that he was to manage for a variable period; at Grignan it was for one year, while at Caudebec he assumed his functions for three to four years, and at Étoile the mandate often extended to five. The management of the hospital resources can be analysed in detail for Grignan, where consular archives can be compared with hospital documents. During his mandate, using the funds and landholdings at his disposal, the recteur made loans and leased land to the consuls, notables of the community, and individuals whom he deemed trustworthy.[80] The sums to be distributed to the poor were derived from the interest payments on these loans and from the annual lease payments received by the recteur. Between 1658 and 1700 almost 5,000 livres were loaned out to individuals from the hospital funds. In addition, the town of Grignan borrowed 4,350 livres between 1654 and 1664 and the neighbouring village of Montségur received 1,030 livres. These loan and lease agreements constituted attractive extensions of credit in a period when access to capital was severely restricted. Once again it was the interest payments on these loans and leases that financed the aid distributed to the poor.[81]

Another patronage opportunity for the recteurs in Grignan came from the grain purchases carried out by the hospital in order to feed the poor during the winter months. There too the close bond, one could even say collusion, between the recteur and the notables was evident. Between 1684 and 1692 the recteur purchased an average of 31 saumées of grain a year, typically paying 298 livres to his suppliers, be they consuls or former consuls, the count's agent, the treasurer of the St-Sauveur chapter, or notables and their families. These suppliers were generally the same members of the elite who occupied the positions of consul or recteur and the same people who donated money to the hospital. On other occasions, they or members of their families negotiated loans or leased land from the institution. It becomes clear that the hospital played a double role: aiding the poorest members of the community with periodic handouts, grain distributions, and temporary shelter and care at the same time that it served the town notables as a "bank" for temporary credit and as a means of extending their landholdings through leases. All the hospitals that possessed respectable endowments played this double role, and in this context they were as important to the rich and the community as they were to the poor.

The success of the dévot movement in implanting essentially urban welfare models in the towns and villages of the kingdom depended closely upon the collaboration of the local elites. The missionaries of the Catholic Reformation, in particular Father Chaurand, insisted upon this cooperation and upon initial contacts with local notables. They were to be convinced first and foremost of the importance of the new measures. They were to be shown the necessity of ending indiscriminate handouts and to be persuaded to channel donations towards a community institution for the poor. Most important, they were to be given key positions in the implementation of the bureaux of charity and the new hospital structures. Chaurand's movement actually proposed to the town elites different ways to reinforce their social prominence and their role in controlling the poorer members of their community. The proposals were based upon those adopted by the large urban establishments: discriminating between "deserving" and "undeserving" poor, turning away the poor and sick from other towns or villages, and forcing the able-bodied to work.

In line with these directives, local leaders tried to concentrate their charitable efforts and resist indiscriminate handouts. This attempt is obvious in most of the communities that at various times during the seventeenth century restricted their poor-relief measures to local residents.[82] In Grignan the revised rules and regulations of the hospice in 1676 contain clear reference to the new principles of welfare distribution. In a series of regulations for the hospital, the bishop of Die and the Comte de Grignan drew up distinctions as to who among the town poor qualified for bread distributions. In a 1686 addition to the regulations, limits were placed on aid to itinerants or vagabonds. The 1676 document ordered that the bureau of the poor carry out an annual visit and inspection of the homes of those requesting the status of *pauvres* and that they grant this status to the physically infirm or those with many children to nourish. The bureau was then to use this list to draw up two rolls: one for the distribution of bread every Sunday for the first five months of the year and the other for money to be given out to invalids

Table 5
Aid distributed to inhabitants and outsiders in Grignan and Étoile towards the beginning and the end of the seventeenth century

	Outsiders (in livres)	Inhabitants (in livres)	Bread distribution (in livres + "charges" of grain)
GRIGNAN			
1600–01	8.95	11.10	3.7 + 6
1680	40.00	220.10	395.1 + 24
ÉTOILE			
1603–04	18.00	20.00	
1667–69	11.00	674.00	

and the sick (who were to be visited monthly to ensure that they still needed assistance).[83] The 1686 addition to the regulations was drafted by the count; he noted the considerable influx of vagabonds into the region, who under such pretences as making pilgrimages were asking to be housed in the hospital and aided by village welfare. Referring to a 1671 royal decree ordering the expulsion of vagabonds from town and village hospitals, the count forbade any future lodging or aid to them.[84]

In fact, since the beginning of the seventeenth century and the increases in charitable donations, most institutions had become more discriminating in their aid to the poor. A clear indication of this new approach can be seen in the distribution made by two of the eight hospitals in this study between the early 1600s and the 1680s (see Table 5).[85] It becomes obvious from both Étoile and Grignan that by the 1660s to 1680s the increased revenues were overwhelmingly distributed to poor townspeople, either in the form of bread or as money. The medieval tradition of handouts to itinerants persisted, but it came to represent a minimal part of hospital operation.

A concrete example of the type of change that occurred in services to the poor in the institutions under study can be seen from a detailed examination of the lists of poor aided by the hospital in Étoile. The recipients of relief changed considerably between 1603–04 and 1667–69. On the hospital roll for the former year, when Louis Tosserand was treasurer, the institution had treated or distributed bread or money to forty-five residents of Étoile and ninety-five outsiders. Among those receiving aid, thirty-four were sick. Most of the outsiders were carried to the hospital on stretchers to be lodged and treated for a maximum of six days before being sent off to neighbouring institutions at Livron, Valence, Beaumont, or La Vache for similar treatment. It was a standard practice in these institutions that outsiders could not be kept for more than four or five days. Claize Mounier was the only resident of Étoile to be treated in the hospital, and she stayed there for sixteen days.[86] By 1667, when Charles Point was treasurer, there were virtually no outsiders receiving significant aid, and the amounts distributed to the recognized town poor had increased to take the form of stipends of 54, 29, or 17 livres. Although most of those receiving aid did not live at the hospital, a caretaker was employed to maintain hospitality, and the bureau of the poor paid a doctor to care for the sick.[87] As the cases of Étoile and Grignan demonstrate, the tradition of maintaining aid to itinerants and outsiders was one of the first victims of attempts by the directors of local welfare institutions to rationalize services along the lines followed by the urban reforms.

While the local elite was conscious of its responsibility in the field of poor relief, it did not hesitate to try to cut the costs of welfare or rationalize services. That it did so can be seen at Seyne in 1656, when the town council took the initiative of merging the two existing hospitals into one institution to avoid duplication of services.[88] The same type of rationalization took place in Auray in Brittany, where the town council in 1777 merged a commanderie of the Order of St-Esprit with one of the hôpitaux-généraux founded by Father Chaurand in order to better utilize space and services.[89] Certainly, the initiatives taken at Étoile, Grignan, Seyne, and Auray demonstrate that local notables often did adopt the welfare reforms proposed by the missionaries and the urban elite.

As long as the changes to poor relief proposed by representatives of the church or state did not conflict with the traditional patterns of the local power structure, they were not opposed. This is the reason why the missionaries, in particular Chaurand, placed such emphasis upon preliminary discussions with local officials and upon the idea that the reforms were to reinforce, not to diminish, their authority. In effect, community elites generally offered no obstacles to the acceptance of the changes as long as their powers were maintained. The problem with the new reforms came in cases where the elite itself was divided or where the new logic behind poor relief threatened existing community structures and the role played by the elite.

Malestroit exemplifies the problematic attitude of community elites towards their charitable institutions. Among the hospitals studied here, it constitutes one of the rare cases where the revenues of an institution actually declined. A profound division in the groups governing the institution seems to explain the Malestroit difficulties. The Hôpital Ste-Anne was a seigneurial foundation, and until the seventeenth century it had always been directed by one of the seigneurial agents, the judge, or the treasurer. In the first part of the century, the nominations of administrators, or provosts, to run the hospital and the inspection of their annual accounts increasingly resulted in struggles between the community and the seigneurial officials. The community scored several important victories during this period. In the case of Jean Crouzil, administrator from 1615 to 1619, town officials obtained the right to be present in 1624 when he brought in and justified his expenses before the seigneurial officials. After 1642 the community was able to add the newly named provost and his assistants (*économes*) to the board of seigneurial judges to examine the accounts of the outgoing provost. That year it took the step of unilaterally naming the provost, Sieur Bocquensue, despite the fact that the seigneurial treasurer argued that the nomination should have been made by the Baron de Malestroit.

Perhaps as a result of these conflicts, the provosts named during this period seem to have been increasingly indifferent to the institution. They rarely completed their four year terms, some, such as François Latoit in 1627–28, serving only one year, others two or three years, among them Gilles Guilhaume, 1628–30, Pierre Theriault, 1634–36, and Maître Michel Nicolas, 1657–1660.[90] In addition, they seldom respected even the calendar year of their nominations, one leaving office after two years and two months and another after a year and ten months. Finally in 1652, the question of who could name the provost, seigneurial or community officials, was appealed to the Parlement of Brittany. On 15 June it declared that the seigneurial officials had not disposed of a monopoly over the administration of the hospital and that the institution should henceforth be directed by a "general assembly of the community" in which seigneurial, community, and religious authorities were represented.[91]

The struggle over the direction of the hospital did not end with the 1652 judgment, and it constantly interrupted the normal functioning of the institution. Unlike at Grignan or Étoile, the Baron de Malestroit was too involved in arguing over administration rights to take part personally in the governing and endowment of the institution. In the eighteenth century the mayor and seigneurial judge became so caught up in the dispute that the general assembly of the hospital did not meet between September 1707 and October 1711.[92] Instead of being headed by the town elite, former councillors, and community leaders, the hospital had more and more difficulty finding provosts, so that younger, less well connected men had to be named to the position. In 1715 a twenty-two-year-old lawyer, Jean Le Manseau, Sieur de Craslon, became provost, and three years later he was reappointed in the absence of any other candidate. In 1722 Le Manseau was replaced by his friend René Géorget, Sieur de La Prevalaye, who had just reached his majority. Between 1727 and 1749 the provost was Sieur Hery Derval, who like Le Manseau was only twenty-two years old when he assumed the position.[93] During this period financial difficulties were more and more frequently mentioned at the meetings of the bureau. By 1719 and 1720 a number of local inhabitants had asked that their grants to the institution be reimbursed. Finally in 1722, amidst this financial crisis and confronted by the announcement that the Order of St-Thomas de Villeneuve was to withdraw the nuns who were staffing the institution, the directors of the hospital did not even meet to deal with the problems.[94]

The case of Malestroit demonstrates the necessity of close community cooperation in building up and maintaining charitable institutions. In the face of the numerous initiatives by crown officials and expanding urban centres to "reform" and shut down outdated or redundant charitable institutions, a small community divided within itself or differing in its welfare priorities was a enticing target for the movements directed by Mount Carmel and St-Lazare, urban hospitals, and crown officials. It is clear that divisions among the elite of small towns, such as the seigneurial-bourgeois dispute in Malestroit, could be particularly crippling to charitable institutions whose operations were being examined in detail for their legality and efficiency.

The local elite's cooperation was necessary if a town was to adopt the new criteria for welfare and the new types of institutions proposed by the urban elite. Town and village notables reacted to these models according to the way that they were proposed and the changes in the local structures that they implied. When the reforms would take away funds from village institutions, as was the case with the St-Lazare interventions in Étoile, Malestroit, and Savenay, the recteurs, consuls, and notables resisted the proposed changes and appealed the decisions. As in hundreds of other small communities, the imposition of "objective" criteria to judge the performance of welfare institutions led to unilateral suppressions and consolidations of hospitals and charitable structures between 1672 and 1700. Far from being preceded by consultation and participation on the part of the local elite, these initiatives diminished the role of local notables and destabilized community structures. Not corresponding to either the traditional structures or the priorities dear to local elites, the "reforms" were greeted with indifference or resistance.

It was clearly in the interest of the community leadership that the hospital appear to be well managed and kept up. In this context, the failure of the hospitals of Étoile, Savenay, and Malestroit to carry out regular reforms of their rules and regulations rendered them vulnerable to the criteria applied by the inspectors and judges of the Mount Carmel and St-Lazare reform. There is evidence that many institutions actually cheated in order to transmit a false image of themselves to crown authorities. Jean-Pierre Gutton has presented the case of the Charité de St-Étienne, where a dual system of admission records was maintained, one set of records being forged to deceive outsiders into thinking that the hospital served far more patients than it actually did.[95] The hospital at Pontorson also seems to have used such a dual system in its book-keeping, and the accounts, or *états*, sent to the provincial administrators often represent only a fourth of the actual revenues taken in by the prior and reported to the father provincial of the Order of St-Jean de Dieu.[96] An even more striking case of duplicity comes from the archives of the Hôtel-Dieu de Beaune, where a text from the hospital of Meursault explains that, having been informed that the commissioners of the Order of St-Lazare were about to visit the institution, its administrators brought in additional beds, in which they installed local peasants to give the impression that the hospital was full. The document notes that the commissioners were satisfied and that the institution continued to operate until the 1764 reform ordered by Turgot.[97]

The shared responsibility of church and community in the direction of early modern poor relief was more theoretical than real. In the wake of the Council of Trent, the French church did try to breathe new life into its poor-relief responsibilities: after some hesitation, authorities participated in efforts to carry forward humanist ideas to rationalize such activity. They attempted to orient alms towards institutions such as confraternities and to create pawnbrokers for the poor, seed banks, and hôpitaux-généraux. However, the success of these initiatives was uneven, and it becomes clear that most of the reformers eventually realized that the principal agents for reforming local poor relief were not missionaries or parish priests, but community notables who were in the most direct control of the bureaux of the poor, the hospitals, and relief agencies.

In a recent article, Alain Croix called for further research to define the characteristics of the local notables, their allies, and their patronage networks.[98] Their role as intermediaries in the chain of command has been underscored by Jean-Pierre Gutton, who saw their power as being whittled away by the regular, unilateral crown interventions in local affairs.[99] On the other hand, Hilton Root, in his study of the exercise of royal power in seventeenth- and eighteenth-century Burgundy, perceived the crown under Louis xv as deliberately readjusting its policies to meet the traditional demands of local notables, reinforcing their position, and trying to appease their opposition to the past intransigence of royal fiscal policy.[100]

This chapter demonstrates that in the field of poor relief, both church and crown officials tried to win over these local elites, attempting to convince them to institute the new welfare reforms. However, the notables' reaction to such solicitation did not allow them easily to be placed either in the camp of those automatically opposed to new, unilateral interventions or in that of the collaborators with the politics of absolutism. What we see instead is the local elites enthusiastically participating in and starting to apply some of the reforms before centralized religious and political authorities even asked for their cooperation. Their donations to the hospitals actually increased several decades before the missionaries began appealing for increased alms giving. It is also clear that local authorities themselves decided to participate in or boycott centralized reform efforts according to their own concerns. The local hospital and welfare structures constituted important elements for reinforcing their economic and social interests. Their management of the revenues and holdings of these institutions procured them substantial economic advantages. They also profited socially by presiding over the distribution of community welfare, deciding who should receive aid and who should not. They generally opposed any effort to reduce these roles by giving priests a larger part in the distribution of aid or the management of institutions of poor relief, and they totally resisted the centralized reforms of local poor relief, which implied closing down or expropriating the holdings of local hospitals. The notables participating in and directing these poor-relief institutions became the principal arbiters of whether or not the new initiatives were in the communities' interests. In this role they were admirably placed to make these decisions in ways that would best protect their own interests.

It is precisely within this context that the bishop of Die met with the Grignan town council in 1736 to discuss how to put "order" into the management of the local institution. The subsequent inspection of the hospital and the drawing up of stringent new regulations for internal and external recipients of aid was left in the hands of the town elite, and in doing so, this authority reinforced its dominant social position. Had church or crown authorities arrived in the town with the intention of closing down or merging the Grignan hospital with a neighbouring institution, it is clear that the count, the bureau, and the councillors would have been uncooperative. Such moves would have cut off the local elite from access to the funds and holdings of the hospital, depriving them of their role as arbiters over who should receive aid and of the social prestige that such power conferred upon them. The Grignan case demonstrates the extent to which the economic and social status of the local elite depended upon their organization of relief efforts for the poorer members of their community.

5 Religious Congregations and Local Hospitals: Women Working in the World

On 3 June 1666 in the town of Malestroit, the assembly of nobles, bourgeois, yeomen (*manants*), and *habitants* met to discuss the deteriorating conditions under which the sick were being treated at the local hospital. They noted that much of the problem lay in the disorder created by the beggars and itinerants who were put up in the institution. The assembly decided by a plurality of votes to accept a proposition that had been negotiated by Sieur Fontano, the recteur, and other town dignitaries calling for the establishment in the hospital of the "damoiselles et filles" from the Hôtel-Dieu at Lamballe.

The damoiselles et filles were the Sisters of St-Thomas de Villeneuve. Having approved the document, the order sent Damoiselles Le Maignan and Laisné to run the Malestroit institution on the condition that the town provide lodging for them and their servants in the hospital, that they have use of the large garden behind the institution for their food, and that they have the right to refuse admission to any unruly girl or woman "so as not to upset the peace of their charitable enterprise." For their part, the damoiselles were committed to accept the sick who were sent to them with admission orders signed by local hospital authorities, provosts, économes, or directors. They were to "nurse them, feed them, and wash their clothes" and receive 4 sous a day for each patient, who was to be cared for as long as the directors judged necessary. Those who were not sick and had received an admission order were to be given bread or food, to be sheltered, and to have their clothes washed. The nuns were to receive 2 sous a day for each of these. Beggars and itinerants were to be kept for no more than twenty-four hours and were to be separated from the sick. No one was to be admitted without an order signed by those responsible for the hospital, and the damoiselles were not to receive or manage any of the hospital funds or properties.[1]

The contract discussed in the Malestroit assembly between the town and the Community of St-Thomas de Villeneuve was typical of hundreds of similar documents negotiated throughout France between the 1650s and the 1750s. Newly created women's religious congregations were established in hospitals and schools everywhere. The enthusiasm generated by the Catholic Reformation led to the creation of a large number of these congregations with a vocation to "work in the world" to save souls. Acceptance of these orders resulted in a radical evolution in the perception of women's place in society. Demand was very heavy for the new sisters, and numerous newly founded congregations had great difficulty meeting requests for their services.

These new orders followed, of course, in the footsteps of a number of men's congregations that had become active in directing French hospitals during the sixteenth and early seventeenth centuries.[2] The best known of these orders, the Brothers of St John of God, had been founded in Spain in 1538. Brought into France by Marie de Médicis in 1602, the order was given a house, Quai Malaquais, from which the brothers moved to rue des Sts-Pères and added the title "Brothers of Charity" to their name. From the time of their foundation in Spain, the order had specialized in hospital service, and once in France they became much involved in the Hôpital de la Charité in Paris and eventually assumed the direction of numerous other institutions in the provinces, the West Indies, and Canada. By 1790 the order consisted of 355 brothers in charge of thirty-eight hospitals, including Pontorson.[3]

However, not enough men were recruited for the Brothers of Charity, and the needs of the hundreds of large and small hospitals were overwhelming. Places such as Malestroit that were trying to improve services to the poor and sick of their communities turned to the new women's orders. In fact, as most hospitals became more conscious of their obligations towards the sick, they began to employ caretakers to look after their patients. In 1690 the administrators of the Caudebec hospital followed this pattern, asking Mlle de Cocquiveau, the daughter of a local notable, to take charge of the institution. She died five years later leaving a considerable sum of money to the hospital, and the bureau set out to try to replace her.[4] After an interim of almost four years, in which the post was filled part-time, the curé noted in 1699 that there was disorder in the institution and that Caudebec should be aware that the crown had undertaken a reorganization of its hospital system, merging small maladreries with regional hospitals. He argued that the Caudebec institution could assume a position of importance in the context of this reform, and he pointed out the need to find another full-time director.[5] A month later the bureau engaged Mme Saint-Martin, who had been proposed by the curé; she served until her death a year later in 1700.[6] Noting the meticulous work of both the previous administrators, the bureau named Mlle de Glatigni to the post in 1700, but she too died within four years.[7] The efforts in Caudebec to find suitable local residents to direct the hospital demonstrate the difficulties of this system. The directors whom they hired were frequently older women or widows who served only a few years, so that upon their death the administrators had to seek out another untrained local woman for the job. Every four or five years the direction changed, with the inevitable hiatus and the difficulty once again of finding a director.

Even worse was the Savenay situation, where the poorly paid caretaker took little or no interest in her responsibilities. This fact is clear from a report by Pierre Pellerin to the bureau of the St-Armal hospital in Savenay in August 1760. He noted that during a surprise inspection of the hospital premises, he had found that the caretaker, Mlle Bouvon, had appropriated almost all the rooms of the institution for her personal use. Although she should have occupied only one of the upstairs rooms, she had in fact taken over a downstairs room and both upstairs rooms for herself, as well as the *grande salle*, the multi-purpose room on the first floor, where she had installed a cow and a calf and where there were even pigs running loose. In the grande salle, where beds for the sick were normally located, there was cow dung and urine all over the floor. Furthermore, on the beds that remained, the linen was only changed when it had rotted completely. The bureau decided that the animals should be expelled and the linen on the beds changed every three days.[8] This incident illustrates the problem of keeping order on hospital premises, in addition to the difficulty in obtaining and retaining responsible caretakers who could maintain discipline while simultaneously caring for the sick and poor. Similar problems had led Pontorson to place its hospital in the hands of the Brothers of Charity in 1644 and Malestroit to bring in the Sisters of St-Thomas de Villeneuve in 1666.

Needing more people to care for the sick and poor, the church radically changed its attitude towards women's congregations and eventually encouraged nuns to work in the hospitals and bureaux of the poor. This chapter discusses this turnabout and the new career opportunities that it opened up for seventeenth- and eighteenth-century women. It shows how new women's religious orders were created to deal with the needy and marginal members of society and how these orders reinforced the management, discipline, and treatments administered in the local hospitals of the kingdom.

Recent studies of early modern women's congregations by Elizabeth Rapley, Marguerite Vacher, and Colin Jones have analysed the long and difficult transformation during the seventeenth century of church attitudes towards nuns "working in the world."[9] Contrary to the arguments of many traditional church historians, it was not the Council of Trent that opened up new possibilities for women. In fact, in an attempt to eliminate scandal, a papal bull of 11 August 1566 dissolved all women's religious communities that did not observe the cloister, and the council fathers formally reiterated the obligation for nuns to follow this regulation. Bishops were ordered to impose cloister upon the nuns under their jurisdiction to keep them chaste in mind and body. No sister, once professed, was to be permitted to go out of her convent, "even for a brief period, under any pretext whatsoever," except with the permission of her bishop.[10]

Initially, there were attempts at greater liberality in the interpretation of these decrees, as when in 1582 Gregory XIII approved the establishment of the Ursulines, whose rules called for them to live in common under simple vows.[11] But by the early part of the seventeenth century, the council decisions were more rigorously enforced, and the Holy See even ordered the suppression in 1631 of one of the first women's teaching orders, the Institute of the English Ladies. Founded by Mary Ward in 1609, the Ladies were to teach the poor and carry out clandestine missionary work in their native England. Despite being accused of aspiring to do tasks reserved for men and of threatening the "natural order," Ward insisted that to carry out their mission, her nuns had to "work in the world" and could not be restricted to monasteries. However, in spite of the initial success and support for her order, the English Ladies were eventually ordered to be dissolved, and Mary Ward was arrested and imprisoned.[12]

The breakthrough in resistance to women's religious orders working in the world began with St Vincent de Paul and his attempts to use women to spread the new church message, especially to the marginal elements of society. Working from Monsieur Vincent's correspondence,

Elizabeth Rapley notes that in 1617, while he was pastor in Châtillon-les-Dombes near Lyon, he told his Sunday congregation that a family living some distance from the village was sick and in need of food. After mass he started out with "a worthy man, a bourgeois from the town," to visit the family; "on the road we found women going out ahead of us, and a little further on, others were coming back. And as it was summer and very hot, these good women were sitting along the side of the roads to rest and cool off. There were so many of them that you could have called them a procession."[13] Seeing the enthusiasm of the parish women to aid their neighbours in need, Monsieur Vincent noted in his journal, "God gave me the thought: could these good women not be brought together and persuaded to offer themselves to God to serve the sick poor? Afterwards, I showed them the way to handle these great necessities with great ease. At once they resolved to do it."[14]

Such women's initiatives became the core of the parish confraternities set up by Vincent de Paul's Lazarists and by most of the other missionary orders. Monsieur Vincent did not initially conceive of this as exclusively female work. As early as 1620, he set up a male bureau of charity, and the following year he encouraged men and women to work together; women were to continue their labours with the sick, while men were to be responsible for corrective action by trying to discipline those who were healthy but unable to care for themselves.[15] The men's charities rapidly dwindled, and the mixed approach never worked out because according to Monsieur Vincent: "Men and women do not get along together at all in matters of administration; the former want to take it over entirely and the latter will not allow it."[16] At the same time as men's participation in charities diminished and eventually collapsed, women's involvement increased significantly, and they eventually became the backbone of the bureaux.

The movement benefited from well-placed friends and patrons of Monsieur Vincent, such as his initial protector, Mme de Gondi, the daughter of Philippe-Emmanuel de Gondi, general of the Mediterranean galley fleet and a member of the family that held the archdiocese of Paris almost as a fiefdom from 1569 to 1660. Philippe-Emmanuel de Gondi was also the father of Cardinal de Retz, coadjutor to the archbishop of Paris from 1643 to 1654 and himself archbishop from 1654 to 1660. Monsieur Vincent's associate in the foundation of the Daughters of Charity, Louise de Marillac, was the niece of the chancellor and leader of the dévot party, Michel de Marillac, and she had been married to Antoine le Gras, *secrétaire des commandements* to Marie de Médicis. The search for funding and organization for Monsieur Vincent's poor-relief efforts was supervised by women related to some of the most important families in France: Mme de Miramion, Mme Villeneuve, Mme Goussault, Mme Foucquet, and the fabulously wealthy Duchesse d'Aiguillon.[17]

At the beginning, this group was essentially a lay organization, formed to provide aid to the poor and the sick. The important and influential women who had initiated the movement eventually became known as the Ladies of Charity (Dames de la Charité). To their ranks were added an increasingly large number of volunteers from among peasant or lower-class city women. The latter were normally uneducated and adapted with difficulty to the new challenges. This was the reason that in 1633 Louise de Marillac offered to take in several of the recruits to form and instruct them to become catechists, to treat the sick, and to aid the poor.[18] With the women of the elite supervising, peasant girls were to be trained to serve the poor and sick and to become the cornerstone of the Daughters of Charity (Filles de la Charité). From this point until the official foundation of the congregation in 1658, Louise de Marillac and Vincent de Paul struggled with the problem of how to create and obtain recognition for a women's religious community that would not be cloistered.

The process of creating the Daughters of Charity was slow and complex; it involved both the internal organization of the order and the external recognition of the women who became its members. Vincent de Paul proposed certain theoretical notions concerning the functioning of the community; however, they frequently had to be adjusted to the reality of their application. Such was the case with the respective roles of the rich and poor women involved in his charities. From the rules and regulations of the bureau of charity of Châtillon-les-Dombes, it is clear that his intention was that all members, rich and poor, should take turns preparing the food and visiting the sick, caring for their dietary needs, and instructing them in their faith. In the evolution of these bureaux, however, it became evident that they functioned best when the wealthiest women concentrated their activities on raising funds, while the poorer women did the work.[19] The same division of labour became associated with the community that eventually was constituted as a religious order. It was left to the Ladies of Charity to direct and manage the organization of the community and to recruit and educate the Daughters of Charity. Poor peasants and town or city women offered to carry out the essential work: the heavy manual labour and the menial chores associated with caring for the poor and sick.

A second factor in the evolution of the community was Vincent de Paul's determination that the women would work in the world and his struggle therefore to unite them within an order. A full-fledged order implied the recognition and protection of a bishop, adoption of a common rule, the taking of perpetual vows, and legal acceptance of the community that would give it the right to receive donations, gifts, and dowries signed over by the families of new nuns. However, Vincent de Paul could not go that far without confronting the problem of the cloister. He can be seen therefore as seeking to unite the women within a "near-order" that could be formally recognized. From 1634 on, they received their first rules – rising time, daily devotions, great silence, obedience. Louise de Marillac was the superior in the mother house; in every other house with more than one sister, a superior was to be appointed. Beginning in 1640 the sisters took vows, but Monsieur Vincent was very prudent about this step, making the community opt for private vows without witnesses, thereby getting around the canon-law provisions that associated vows with cloisters. On all these questions, Louise de Marillac and the sisters of the community continually pushed Monsieur Vincent to seek more explicit recognition of their status. By 1645 they had five houses, but he continued to define them as a simple confraternity, like the bureaux of charity where the sisters had, in fact, often been recruited.[20]

The community prospered, and by 1658 there were eight hundred members and sixty to seventy houses. The problem posed by this expansion, however, was that the order ran up against new ecclesiastical obstacles. To that point, all the new houses of the Daughters had been founded in the diocese of Paris, where the congregation had high-placed friends and protectors. The decrees of the Council of Trent had given each bishop responsibility for all the nuns in his diocese, and the corollary to this type of control was that it became impossible to ensure a centralized direction and common rules and regulations for a community that worked in the world and actually operated in several dioceses. Any one bishop could refuse to recognize orders coming from the nuns' mother house and simply order the Daughters of Charity to return to their cloister. It was at this point that Louise de Marillac intervened personally to assure the status of her nuns. At her request, the queen mother petitioned the pope to place the confraternity under the perpetual direction of its superior general. Rome eventually granted this request in 1655, thereby conferring on the confraternity what no women's religious congregation had previously achieved in France: centralized direction and a partial exemption from local episcopal control.[21]

The Daughters of Charity continued to expand throughout the Ancien Régime, so that they were associated at one time or another with nearly 400 institutions of charity, about 160 of them hospitals.[22] In addition to the large city institutions, such as the Hôpital-Général de Paris, they continued to serve in small hospitals and charitable establishments; Colin Jones has identified over half the hospitals with which they signed contracts as small-town or semi-rural establishments.[23] Once the Daughters of Charity had created a model for women's religious congregations to work in the world, other orders were founded to follow in their footsteps.

None of the eight local hospitals treated in this book signed contracts with the Daughters of Charity, but most of them brought in nuns to staff their institutions. As mentioned at the beginning of the chapter, Malestroit signed a contract with the Sisters of St-Thomas de Villeneuve in 1666. At St-Vallier, the Sisters of St-Joseph began serving in the town hospital in 1683. Lower down the Rhône valley, Grignan obtained the services of the Congregation of the Holy Sacrament in 1764 after failing to negotiate a contract with the Grey Nuns.[24] At Caudebec in 1726 the bureau engaged three nuns from the Rouen branch of the Filles de la Croix after the failure of an attempt to bring in the Sisters of Providence.[25] And finally, in 1778 Savenay gave the contract for its hospital to a group of local women who had organized themselves into a religious community to care for the institution's patients.[26] Seyne and Étoile continued the tradition of engaging older local women to serve in their hospitals.

The archives of most of the religious communities staffing these institutions suffered enormously during the Revolution: the orders themselves were suppressed, their houses shut down, and their documents confiscated. Sufficient material escaped destruction to permit a relatively thorough treatment of the congregations active in three of the eight hospitals under study: the Congregation of St-Thomas de Villeneuve, the Sisters of St-Joseph, and the Sisters of the Holy Sacrament. They are studied comparatively here in terms of the differing circumstances of their foundation, the internal functioning of their order, and their work in the hospitals they staffed.

Despite the fact that Vincent de Paul and Louise de Marillac had produced a clear model of the steps to take in creating a women's religious order that could work in the world, the foundation of each of the subsequent women's orders demonstrates a mixture of emulation and differentiation. In each case, the founder was a priest, more or less involved in spreading the message of the Catholic Reformation. The majority of these new orders placed overwhelming emphasis upon the role of the traditional "father figure," who, like St Vincent de Paul, was seen as organizing and recruiting the nuns, inspiring their rules and regulations, and laying the groundwork for the eventual recognition of their order. Under closer scrutiny, the role of these "founders" is frequently discovered to have been overemphasized in Catholic historiography, since the women who entered the orders played a much larger role in establishing their congregations than has often been believed. In fact, the founding father and the sisters whom he recruited did not always agree. During the period of establishment, there was always a certain tension over questions about rules and regulations for the community, a distinctive habit for the nuns, and the pronouncement of vows. While the founder's role in starting up the new communities was somewhat spontaneous, the nuns who joined the new orders rapidly became interested in assuring the permanence and continuity of their congregation.

Even before the three women's congregations that are studied here received their official recognition as a religious order, elements already existed as groups of devout women living in community and serving the poor and sick. Marguerite Vacher has shown that as early as 1646 some of the women who were to become the core of the Sisters of St-Joseph five years later had formed a community in Le Puy as a women's branch of the local Company of the Holy Sacrament.[27] Like others founded by the company, this community was bound to secrecy. Its rules and regulations were written by a Jesuit priest, Father Jean-Pierre Médaille, an administrator of the Collège de St-Flour, who was active in directing the Company of the Holy Sacrament. According to early texts, the goal of this initial community was to work in close liaison with the company to aid the poor; it was to intervene in cases brought to its attention by the company and to report back constantly on the results of its actions.[28] In 1644 the bishop of Le Puy, Henry de Maupas du Tour, an active supporter of the work of the company, had asked a group of "sisters" from this community to take over the direction of his Hôpital de Montferrand, and three years later Françoise Eyraud, one of the women who were to become members of the founding group of the Sisters of St-Joseph, was among those attached to the hospital.[29]

The research of Marguerite Vacher demonstrates that the embryo of the Sisters of St-Joseph existed at work in the community, with some members serving in the hospital at Le Puy, at least three to four years before 1651, when the six founding members of the congregation met with Father Médaille officially to begin the order. As the group expanded, it took in groups of women linked with the Company of the Holy Sacrament in other towns and parishes. At Chambon, for example, a community of women founded in 1650 by Gaspard de Capponi, a local nobleman associated with the company, seems to have been incorporated into the Sisters of St-Joseph eight years later.[30] The order, a veritable federation, appears to have been built up by bringing in such local groups and by founding new communities in towns where Jesuit missionaries linked with Father Médaille and the Company of the Holy Sacrament were particularly active.

The beginnings of the Sisters of St-Thomas de Villeneuve in Brittany can be traced to a similar group of local women who were working together before the official foundation of their order. The first three founding "mothers" were members of a charitable confraternity begun at Lamballe around 1650. Inspired by the model proposed by Monsieur Vincent, this confraternity grouped together the wives and daughters of local notables in order to carry out charitable works: visiting the homes of the poor, furnishing them financial and material aid, and taking care of the poor and sick in the hospital. The group was affiliated with the Third Order of St Augustine, and the local Augustinian monastery gave it spiritual direction.[31] Father Ange Le Proust, the Augustinian superior between 1658 and 1660, convinced four women from this group to join together to form a religious community specifically designed to serve the sick and the poor.

Arriving in Lamballe in 1652, Father Le Proust is said to have been influenced in his initiative by the canonization six years later of St Thomas of Villa Nova, a sixteenth-century Augustinian who had dedicated his life to the service to the poor.[32] It is also evident that he was inspired by the Daughters of Charity, for he offered the same reasons as Monsieur Vincent concerning the "religious" nature of the community. In an obituary for Father Le Proust in 1697, it was noted that he had founded what were initially known as the *Augustiniens hospitalières* "to care for the sick poor, with women's hearts and hands all consecrated to God and to his poor; they [the sisters] will live with them [the poor], leading a life similar to that of nuns, but without officially appearing as such."[33]

The four women selected were to take charge of the hospital of Lamballe. They signed a contract on 6 February 1661, a document referred to by Father Le Proust as the "act of foundation" for the order. The contract specified that the confraternity and the hospital were to unite their funds for the "service and assistance of the poor," that the confraternity would designate several of its members to live in the institution "without using either the revenues of the hospital or of the charity," that the four selected women were to be named sisters of charity in the institution, and that to carry out their mission, "[they] could recruit the girls whom they deem useful for service to the poor."[34] Among the four founding members of the order, one, Renée Lorans, Dame de Breil, was the daughter of an administrator of the Lamballe hospital, and she received the mandate to educate the girls to be added to the initial contingent.[35]

In the case of the Sisters of the Holy Sacrament in the Ardèche region, it was the women who took the initiative in proposing the foundation of the new order. The beginnings of the community can be traced to four women from villages surrounding Boucieu-le-Roi, the parish of a local missionary priest, Pierre Vigne. A member of a Lazarist group called the Missionary Society of Valence from the time of his ordination in 1694 until his death in 1714, Father Vigne spent his life on the road preaching to and evangelizing in out-of-the-way villages and former Huguenot strongholds along the Rhône valley and in the mountains of Dauphiné and Ardèche. His experience as a preacher led him to trans- form or at least dilute the austere and essentially urban doctrines of the Catholic Reformation, just as the Brittany missionary Father Le Maunoir had done. Vigne used objects of piety, such as the monumental thirty-nine Stations of the Cross that he constructed at Boucieu-le-Roi in 1712, to serve as an attraction for pilgrimages and for his evangelizing activities.[36]

Impressed by his approach, Marguerite de Nozière, Catherine Junique, Louise Bouveyron, and Jeanne Rouvère offered to accompany pilgrims along the route to the reconstituted Calvary and to serve as spiritual guides at the stations. To carry out this work, Marguerite de Nozière, who seems also to have been very well versed in the domestic arts, rented a house where she began teaching spinning, carding, and weaving to the village girls.[37] Catherine Junique came to live with her in 1714 and joined her enterprise "to teach the youth" of Boucieu.[38] Their work in hospitals with the sick and the poor was a later extension of their missionary conception, since catechizing was the initial purpose of the order and Father Vigne came to see the activity of these women as an extension of his missions and retreats. Clearly oriented around his concern to preach and promote devotion to the Stations of the Cross, the new group consisted of seven women in 1715 and was initially known as the Sisters of Calvary.[39]

As with the other new orders, fusions and regroupings of pre-existing women's communities marked the beginnings of the Sisters of the Holy Sacrament. As a result of the continuing parish visits and missions of Father Vigne, women's communities in neighbouring villages asked to be integrated into the new order. Rochepaule was one of the places where he had concentrated his activities. There in 1708, even before he had arrived in Boucieu, he had constructed three crosses to symbolize Calvary. When he returned to the village in 1715 to preach a mission, a group of local women had asked his help in forming a community and living under a common rule. By 1722, when the official document organizing the Congregation of the Holy Sacrament was prepared, the twelve sisters from Boucieu and the six from Rochepaule decided to live together under a common rule. The document founding the new order also specified that the group would welcome the adherence of two existing communities in Macheville and La Batie.[40]

The steps leading to the foundation of these orders reveal that everywhere in France the missionary activities of the Catholic Reformation and the promotion of aid to the poor and sick seem to have influenced women of all social classes to form small communities to aid those in need. The new religious orders often combined these pre-existing communities under common rules and regulations, as has been seen at Le Puy, Lamballe, and Boucieu-le-Roi. The lifestyles resulting from these new living conditions for women, neither in family units nor in cloistered communities, prompt the questions of exactly what type of woman was attracted to this new life and what were the reasons for their attraction.

The women who made up the communities eventually integrated into the new orders came from very diverse social origins. They did not only consist of the devout peasant women praised in the correspondence of St Vincent de Paul. Of the six sisters mentioned in the 1651 contract of association for the Sisters of St-Joseph, Françoise Eyraud, Claudia Chastel, and Marguerite Burdier came from families of the regional robe or bourgeois elite: solicitors, lawyers, or merchants. Anna Vey was apparently from a fairly well-to-do background, for her father promised the order a dowry of 125 livres, while Anna Brun was, it seems, an orphan, and Anna Chaleyer's origins are not mentioned. Half the group was composed of older women; Claudia Chastel was a widow who died four years after the formation of the order; Anna Chaleyer was forty-seven years old in 1651, and Françoise Eyraud forty. Among the younger recruits, Marguerite Burdier was probably twenty-five at the time of the contract of association, Anna Brun fifteen, and Anna Vey most likely a minor, for her contract alluded to permission from her father.[41] Of the initial group, only Claudia Chastel was able to read and write.[42]

Specific data are available about professions taken at the Vienne house of the Sisters of St-Joseph, and this information permits an overview of the demographic characteristics of the women who entered one of the most active houses of the congregation during the Ancien Régime. Like the founding sisters, most of the eighty women who joined the Vienne house between 1681 and 1792 were relatively old: the average age of entry was twenty-six, one of the youngest recruits being Claudine Jacquin an eighteen-year-old from Lyon. For the fifty nuns whose records indicate such details, fifty-nine was the average age at death. A good percentage of the nuns died relatively young – several thirty, thirty-three, and thirty-five – and of the fifty sisters who can be traced, only twenty-three lived beyond sixty-six. As could be expected, the vast majority of these women came from Vienne or outlying regions, such as the Lyonnais, Le Puy, Forêt, or Vivarais. The exceptions were two who came from Sisteron and one each from Franche-Comté and Avignon. Most of these novices spent their years of training at the Vienne hospital, although some also frequented the houses and hospitals of St-Vallier, Condrieu, and Lyon.[43]

Unlike the disparate group that founded the Sisters of St-Joseph, the four founding sisters of the Congregation of St-Thomas de Villeneuve in 1661 were from more homogeneous backgrounds. All of them were far removed from the image of the young peasant woman. Gillette le Bohu de la Pommeraye was of minor noble extraction, while her friend and collaborator in the beginnings of the community, Renée Laurans du Breuil, was the daughter of an important notary in Lamballe and a magistrate and administrator of the hospital. The third "founder," Anne Le Maignan du Canton, was also the daughter of a Lamballe notary who had served as first consul of the town and administrator of its hospital. The fourth woman was Jacquemine Gueheneuc, about whom little is known and who, furthermore, did not remain part of the community. She returned to her home, but nevertheless continued to support and aid her former colleagues.[44] The strikingly elitist profile of the founding nuns of the congregation was reinforced by the early recruits, who were daughters of local nobles, parlementaires, lawyers, notaries, and regional dignitaries.

In 1698 the congregation began accepting peasant girls into its ranks, and just as in the case of the Ladies and Daughters of Charity, it made a fundamental distinction in its membership between "mothers" – the women from the elite society – and the "sisters": lower-ranking lay nuns (*sœurs converses*), a new category for peasant girls. In addition to the absence of peasant girls among the founding members of what was originally called the charitable confraternity of Lamballe, few of the women founders were particularly young in 1661. Anne Le Maignan was twenty-seven, and she died nineteen years later in 1680. If the ages of the others are not known, it can be assumed that they were even older, for both Renée Laurans du Breuil and Gillette le Bohu de la Pommeraye died in 1669, only eight years after entering the community.[45]

The archives of the Sisters of St-Thomas contain no registers of professions or entries into the order; instead, they retained death records for their nuns. This practice, common to many religious congregations, came from a tradition of sending short statements announcing the death of a nun to the other houses of a community.[46] The notices sometimes included a short account of the life and the qualities of the deceased (*nécrologies*); resumés of the notices were also sometimes entered into the *annales*, or chronological accounts of the major events affecting each house. For the Sisters of St-Thomas, the death notices preserved are more succinct than is often the case, and they rarely indicate the age or birth date of the deceased. More important was the profession, the date on which each woman became a nun, and in rare cases, the notice mentions her birthplace, her status, for example, as a widow, and the positions that she occupied in the order. The dates of their profession as nuns are available for twenty-four of the first fifty women who died as members of the order. This information shows that the period of service was very short for the initial women recruited. The first fifty nuns died between 1668 and 1708. The twenty-four of them for whom statistics can be calculated lived an average of only twelve and a half years after taking their vows. However, this average is actually lengthened by four nuns who served the order twenty-four, twenty-seven, thirty, and thirty-nine years because the median period of service for these nuns was only eight years.[47]

Why did the early Sisters of St-Thomas have such short life spans? There are two possible answers. First, they may have died unusually young because of the illnesses and contagious diseases to which they were exposed in their work with the sick and poor. It is obvious from the death notices that certain years – periods of widespread epidemics – were more devastating than others. In 1669 and 1670, shortly after the foundation of the order, six nuns died during an outbreak of dysentery.[48] The other factor to be considered is the age of the women. Just as with the Sisters of St-Joseph and the founders of the Sisters of St-Thomas, recruits into the order were probably not very young. While we do not have any overall data on their ages, a 1790 listing of sisters in the Paris houses of the order indicates that, as with the nuns in the Vienne convent of the Sisters of St-Joseph, there were few young recruits. The Paris list was drawn up by Mother Walsh at the request of the Revolutionary authorities. For the eighty-four nuns, lay nuns, and novices included, the average age was 47.7, and even if the mother house, where many of the older and more sickly nuns were cared for, is removed from the list, the average age for those active in the Paris region still remains as high as 45.3. Nevertheless, the novices listed were always in their 20s, leading us to believe that the pattern observed for the early members of these communities, recruiting among spinsters and widows, seems to have continued throughout the Ancien Régime.

The social origins of the founding nuns of the Congregation of the Holy Sacrament corresponded more closely to Monsieur Vincent's category of peasant women. Marguerite de Nozière, the first to offer her services to Father Vigne, was from that background. However, soon after she had been joined by Catherine Junique, she abandoned community life. The group who came to constitute the founding nuns formed around Catherine Junique, Louise Bouveyron, and Jeanne Rouvère. According to an early unpublished history of the order written by Sister Antoinette Ponthier, Father Vigne's niece, the three initial sisters "rented a house to begin to live together … practising all the virtues known to women of their sex, prayer being their most all-encompassing occupation."[49] The group was joined almost immediately by four widows, Marie Spéliat, Marguerite Rouveure, Marie Bost, and Jeanne Lalaye, but Rouveure dropped out before the widows took their vows.[50] All the members of this initial group seem to have come from peasant backgrounds. None of them brought money in the dowries turned over to the order: Louise Bouveyron arrived with a spinning wheel, and Marie Spéliat, the daughter of a carpenter, brought with her a cow and eggs.[51] The parents of Marie Forite, a later recruit, promised yearly contributions of three *setiers* of rye (1.8 hectolitres), ten pounds of butter, and a monetary contribution of 5 livres, and one of the wealthiest later recruits, Sister St-Joseph Gay, who entered the order in 1736 as a minor, was to inherit 1,000 livres at her majority.[52]

As was the case in the other orders, the majority of the six initial sisters were not apparently very young: we know that the widow Marie Spéliat was fifty at the time of her vows, but in the absence of parish registers, the ages of her colleagues cannot be determined. The notarized documents indicate only that all the women were "free and emancipated," indicating that there were no minors among them.[53] The congregation archives contain a register of the nuns' professions indicating the dates of their vows, generally including those for their deaths, but rarely noting their birth dates. If we can base any conclusions upon their short span of service in the order, these notices again tend to confirm that few of the new recruits were very young: Louise Bouveyron died after only four years in the order, Jeanne Rouvère after three years, Marie Spéliat after six years, and only Marie Junique, Catherine's younger sister, who entered the congregation late in 1722, lived as long as forty-six years after becoming a nun.[54]

As with the other orders examined, the Sisters of the Holy Sacrament do not possess documents giving complete data on their nuns. There is an incomplete listing of 132 sisters detailing the dates of their religious profession and a document that contains spotty dates of birth and death. More interesting is a collection of forty-three wills left by nuns who entered the congregation between 1723 and 1788. While obviously constituting no more than a random sample of the women who joined, it does indicate that the average age of recruits in the sample was 25 and their median age 27.7. The ages at which they died changed little between the 1730s and the 1780s, with the youngest nun, Marie Roselie Descour, having been received in 1775 at 18 and the oldest, Ursule Eynard, having taken her vows in 1728 at 62 years of age.

The demographic profile of the women who joined these three orders reveals both similarities and striking contrasts with the recruits to the cloistered communities examined recently by Elizabeth Rapley.[55] In analysing the death notices of the teaching congregations of the Ursulines and the Congrégation de Notre-Dame, Professor Rapley demonstrated that girls from "noble" or "honourable" families tended to have their futures decided when they were much younger, since their families planned strategies for maintaining or enhancing their social position. Because the dowry attached to entering a religious order was less onerous than that required for a good marriage, placing younger daughters in

these orders at an early age became common: 572 out of the 776 presti-
gious "choir" nuns joined the communities in question between the ages
of fourteen and twenty.[56] On the other hand, the girls who became lay
sisters in the two orders tended to come from more modest backgrounds,
and for their parents the dowry necessary for admission represented a
considerable sum of money. For this reason, the lay sisters tended to
enter the Ursulines and the Congrégation de Notre-Dame much later:
66 per cent of the 80 lay sisters in the study were admitted between
twenty-one and thirty.[57]

The profile of the nuns who joined the Sisters of St-Joseph, the Sisters
of the Holy Sacrament, or the Congregation of St-Thomas clearly
resembled the itinerary of the lay nuns described by Elizabeth Rapley.
The hospital work assigned to these women was closer to the menial
tasks carried out by lay nuns than the more exalted positions held by the
choir nuns of the cloistered orders. This fact is demonstrated by correspondence between Mother Dunoyer, the superior of the St-Vallier
house, and Sisters Madelaine Servant and Catherine du Faure towards
the mid-seventeenth century. The superior refused to keep the young
postulates, for she noted that they were weak and unable to carry out
the chores demanded of a nun.[58]

Other differences between the women who joined the congregations
working with the sick and poor and the cloistered teaching orders revolve
around the reasons for their entry into religious life. Elizabeth Rapley
uses death notices to identify several different routes followed by these
women. These documents, of course, were aimed at influencing new
recruits; specific mention was made of the vocational motivation of the
nuns, as it was noted that they came from devout families with uncles
as priests and aunts as nuns. Furthermore, following their placement in
convent boarding schools, they were said to have been influenced by
their teachers. The documents also underline the cases of girls so convinced of their vocation that they refused to accept their parents' designs
for their futures.[59] While we can suspect a certain amount of propaganda
in these descriptions, other, more down-to-earth reasons for entry can
also be gleaned from the documents. There were, for example, health
reasons; Elizabeth Rapley shows that 14 per cent of the 856 nuns in her
sample were described as "sickly." In other cases, women seem to have
joined in order to escape strained family situations or recover from
broken love affairs. Finally, there were the forced vocations, cases where
parents placed rebellious girls in the communities to break their "tor-
tured" spirits.[60]

Although some of the women entering the communities that were working in the world may have corresponded to the "sickly" recruits in the cloistered orders, the overwhelming majority of them were much older than the postulants for the cloister, and they probably did not reflect the spontaneous, naive motives of the younger women. One suspects that the sisters working with the sick and poor had joined their orders either out of personal conviction or because, as older, unmarried women or widows, they saw the congregation as a haven of security.

From the very beginning of each of these orders, widows were among the earliest candidates for admission. In the case of the Sisters of the Holy Sacrament, Pierre Vigne hesitated to accept the four widows who asked to be admitted in 1714, and his reluctance was not unique. The church attitude towards widows was decidedly ambivalent: women entering into religious life were seen as "dying to the outside world." They were to cut all ties with family, friends, and worldly possessions and to consecrate themselves entirely to God. Within this context, widows were looked on with suspicion since they often left children behind and they remained involved with the inheritance to be passed on to their offspring. Some of the newer orders had confronted and resolved this problem: the Ursulines had accepted widows, and the Baronne de Chantal, co-founder with François de Sales of the Visitation nuns, was herself a widow. Of course, Monsieur Vincent's argument that his Daughters of Charity was not, strictly speaking, a religious order certainly removed some of the ecclesiastical arguments against widows, and the founding fathers of each of the three orders examined here took great pains to avoid having "his" congregation identified as a fully recognized religious order.

The attraction of widows and older women towards these new orders was certainly a result of their interest in the movements of piety promoted by the Catholic Reformation and in the links made between piety and service to the poor and sick.[61] Besides this spiritual attraction, however, the new orders offered clear material security to older single women who had difficulty fitting into traditional family structures or the monastic tradition. Historical demographers have always emphasized the fragile position of widows in early modern European society. With the disappearance of their husbands, these women lost their major source of revenue, and often, being burdened with young children, their chances of a second marriage were limited.[62] Contrary to popular belief, their older children frequently refused to take them in, and Jacques Dupâquier has argued that the chances of widows or older women finding mates declined dramatically in the eighteenth century, when there was a disproportionately larger number of women than of men.[63] Perceived as burdens to their families, these women often finished their lives interned in one of the disappearing local hospitals, rejected by kin and community. The new religious communities offered not just security to them, but also the possibility of occupying a position of responsibility and often a certain social status.[64]

Traditional historiography has always placed great emphasis upon the primary role of men, the "father founders," in starting these new women's orders, yet the women who were involved in setting them up were not entirely absent from the decision-making process. Far more than the father founders, they seemed to have been preoccupied with ensuring the continuity of the communities that they had entered. The father founders are often seen as the source of the communities' organization, constitution, and rules and regulations, but upon close examination, it is evident that the women who became members of the new communities were often the ones who prodded their founders to produce the structures necessary for the new orders, and in some cases they themselves took the initiative in seeking official approval for their communities.

Like Louise de Marillac, the nuns of all three congregations under discussion constantly encouraged the priests who were responsible for them to seek more official status for their groups. Father Ange Le Proust was named visitor to the Sisters of St-Thomas de Villeneuve in 1662, but he was always reluctant to obtain permanent, official recognition for the nuns. This approval seems to have come more through the connections of the nuns and their relatives with church and crown power structures. The order had always remained closely tied to the royal court and the provincial elites. From the very beginning, the position of *procuratrice générale* and one of the directors of the community had been given to Mme Rouxel de Thierry de St-Brieuc, a woman chosen outside the ranks of the congregation. In this nomination the Sisters of St-Thomas followed the practice of the Daughters of Charity, who had also named an outsider as one of their directors, giving her the task of representing them in civil suits and in administrative matters.[65] They thus preserved the often-false idea that the sisters, as women consecrated to God, did not become involved in material and administrative affairs. In 1671, through the intercession of their procuratrice, the Sisters of St-Thomas obtained recognition from the queen mother, Anne of Austria, for their order and particularly for the contract of 12 January 1669 containing the statutes and regulations of the community and the clause recognizing Lamballe as its mother house.

These important links with provincial and crown officials were again evident in 1697 when the new procuratrice, Hélène de Vaulavie, Dame de la Bois de la Roche, sought royal permission to move the mother house of the Sisters of St-Thomas to Paris; she pointed out that the nuns served in over twenty-five hospitals in different provinces and under the authority of different parlements, and she declared that "the mother house is not located in a place of easy communication ... and secondly, its distance ruins both the economy of the order and the health of the nuns, who are obliged to pay considerable sums of money and undertake long trips [to communicate with their superiors]."[66] In the new structure of the order, the mother house in Paris, with its annex in Vaugirard, was to preside over a seminary in Beauce and houses in Charantain and Normandy. Provincial houses were recognized in Rennes for Brittany and in Loudun for Poitou, Anjou, and Berry. According to a recent study by Claude Langlois, this move, supported and encouraged by Father Le Proust, entrenched the Sisters of St-Thomas in the circles of royal favour and marked the movement of the order towards the lucrative field of teaching women of the elite and running convent schools in addition to maintaining their hospital involvement.[67] The congregation histories all present this change as having been initiated by Father Le Proust, although the new field of the sisters was far from the goal of working with the poorest and most desolate elements of the population that the same literature identifies as his original mission for the order.[68]

With the move to Paris and the new orientation towards convent schools, the order was on its way to becoming one of the twenty-five richest women's congregations in France in the period after the Revolution.[69] By the time of the Revolution, the three provinces of the Sisters of St-Thomas de Villeneuve had thirty houses, but the exact composition of only the Paris institutions is known. The mother house on rue des Sèves was occupied by 24 nuns, 9 lay sisters, and 4 novices; the convent school at St-Germain-en-Laye included 7 nuns and 3 lay sisters; and the convent school for poor girls at rue de Sèves contained 6 nuns, 8 lay sisters, and 2 novices. The five other Paris houses were smaller, lodging from 3 to 9 nuns and lay sisters.[70] The 84 nuns in the diocese of Paris probably represented an important segment of the order, for according to the annals left by the nuns in each community, most of the local houses of the order seem to have been made up of 3 to 5 sisters; in addition to the provincial houses in Rennes and Loudun, they possessed twenty-eight local houses in Brittany, Normandy, and Poitou (see

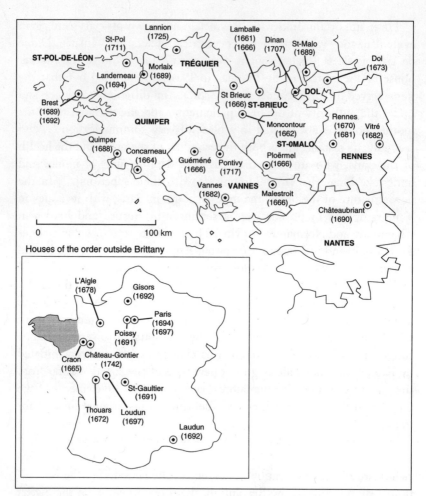

Map 8   Foundations of the Sisters of St-Thomas de Villeneuve in Brittany before 1789

Map 8), representing possibly another 100 to 160 nuns, bringing the total to around 220.

The Sisters of St-Joseph were a very different type of organization. The order was essentially a federation, a patchwork of communities, often with their own rules and regulations and without centralized direction. Father Médaille had conceived of "his" nuns as a community of communities without a mother superior. He had not in any way sought to limit the control of local bishops over the order as had Louise de Marillac when she pursued a centralized organization for the Daughters of Charity or as had the procuratrice of the Sisters of St-Thomas when in 1671 she persuaded Anne of Austria to obtain crown recognition for the centralized structures of her order.[71] Marguerite Vacher has argued that the early statutes and regulations of the Sisters of St-Joseph were actually inspired by Jesuit structures, but it is clear that such was not the case, for the hierarchical organization – the local bishop together with the superior of each house – constituted a shared source of authority.

At the time, this decentralized structure seems to have pleased ecclesiastical authorities, who enthusiastically called for the creation of new houses of the Sisters of St-Joseph. In the dioceses of the region, during the first twelve years of their existence, the sisters set up over twenty houses: sixteen in the diocese of Le Puy, three in the diocese of Vienne, one in Lyon, and one in Clermont.[72] Vienne became one of the most dynamic elements of the order. Bishop Henri de Villars brought the sisters from Le Puy to work in the Vienne hospital in 1668, and Mother Marguerite Burdier, one of the six "founding" nuns, was sent to set up the new house. Under her leadership, eight new convents were opened in the diocese, including St-Vallier, and outside the diocese, Vienne was responsible for founding the house at Gap in 1671, Sisteron in 1688, Grenoble in 1694, and Lyon in 1696, all of them serving local hospitals (see Map 9).[73] By the end of the Ancien Régime there were more than fifty houses in the diocese of Le Puy and about thirty in each of the dioceses of Clermont and Lyon, while Vienne counted about twenty (see Map 10).

The decentralized organization of the order constituted both an advantage and a disadvantage. Although it was a formula favoured by ecclesiastical authorities, it posed problems as more and more houses were founded and the nuns came to require more developed structures. Eleven years after the establishment of the order, in the absence of a mother superior and in the face of differing interpretations by the bishops under whom the order was operating, there seems to have been a problem ensuring uniformity. A conference was held in 1661 at which the affiliated houses were divided into districts, with certain urban communities being given responsibility over the more rural convents. At the same time, habits were adopted to distinguish different nuns, novices, and associates in the order.[74]

The loose framework of the Sisters of St-Joseph had to be regularly adapted to the new situations posed by the spectacular expansion of the order. In the initial conception of Father Médaille, his sisters were merely a step beyond a women's confraternity and adhered to the structures and

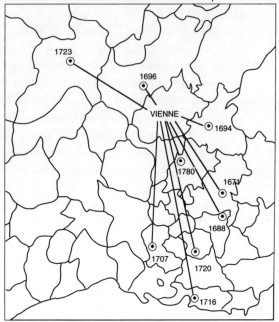

Extensions of the Vienne house of the Sisters of St-Joseph into other dioceses

1723
1696
VIENNE
1694
1780
1671
1688
1707
1720
1716

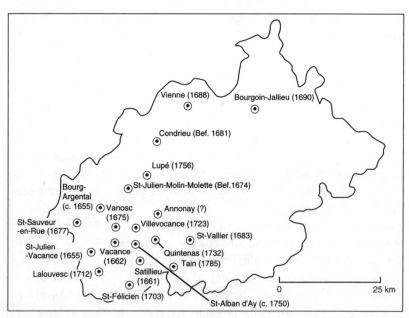

Vienne (1688)
Bourgoin-Jallieu (1690)
Condrieu (Bef. 1681)
Lupé (1756)
St-Julien-Molin-Molette (Bef.1674)
Bourg-Argental (c. 1655)
Vanosc (1675)
Annonay (?)
St-Sauveur-en-Rue (1677)
Villevocance (1723)
St-Vallier (1683)
St-Julien-Vacance (1655)
Vacance (1662)
Quintenas (1732)
Lalouvesc (1712)
Tain (1785)
Satillieu (1661)
St-Félicien (1703)
St-Alban d'Ay (c. 1750)

0   25 km

Map 9   Foundations of the Sisters of St-Joseph in the diocese of Vienne, 1668–1785

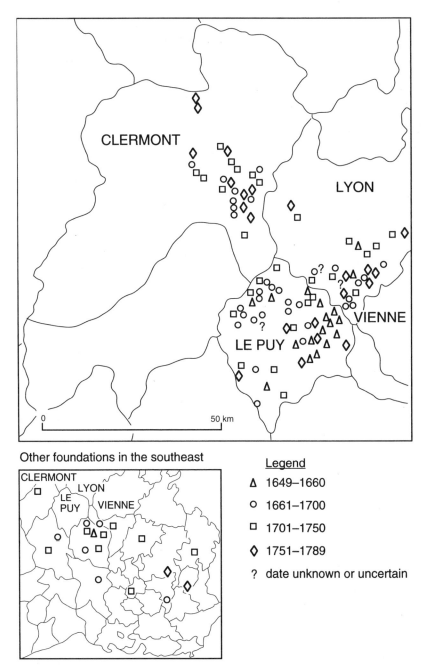

CLERMONT

LYON

VIENNE

LE PUY

0   50 km

Other foundations in the southeast

CLERMONT
LYON
LE PUY   VIENNE

Legend

△ 1649–1660

○ 1661–1700

□ 1701–1750

◇ 1751–1789

? date unknown or uncertain

Map 10   Foundations of the Sisters of St-Joseph in the dioceses of Clermont, Lyon, and Le Puy during the seventeenth and eighteenth centuries, in addition to houses founded in Vienne

preoccupations of the Company of the Holy Sacrament, but did not claim to be a full-fledged order. As the number of houses grew, the nuns and superiors of the order required a more structured framework and better legal protection for the holdings that the order began to accumulate. These attempts to improve the organization of the order took place without any fundamental revision of the decentralized structure and without any apparent move to create a central administration responsible for all the houses. Certainly, the decentralized structure had its merits, and Claude Langlois, treating the rapid expansion of the Sisters of St-Joseph in the post-Revolutionary period, argues that it was precisely their decentralized status that best protected them from the excesses of the Revolution, placing them closer to the local towns and villages that supplied the community with important new recruits and material resources.[75]

The Sisters of the Holy Sacrament were profoundly influenced by the experience of the Sisters of St-Joseph. Despite the fact that Father Vigne's nuns were more centralized, having a mother superior from the very beginning, the practices of the nuns from Boucieu were often inspired by the Sisters of St-Joseph. In her early history of the order, Antoinette Ponthier noted that their habits were copied from the Lyon sisters and that Father Vigne adopted the idea of organizing his nuns as a legal "association," avoiding reference to their status as an order and imitating the formula used by Father Médaille.

Just as in the other orders, the women who actually joined the Sisters of the Holy Sacrament were the ones who pressured Father Vigne to make the necessary contacts and to seek their official recognition. According to Antoinette Ponthier's account, Marie Spéliat, a fifty-year-old physically handicapped widow who joined the other sisters in 1722, was the first to encourage him to give them statutes and rules to guide their community life, and Father Vigne noted in his journal that he visited the Sisters of St-Joseph in Lyon to get a copy of their statutes.[76] In 1721, when he was still hesitant to seek official recognition for their order, Louise Bouveyron, the first superior of the congregation, had written to Jean de Catellan, bishop of Valence, to request recognition. The bishop replied evasively, asking the sisters to continue to "observe their rules" and to "faithfully carry out all that Father Vigne asks of you."[77] He seems to have remained unconvinced that recognition was necessary; indeed, the congregation was not recognized for another thirty years.[78]

Just as the sisters played a major role in encouraging Father Vigne to seek recognition for their order and give them rules and regulations, so their independence is shown in another major initiative of the sisters – a decision that seems to have gone against the directives of their "father founder." The nuns, under the leadership of Antoinette Ponthier, third superior of the order and Father Vigne's niece, purchased the luxurious Château de Boucieu for their mother house. With this acquisition, a community founded to serve and catechize the poorest peasants was established in the splendour of the local chateau. The sums involved in the purchase left the sisters with a considerable debt. Father Vigne was in the last years of his life when the acquisition was made, and there is no indication of his reaction to his niece's decision. Nevertheless, general criticism of the transaction led Antoinette Ponthier to leave the order shortly after.[79]

There was a major evolution in the activities of the order when, in 1737, in addition to continuing to teach poor girls, the nuns agreed to care for the sick in the hospital at Die. This time it is clear that Father Vigne consented to the change. The first signs of the new role to be given to the nuns had come in 1731 when he noted in his journal that a rich woman had left the order a legacy under the condition that the nuns continue to respect their rules and lifestyle and that they become involved in treating the sick.[80] He added that the châtelain and other local notables had indicated to him that they were ready to turn over the hospital to the sisters. Written during Vigne's mission in Pont-en-Royans, this passage probably refers to discussions with the local directors of the Die hospital, which was the first to be placed in the hands of the sisters. They subsequently accepted service in the Grignan hospital in 1764, at Nyons in 1773, at Buis-les-Baronnies in 1773, and at the Hôpital-Général in Valence in 1787.

The Sisters of the Holy Sacrament always remained a much smaller and more modest congregation than the other two treated here. At the time of Pierre Vigne's death in 1740, they had eighteen houses concentrated in the Ardèche region of the diocese of Valence and scattered communities in the Vivarais, the Valentinois, and the Diois. By the end of the Ancien Régime, the order, officially recognized by royal letters patent in 1787, controlled a network of thirty-nine houses active in teaching and in hospital service (see Map 11). The number of members of the congregation is difficult to determine. In 1730 Antoinette Ponthier wrote to one of the order's patrons that there were eleven nuns in the mother house training sisters to be sent to fourteen different parishes.[81] Félix Vernet, historian for the order, notes that by 1740 they were three to a house, and he estimates that there were almost a hundred nuns in

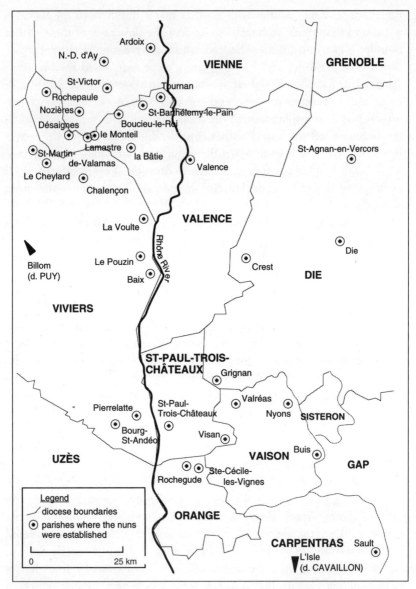

Map II   Foundations of the Sisters of the Holy Sacrament in the southeast before 1789

the congregation.[82] It is clearly incorrect to argue that with fourteen houses having three nuns each, the order could have consisted of a hundred nuns. It is more probable that by the 1770s to 1780s, when the order had increased to thirty-nine houses, the sisters could have approached a hundred. We do know from a 1790 list of members of the congregation that there were sixty-three nuns in the order at the beginning of the Revolution, but then too the results of the "dechristianization" movement in the latter part of the eighteenth century may have reduced the number of sisters.[83] It is clear that they were a local order made up of women of more modest backgrounds than either the Sisters of St-Thomas or those of St-Joseph.

What was the effect of these new orders on the hospitals in the areas that they served? To what extent did they transform services to the sick and the poor? First, it is clear that their experiences varied. The hospital at Pontorson, which was under the complete control of the Brothers of Charity, demonstrated the most radical change. According to the 1644 contract under which the brothers took charge of the hospital, they were obliged to continue the tradition of "lodging poor itinerants [*passants*] for only one night unless they were sick." As in larger establishments, the brothers began physically to separate this group from the sick to prevent the spread of infectious diseases. By 1656 the "pauvre passants" were lodged in a room reserved for them in a separate house facing the hospital.[84] In 1665, when the new hospital was completed, itinerants were placed in the old building. Men and women were accepted without discrimination, and despite the presence of a caretaker, the brothers argued in 1739 that mixing the sexes had regularly led to abuse of their hospitality.[85] This situation, together with a general disapproval of roving itinerants, appears to have led hospital officials progressively to reduce access to them: the four straw mattresses available to this group in 1665 were reduced to three in 1693 and to two in 1720.[86]

Separating the long-integrated functions of the hospital, "caring for the sick and service to the poor," the brothers at Pontorson concentrated more upon improving the treatment of the ailing and the injured. The registers of admissions to the hospital, available for the period from 1665 to 1781, stand in stark contrast to the summary documents that exist for the other institutions studied. These registers give the dates of admission, names, ages, parents' names, towns or villages and dioceses of origin, and clothing taken in charge by the institution, as well as a summary diagnosis of the injury or sickness for which the patients were to be treated. In the margins, the deaths or dates of release are entered, along with notes concerning any relapses that might have occasioned further hospitalizations.[87]

These registers shed considerable light upon the debate over the state of hospital services to the sick during the Ancien Régime. Certainly, hospitals have not been well treated by the traditional historiography dealing with the period. Diderot, a contemporary, transposed the case of the Hôtel-Dieu in Paris to the other institutions of the kingdom when he wrote his entry on the "Hôtel-Dieu" in the *Encyclopédie*: "three, four, five or six [patients] often share the same bed; the living are placed beside the dying and the dead; the putrid air breathed out by this multitude of sick bodies infects each other with the germs of their respective diseases; and the spectacle of the pain and the agony is offered and received on all sides. That is the hôtel-Dieu."[88]

In discussing the mentally ill during the great confinement movement, Michel Foucault has selectively used examples from the Hôpital-Général or the Salpêtrière in Paris to confirm and even go beyond many of the contemporary assessments of the "horrors" of hospitalization. He uses reports such as those of Jacques Tenin or Coguel in the late eighteenth century to stigmatize the hopitaux-généraux as virtual prisons where the mentally ill, along with the sick, the vagabonds, and their children, were crowded into dirty, smelly, and unhealthy quarters, often chained to iron bars and subjected to torture and forced labour.[89] Jean Meuvret also reflected the contemporary accounts of hospital horrors when he argued that death rates in these institutions far exceeded those of society in general and that in 1740–41 over 15,000 died in the Paris Hôtel-Dieu alone.[90] These authors contributed to what Colin Jones has called "the black legend" concerning eighteenth-century hospital conditions.

The registers for the entry and discharge of patients at the Caudebec hospital show that it is incorrect to generalize about hospital conditions and death rates based upon Paris examples. At Caudebec, death rates even dropped in the course of the eighteenth century: out of 1,338 sick and poor admitted to the hospital between 1725 and 1754, 9.8 per cent died in the period from 1725 to 1734, 10.8 per cent between 1735 and 1744, and 7.1 per cent from 1745 to 1754.[91] At Pontorson, too, registers permit the death rate to be calculated for certain years, and again it was surprisingly low. Even in 1676, the year of a dysentery outbreak, only 13 patients died out of the 97 admitted. Ten of the 13 had been diagnosed with dysentery, and they represented about a third (10 out of 27) of the patients admitted with the disease. Of the others taken in, 15 had been injured in accidents and 32 suffered from high fevers.[92] Neither of these hospitals confirm the exceedingly pessimistic vision of Ancien Régime institutions.

It is true that at Pontorson, Grenoble, the Hôpital de la Charité in Paris, and elsewhere, the hospitals directed by the Brothers of Charity were well ahead of most French institutions in their treatment of the sick. Upon their acquisition of Pontorson in 1644, the brothers had set up a small pharmacy in the common room that served both as a kitchen and as a library. In the new buildings for the hospital, completed in 1649, there was an infirmary containing six beds, a pharmacy, a refectory, and a kitchen on the first floor, and on the second was the prior's room, a dormitory for five brothers, a separate infirmary for the brothers, and a chapel.[93] The existence of the pharmacy demonstrates the interest of the brothers in producing remedies to treat the sick. While there are no indications of the specific nature of these *drogues*, we do know that the Brothers of Charity provided training for pharmacists at their Hôpital de la Charité in Paris and that from 1661 on, young apprentices in pharmacy were sent to Pontorson.[94]

Pontorson was also a training ground for apprentices in surgery. They too generally began their practice at the Hôpital de la Charité in Paris. That institution had an enviable reputation for its surgical innovations. Operations to remove kidney and liver stones (*taille*) were specialties of the brothers, and at La Charité they claimed to have carried out 1,310 such operations between 1701 and 1724, with only 308 deaths.[95] At Pontorson, too, the removal of stones was one of the principal operations: between 1716 and 1721, 35 such procedures were carried out, 28 of them on children, with only 8 deaths resulting from the surgery.[96]

The success of the brothers in these operations and in attracting students (*garçons chirurgiens*) to their school of surgery at La Charité eventually drew the criticism and opposition of the master surgeons of Paris. The brothers claimed to have the right to practise surgery in virtue of letters patent dating from September 1699. This right was first challenged in 1715 by the Order of Surgeons of Paris, who claimed that only they had the right to practise surgery and to accredit surgeons. The case went before the Parlement, where Brother Maximin violently denounced the incompetence of the Paris surgeons, noting that one of them, Guérin, had performed 84 operations since 1710 and that 72 of his patients had died, 7 had had limbs amputated, and only 5 had fully recovered. In contrast, according to Brother Maximin, the patients of La Charité had been admirably treated and the mortality rate was very low.

The final decision, pronounced by the lieutenant of police on 3 December 1715, maintained the right of the brothers to continue practising surgery. The surgeons, however, appealed the ruling, and on 31 September 1721 the brothers were ordered to call in an accredited surgeon for operations, and letters patent issued in September 1724 forbade them to perform operations.[97] Appealing this decision in 1758, the Brothers obtained certain concessions three years later giving their prior the right to select his chief surgeon and permitting the brothers to take courses in surgery and, in cases of necessity, to operate on patients.[98] This controversy and the restrictions placed on operations in Paris had little effect on Pontorson, where the brothers' right to practise medicine was never challenged.[99] In other local hospitals, including Montmorillon in Poitou, surgeons such as the Augustinian friar Jean Rozet practised medicine, performed operations, and prescribed such treatments as the use of cinchona for purgations and opium as a soporific, both of which were innovative for the early eighteenth century.[100]

The experience of the women's orders in the field of hospital service was decidedly more limited. To begin with, they never took over the direction of an institution as was the case with the Brothers of Charity. Nuns were not to come in contact with the "worldly" aspects of hospital work such as administration or accounting. In all the contracts signed, the different orders of nuns were always to work under the authority of the hospital directors or the recteurs of the poor. As is made evident in the contract between the Sisters of St-Thomas de Villeneuve cited at the beginning of this chapter, the responsibilities of the nuns were established by the bureau of the hospital. The order was paid to furnish sisters to care for the poor and the sick according to the directives of the hospital administration. At the same time, however, the nuns had a certain leverage since the demand for their services was great; hospital directors had to be careful not to alienate their nuns, for it was not always easy to obtain the services of another order.

This situation clearly imposed limits upon the capacity of hospital administrators to dictate their agendas to religious congregations, a fact that was especially evident at Caudebec. In 1719 the directors of the hospital proposed that Mme de la Marc, a local woman, be made responsible for the production of wool in the workshop, and at the same time, they hoped to obtain a nun to be placed in charge of the spiritual instruction of the sick and poor and of the overall discipline of patients and inmates.[101] That same year the bureau signed a short-lived contract with the Sisters of Providence from Rouen, and on the 28 April the order sent Sister Bullée to serve in Caudebec. Five years later, on 22 September 1724, she appears to have been recalled; the administrators noted that Mme de la Marc was aging, and they announced that they had written to Mme de la Coudraye, superior of the Hôpital-Général of Rouen, and to Mme d'Ambray, superior of another Rouen community, to try to obtain nuns to serve the hospital.[102] This time it was clear that the administrators wanted more than one nun, and when Mme d'Ambray offered three sisters, the hospital accepted. However, the three women who arrived were hardly able to cope with the responsibilities of the institution. The hospital deliberations note that the superior was ill when she arrived and that she died in the hospital shortly thereafter; as well, her two assistants immediately fell ill with malignant fevers and were recalled. One nun was sent to replace the initial three, and in response to the directors' protests, Mme d'Ambray replied that she would be just as happy if they found another order to take charge of the institution, which contained over one hundred poor and sick patients.

It was in this context that the directors returned to Mme de la Coudraye, and on 25 November 1725 signed a contract with her Filles de la Croix agreeing to pay her 100 livres a year for two sisters.[103] These contracts and the sums of money that the nuns demanded for their services were the sources of frequent disputes. In effect, Caudebec cancelled its contract with the Filles de la Croix in 1772, hoping to find an order that was less expensive. On 29 July the directors wrote to Mme de Ruffell, first assistant of the superior general of the Sisters of St-Thomas de Villeneuve, and to Mme de Rosemboir, superior of the hospital at Le Havre, asking them to supply nuns for the hospital.[104] They received negative replies from both the orders contacted, and they were finally obliged to renegotiate their agreement with the Filles de la Croix in 1774.[105]

There were several different approaches to the contract negotiations between the different congregations and the hospitals. Mme de la Coudraye's Filles de la Croix signed an open contract with the directors of the Caudebec hospital by which they agreed to serve the institution in return for the payment of 50 livres a year for each nun.[106] The same type of contract linked the Sisters of St-Joseph with the hospital at St-Vallier, where the order received 150 livres for each nun. In the case of the Sisters of the Holy Sacrament, who were brought to the Grignan hospital, each of the two sisters received 250 livres a year.[107] The financial aspects of these agreements closely resembled the hiring practices of hospital directors who had brought in local caretakers and administrators

Table 6

Contracts negotiated with hospital directors by the Sisters of St-Thomas

Date	Place	Type of institution	Staff		Lodging furnished	Food furnished	Wages¹	To be responsible for			To supervise work for poor	Contagious illnesses excluded
			Demoiselles	Sisters				Nursing	Teaching	Work		
1661	Lamballe	hôtel-Dieu			•	•		•				
1662	Moncontour	hospital			•	•		•				
1664	Concarneau	hospital		1	•	•	5 s/day	•				•
1665	Craon	hospital	2		•			•		•		
1666	Lamballe	hôpital-général	2		•	•	4 s/day	•				•
1666	Malestroit	hospital	2	1	•		4 s/day	•		•		•
1666	Ploërmel	hospital	2	1	•		4 s/day	•				•
1666	St-Brieuc	hospital	3	1			4 s/day	•		•		•
1669	Moncontour	hôpital-général	1	1				•				
1672	Thouars	hospital	2	1				•				
1673	Dol	hospital	2	1	•	•	4 s/day	•				
1673	Buzançais	hospital	2		•	•		•	•	•	•	
1681	Rennes	hôpital-général	2	1	•	•	50 l/year	•		•		
1682	Rennes	hospital	2	1	•	•	50 l/year	•		•		
1682	Vitré	hospital	2	1	•	•		•				
1688	Quimper	hospital	2	1	•	•		•		•		
1689	Morlaix	hospital	2	1	•	•		•		•		
1689	St-Malo	hospital	1	1	•	•		•		•		
1690	Chateaubriant	hospital	1	1						•		
1692	Gisors	hospital	2	1						•	•	
1692	Loudun	hospital		2			60 l/year					
1693	Dol (renewal)	hospital					60 l/year					
1694	Landerneau	hospital	2	1	•	•		•		•	•	
1735	St-Méen	hospital	1	2	•	•	50 l/year	•		•		

¹ s = sous; l = livres.

before turning to religious congregations. Savenay, Étoile, and Seyne continued to function using local women: Savenay paid Damoiselles Rose-Marie Alezeron, Jeanne Bouron, and Jeanne Allain 50 livres a year;[108] Étoile hired Mlle Borne in 1768 for 30 livres a year;[109] and in Seyne, Mlle Anne Daniel received 18 livres a year between 1758 and 1782.[110]

It is clear that it was often far more expensive for the hospitals to bring in religious orders rather than rely on local women. Nonetheless, the nuns were able to ask for such remuneration since they possessed training in the care of the sick and some experience in hospital administration. At the same time, the shortage of nuns to carry out hospital work probably explains the important discrepancies between the amounts paid to the different orders and notably the 500 livres a year that Grignan had to promise to obtain two nuns from the Sisters of the Holy Sacrament.

A totally different legal approach to internal hospital administration came with the rigorously defined contracts that the Daughters of Charity of St Vincent de Paul introduced and which were used by most of the other orders. These documents show the dynamism of hospital orders and illustrate the various fields of responsibility accorded to nuns working in eighteenth-century hospitals. Colin Jones has analysed the contracts for 161 provincial hospitals and 4 Parisian institutions controlled by the Daughters of Charity. They show who brought the nuns to the institution, the type of hospital, what the directors had agreed to supply to the nuns, how many nuns were to be provided, and what their responsibilities were.[111] For the Sisters of St-Thomas, a similar series of contracts has been conserved, and I have analysed 27 of them in comparison with the data available for the Daughters of Charity (see Table 6). As to the communities served, almost half the hospitals attended to by the Daughters of Charity were situated in small or medium-sized towns (40.4 per cent), the majority of their nuns were placed in the hôtels-Dieu or medically oriented institutions (43.6 per cent), and only 16 per cent worked in the hôpitaux-généraux or charitable institutions frequented primarily by the able-bodied poor.[112]

Likewise, out of the 27 contracts analysed for the Sisters of St-Thomas, the vast majority were signed with small and medium-sized towns; only Rennes was an exception.[113] In addition, most of the agreements were concluded with institutions that took care of both the sick and the poor, for the sisters staffed only three hôpitaux-généraux: in Rennes, Lamballe, and Moncontour. In the majority of these contracts, the nuns were responsible both for administering care (soins) to the sick and for overseeing workshops to occupy the poor and teach them skills (*travaux*). Only in the Hôpital-Général de Rennes were the nuns exclusively concerned with organizing work for the poor, while in Buzançais they administered care and catechized children, and in Concarneau, Dol, Lamballe, Malestroit, Moncontour, St-Brieuc, and Thouars, they were exclusively responsible for treating the sick.

As could be expected, the number of nuns supplied to these institutions by the Sisters of St-Thomas was far smaller than the staff sent to the hospitals controlled by the Daughters of Charity. The Daughters generally sent three or four sisters to their hospitals and two or three nuns to their hospices or smaller institutions.[114] The Sisters of St-Thomas, however, rarely assigned more than one nun, accompanied by one, two, or three demoiselles, who were generally lay nuns or novices. As Colin Jones has argued, the question of the payment of these sisters was a constant preoccupation of the hospital directors, who tried to keep remunerations as low as possible. In the case of habits or uniforms for the Daughters of Charity, the directors often cut back on the initial offers. At Angers, where in 1640 the congregation had negotiated for the hospital to pay for the nuns' habits, the directors had changed this practice by the 1670s, giving them a set stipend to buy and keep up their own clothes.

The same type of negotiation marked the questions of residence and meals for the Daughters of Charity. Although they were almost universally lodged in the institution, there was frequently a question as to whether separate, closed-off quarters should be provided. As for meals, while the initial contracts in the 1670s specified that the nuns would be fed, later agreements stipulated that the 60 to 80 livres allotted for each sister should be used to pay for her meals.[115] The same type of debate occurred for the Sisters of St-Thomas. With ten exceptions, the contracts specified that the nuns be lodged by the hospital direction. At Malestroit it was stated that "they will have use of the houses and the large garden of the hospital, and an inventory of the premises will be carried out by the sisters to evaluate the holdings."[116]

The stipulation that meals be provided was even rarer. Ten contracts did not mention meals, and of the remaining seventeen, three specifically stated that they were not to be provided. In eight hospitals the directors agreed to feed and house the servants working in the institution. It was clear that for the Sisters of St-Thomas, just as for the Daughters of Charity, the negotiations for all these "fringe benefits" became more difficult as they asked hospital directors for larger annual fees.

The annual payments made to religious communities for their sisters varied considerably, and even the terms were not standard. The early contracts of the Daughters of Charity with Montpellier in 1668 specified a payment of 40 livres for each nun, while the 1670 contract with Pithiviers asked for 25 livres, and the 1671 Montluçon agreement was for 36 livres.[117] The documents signed with the Sisters of St-Thomas were even more diverse. First, the payments negotiated varied considerably. The earlier contracts with Concarneau (1664), Lamballe (1666), Malestroit (1666), Ploërmel (1666), St-Brieuc (1666), and Dol (1673) were all negotiated on the basis of daily payments. The sisters received 4 or, in the case of Concarneau, 5 sous for each day of service. The congregation replaced this type of clause in the 1681 contract with Rennes, when they asked for 50 livres a year for each nun, a tariff base similar to that received by the Daughters of Charity. At Loudun (1692) and at Dol (1693), just as was the case with the Daughters of Charity, the Sisters of St-Thomas sought for increases in this annual payment to 60 livres per nun.

The principal contribution of the Sisters of St-Thomas and the other smaller orders was to extend the techniques of hospital organization pioneered by the Daughters of Charity to the province of Brittany and more particularly to smaller towns and outlying areas. At the same time, the services of these nuns were considerably more expensive for the directors than the more traditional solution of hiring local caretakers and servants. Why then did they bring in these new orders? A few of the preambles to the hospital contracts give a partial explanation. That of Malestroit mentions specifically that the inhabitants of the town were "influenced by the dilapidated state [*mauvais état*] of the hospital and the need to procure better care [*soins*] for the sick and to eliminate the disorder caused by the beggars and itinerants who are sheltered there."[118] In the contract with Moncontour, the hospital buildings ("in ruins") were transferred to the sisters, and it was specified that they could erect a new building "at their expense."[119] The same context had been evident at Lamballe in 1661 when the bishop of St-Brieuc asked Father Le Proust "to oversee a reorganization of the Hôtel-Dieu."[120] As is evident in all the contracts, the management and organizational skills, as well as the political contacts, of the nuns were clearly recognized by hospital directors.

An example of the nuns' approach to hospital organization is furnished by a report submitted to the directors of the Caudebec hospital on 17 June 1725. The institution was negotiating with the Filles de la

Croix from Rouen for the services of two nuns, and the order sent one of its representatives to inspect the buildings and premises. At their meeting the directors discussed the different recommendations that the nuns had made, all of which are perfect illustrations of the types of reorganization carried out by the nuns in the hospitals they served.

The first concerned the poor who were lodged in the institution. It stipulated that the two sexes be separated, that the poor should have individual beds rather than being placed two to a bed, and that to that end, twenty new beds should be built by a carpenter and blankets acquired for them. The second recommendation concerned cleanliness in the institution. The nuns' report began by noting that "cleanliness is a basic requirement for health," and it indicated that the unsanitary conditions observed in the hospital contributed to communicating disease. The sick should no longer be placed two by two in beds, and it would be useful to use wet lime to whitewash the kitchen, the refectory, and the dormitories, where the walls were partly composed of earth, and to pave the two small rooms near the entrance, one to become a receiving parlour and the other the nuns' refectory.

Finally, concerning meals, the report asked that the directors furnish a *quateron* of meat (22 livres) each day, a quantity that would be sufficient to feed the three sisters, the servants, and eighty poor and sick inmates. From this meat, broths would be prepared for the sick, resulting in reduced expenses. Soups would be prepared with peas, beans, and other vegetables, which would have to be purchased in order to feed inmates on the days when meat would not be served. The report noted that, in any case, "soup was better sustenance and more likely to maintain the poor in shape for work." After discussing this report, the hospital directors ordered that its recommendations be carried out.[121]

As is clear from the Caudebec report, the nuns' contribution was primarily in the field of organization and the application of fundamental sanitary principles to the often-neglected small-town hospitals. Despite the fact that, unlike the Brothers of Charity, the nuns were not a threat to any of the groups involved in the hospitals, their integration often resulted in friction. Everywhere the members of the hospital board were drawn from the ranks of doctors, surgeons, pharmacists, and priests as well as other local notables. Even before the nuns arrived on the scene, there was frequent feuding between these groups, and after their arrival the sisters were often caught in the middle. Such was the case at Caudebec, where the powerful pharmacist Louis-Philippe Falloppe was often at odds with the doctors. In July 1719, three months after her arrival in Caudebec, Sister Bullée of the Sisters of Providence in Rouen became embroiled in one of these controversies. Doctor Le Brunent, who had been named several years before to serve as surgeon to patients in the hospital, was opposed by Falloppe.[122] Le Brunent had furnished several "drogues" to the patients he treated, and Falloppe had subsequently insulted the surgeon, challenging his right to sell remedies to the institution. The administrators decreed that in the future neither Le Brunent nor Falloppe could enter the hospital without the permission of Sister Bullée.[123]

More frequent were the conflicts between the nuns and the directors of the hospital; almost all these feuds revolved around financial considerations. At Caudebec in 1729 the board contested the arrival of an additional nun and two servants over and above the number that they had approved five years earlier. They argued that the additional stipends required to pay the new arrivals would have to be deducted from the money for the poor, and such expense would be prejudicial to the very people whom the institution was created to serve.[124] Similar financial disputes occurred elsewhere. At St-Vallier in 1724 the directors noted that the sisters had been taking up collections in the parish that amounted to close to 600 livres a year and that they were not reporting this revenue to the bureau.[125] Seven years later the directors refused to pay the funeral expenses of the late Sister Porchas, informing the superior of the community, Sister Molle, that the family of the deceased should pay the bill.[126]

At Malestroit, problems arose between the directors and the Sisters of St-Thomas from 1715 on, when every meeting of the board was confronted with the financial problems of the institution. That year, as the conflicting interests between town and seigneurie continued to divide community support for the hospital, the meeting noted that the income from house and property rentals had declined as a result of the devaluation of the currency, that there were repairs to be made to the houses and buildings owned by the institution, that the revenue from the annual *papegault*, or shooting competition, was not being paid, and that the hospital buildings were deteriorating.[127] In this context, the Sisters of St-Thomas submitted a proposal to the directors noting that they wanted to increase the capacity of the institution and the number of nuns attached to it. They asked for permission to construct a new building near the old hospital at their own expense to enable them to house the new nuns who would be needed. Meeting very infrequently, the board procrastinated, forwarding the request to the mother superior of the order and to the Baron de Malestroit, who, they felt, should grant permission. However, they reserved for themselves the right to the final decision: "we will see what should be done in the best interests of the poor."[128] The relative indifference of the directors to the nuns' request and the continuing financial difficulties of the institution seem to have convinced the order to withdraw from the institution. By 1721 there was only one nun working in the hospital, yet the board did not meet even once. By July Anne Dubois, mother superior of the order, directed the remaining nun, Sister Rose du Bignon, to leave Malestroit. The directors, having no replacement, refused to let her go; not until April 1723 did they finally agree, thus acknowledging that the 1666 contract with the Sisters of St-Thomas had become nul and void.[129]

It is clear that the principal services of the nuns in these small, local hospitals were to restore order and authority, to adopt new and strict sanitary standards, and to oversee the "nursing" function of healing the sick and caring for the poor. Jean-Pierre Gutton has shown that their main contribution to hospital services during the eighteenth century was to initiate "bedside treatment" for their patients. Rather than bringing new medical skills to the hospitals, the women's orders introduced an approach that emphasized individualized treatment for the inmates. They had been taught to see the sick and poor as representations of Jesus Christ and to treat them accordingly. This attitude explains their insistence upon individual beds, the new sanitary regulations for wards, the appearance of registers for prescriptions given to the sick and for special diets, and the charts attached to each bed on which the patient's progress was indicated.[130]

Closely linked to the nuns' conception of their role in caring for and healing the sick was the widespread adoption in the hospitals of medicinal plants from the herb gardens that became a characteristic of the new orders.[131] The sisters sent out by these communities rarely had any advanced medical training, but they drew lessons from the traditional use of these plants and herbs by monasteries and men's hospitaller orders. The hospitals under their direction seem to have applied what François Lebrun described as "empirical medicine" or local remedies, usually made from herbs.[132] In the contracts signed with most hospitals, the sisters were provided, as in Malestroit, with land for a garden. A part of these gardens was always devoted to the production of herbs as remedies for the sick. This fact is clear in the contract between the Dol hospital and the Sisters of St-Thomas, in which a herb garden "for treating the poor of the hospital" is specifically mentioned.[133] At St-Vallier in 1697 the

Sisters of St-Joseph were given "a small garden to raise pharmaceutical plants."[134] Colin Jones notes that from the seventeenth century onwards the Daughters of Charity had become versed in herbal treatments for their patients and that by the early 1700s each of their houses was equipped with a copy of Mme Foucquet's folkloric compilation of remedies, the *Recueil de remèdes charitables*.[135]

At the same time, the proximity of the nuns to their patients and the conviction that they dispensed remedies to treat the sick often made them sceptical of the new types of medicine introduced during the Enlightenment. Colin Jones has shown how the Sisters of Charity often stood up to Enlightenment doctors, who were anxious to gain freer access to bedside observation and medical examinations of the sick. The nuns regularly rejected the use of apprentice surgeons to treat those who were ill as part of their training, the dissection of corpses to advance clinical knowledge, and doctors' criticism of certain types of hospital food, which they argued were not adapted to the patients' needs.[136] The sisters' close individual contact with patients led them to defend the rights of the sick and the poor against what they saw as exaggerated intrusions and experiments of eighteenth-century physicians and surgeons. In addition to their role in reorganizing the structure and improving the sanitary conditions of the hospitals in which they served, they came to have a say in the preparation of remedies and the care of the sick, even to the point of intervening in the applications of new medical treatments.

The changes in church attitudes towards women working in the world had opened the floodgates for the integration of thousands of women into the organization, administration, and healing process of the small, local hospitals of France. From the small communities of women grouped around the Company of the Holy Sacrament and other dévot organizations, the new women's congregations were born. Made up to a great extent of older women and widows, the orders bore the mark of their experience in organization, the application of empirical treatments to the sick, the use of herbal remedies, and attempts to ensure the permanence of their order. These new groups accepted contracts with the thousands of small hospitals serving the sick, the poor, and the marginal social groups of seventeenth- and eighteenth-century France. Many of these institutions, such as Moncontour, taken over by the Sisters of St-Thomas in 1661, were little more than ruins, and it was up to the nuns and the local communities to raise funds, renovate buildings, reorganize services, and improve the treatments accorded to patients.

Most of the time, town notables collaborated in these enterprises, although in some places, such as Malestroit, conflicts and the indifference of local leaders to the needs of the sick and poor eventually led the nuns to abandon the institutions. The new women's orders improved the physical installations, the internal organization, the morale, and to some extent the medical treatment offered by small, local hospitals that otherwise would have been candidates for closure and expropriation. They transformed the manner in which the sick and the poor were treated and the ways in which small and large hospitals functioned.

6 The State and Hospital Reform in the Eighteenth Century: New Direction or Continued Improvisation?

On 10 December 1774 the directors of the Caudebec hospital received a letter from the subdélégué in the town asking for information about the institution as part of a general inquiry into charity launched by Controller General Turgot. The directors named their colleagues Gueret and Falloppe to collaborate with hospital administrators in replying to the questions posed.[1] In the documents published from the replies sent to the intendant from all the hospitals in the généralité, the Caudebec data indicate that the St-Julien hospital had been founded in 1200, that its charter and founding documents no longer existed, that the institution concentrated on the "soulagement des pauvres malades," and that its patrimony and *rentes* produced annual revenues of 2,025 livres, 11 sous, 5 deniers.[2]

The 1774 inquiry to which Caudebec contributed was one of the major elements in a series of reports, discussions, and debates that took place within eighteenth-century French society over the role of hospitals and the responsibility of the state in reforming them. Muriel Jeorger has identified nine of these "national" inquiries launched between 1721 and 1789 to obtain information on health services, poor relief, aid to abandoned children and the elderly, and the physical state of hospital buildings and related facilities.[3] Most of these calls for information were directly related to crown projects to intervene in one of the areas of hospital responsibility.

Two distinct tendencies can be observed in these efforts at intervention. The letters, requests for information, and inquiries of the years 1721–74 reflect mainly financial preoccupations. They sought to collect information on the budgetary situation of hospitals with the eventual goal of using their facilities. All the inquiries were launched in connection with crown attempts to arrest beggars and vagabonds and to ensure that there were financially stable institutions to contain them. For this reason, the questionnaires asked about the revenues of each institution, details on the management of their budgets, the possibilities of "uniting" hospitals to form larger, more stable establishments, and finally the possibility of placing more importance on local relief.[4]

The second tendency that can be identified was the attempt, after the Turgot inquiry in 1774, to place greater emphasis upon specializing assistance by segregating those who were sick and were to be directed towards more medically oriented institutions from those who were poor and were to be "reformed" through work projects. The requests for information by Controller General Necker in 1778 sought specific data on the population of each city, town, or village, the number and types of hospitals, the number of beds, how many poor there were in the institutions on 1 January 1776 and how many were received in the course of that year, and the total number who died in the institutions in 1776. Controller General Calonne in 1785 concentrated his request for information more specifically on the hospitals "established for the sick."[5] All these interventions were directly linked to crown attempts to prepare laws better to deal with separating the sick from the poor and to regulate areas of hospital jurisdiction.

Historians have long debated the question of state attempts to carry out reforms of public welfare during the eighteenth century. Camille Bloch, in his 1908 book *L'assistance et l'état en France à la veille de la Révolution*, argued that in the last century of the Ancien Régime, legislation was enacted and structures adopted to create a system of public welfare that was passed on to and transformed by the Revolutionary governments.[6] In effect, he tried to demonstrate that the ideas proposed by crown officials from the middle of the eighteenth century on had been influenced by debates among writers, officials, and statesmen influenced by Enlightenment ideas. Bloch noted that after the failure of the 1724 crackdown on vagabonds and beggars and an abortive attempt in 1750 to reintroduce measures for the internment of beggars in the hôpitaux-généraux, crown projects sought new and more direct ways to control hospitals. From 1764 on, discussions tended to propose that royal authority over these institutions be reinforced to correct what were perceived as errors in the management and objectives of public charity, and for Bloch, this perception "legitimized the more and more marked interventions of the state in the administration of charity."[7]

One of the first concrete measures that he cited to prove such crown intervention was a piece of legislation dealing with vagabonds, proposed in 1764 by a new controller general, Charles-Clément-François de Laverdy. The eventual law ordered that beggars and vagabonds be shut up in new institutions, the *dépôts de mendicité*, and that the sick and crippled poor be sent to hospitals. It cited the failure of traditional hospitals adequately to carry out the 1724 provisions to intern beggars and noted that this was one of the reasons for the creation of the dépôts. The legal framework for these new institutions was eventually approved in 1767, and eighty-eight of them were set up under the direct control of intendants. Somewhere between a prison and a workhouse, the dépôts depended for their operation upon the initiative of the intendant who was in charge.[8] The legislation also confronted the problem of preventing vagabondage by stipulating that local charity should be reinforced to deter the poor from migrating to towns and cities in search of handouts. To that end, it directed that bureaux of charity be set up in each locality.

The second major intervention noted by Bloch also came from a new controller general, Anne-Robert-Jacques Turgot, Baron de l'Aulne, who was appointed by Louis XVI. In 1774 he undertook a broad-based review of the measures relating to mendacity and in particular to the work of the dépôts. Bloch has seen this administration as representing a turning point in the welfare philosophy of the Ancien Régime.[9] The essential features of the policy were articulated around three major elements. The first was the holding of a conference on welfare relief to bring together the most important proponents of new solutions to the problem. The second element was the preparation of a report on possible new orientations for welfare, a project that Turgot confided to Lomélie de Brienne, archbishop of Toulouse. Thirdly, the new controller general ordered an inquiry into local facilities available throughout the kingdom for dealing with the sick and the poor. It was the reply to this inquiry that the directors of the hospital at Caudebec had discussed at their December 1774 meeting.

Turgot was not in power long enough for his initiatives to produce new legislation, and Bloch's principal interpretation of his plan comes from a series of letters written by Turgot to intendants after his nomination as controller general. In these documents he was generally hostile

to the dépôts, arguing that they differed little from the type of internment organized in 1724. They were overcrowded and underfunded, rarely
organizing their inmates into the work detachments that he and most
physiocrats saw as the ideal means to inculcate a work ethic in the poor.
This opinion led him to order the closing of all dépôts in 1775 and, in
the face of public outcries, to reverse himself and reopen a selected
number a year later.[10] In place of large institutions of incarceration,
whether they were hôpitaux-généraux, dépôts de mendicité, or the medically oriented hôtels-Dieu, Bloch argued that Turgot favoured a more
local approach to charity.

Just as Laverdy had done in 1764, Turgot emphasized the need for an
efficient, organized structure of local bureaux of charity. Bloch notes that
this solution was clear in the 1751 article on "Foundations" that Turgot
wrote for Diderot and d'Alembert's *Encyclopédie*, and he argues that it
constituted the basis of the new policy that the controller general would
have implemented. The bureaux would have been responsible for taxing
local residents, with part of the money collected going to aid the poor;
they would then supervise the distribution of the remaining funds to the
sick, the mentally and physically handicapped, and the aged residents
who could no longer work. Ideally, these persons were to receive aid in
their homes or in those of local residents, who would be paid to care
for them. Turgot's entry argued that the able-bodied poor should not
be helped since such alms distributions only made them lazy, confirming
them in their vagabondage. Instead, the bureaux should see that they
were organized into work detachments with quasi-military discipline.
These detachments, or *ateliers*, should be set up in each province to build
roads or carry out public projects such as canals. The wages that the
poor earned by their work should, furthermore, enable them to support
themselves and their families.[11]

The third major innovation that Bloch saw as comprising the "system"
of Ancien Régime welfare was instituted during Necker's term as con-
trollor general. Coming to power in 1777, he was more critical than
Turgot of the underlying economic situations that produced poverty. For
the physiocrat Turgot, if the market forces were sufficiently liberalized,
enough jobs would be created to eliminate poverty. Necker, on the other
hand, felt that the social and hierarchical organization of the kingdom
was such that even if the poor worked a full year, once their taxes and
gabelle payments were deducted, they generally would not make enough
money to pay for their needs and those of their families. Despite that
premise, Necker's solutions were not much different from those of

Turgot, and he also saw the necessity for a decentralization of welfare structures. Shortly after coming to power, he proposed to abolish begging. An ordinance issued on 27 June 1777 directed beggars to return to their places of birth and the sick, crippled, and elderly who could not work to be sent to the hospitals. The others should be employed. To enforce this legislation the dépôts de mendicité were reopened and intendants ordered to arrest and intern all beggars, including those with certificates or passports giving them permission to beg.[12]

This legislation in 1777 led to the re-establishment of dépôts de mendicité for the arrested beggars and the creation of bureaux of charity to help those who returned to their native towns and villages. But for Bloch, Necker's essential contribution to this new "policy" was the creation of a series of model institutions that he hoped others would emulate. He set up a model dépôt at Soissons, near Paris, where internees were put to work polishing glass, weaving, knitting, and producing clothes. For their work they received wages that were turned over to them at their release. At the same time, a model bureau of charity was set up at Châteauroux in 1778. Organized by Mme Necker, this establishment drew up a list of local families to be helped, indicating the type of aid to be furnished: monetary aid, food, clothing, or medication. The bureau organized lessons to teach spinning to poor girls, orphans, and illegitimate children, and it set up a special committee to defend the poor before justice officials. Finally, with the help of municipal officials, ateliers were created to put the able-bodied poor to work on local projects.[13]

Necker's other major initiative in welfare reform was what Bloch saw as his effort to modify hospital organization. On 17 August 1777, Necker created a commission to study the problem. In his writings on welfare reform, the new controller general agreed with the eighteenth-century diagnosis of the large urban hospitals. He saw them as obstinately opposing any attempts to reform their functioning and as maintaining the poor in their laziness. The new commission was to study the overcrowding at the Hôtel-Dieu in Paris, but its conclusions extended beyond that specific problem. On 22 July 1778, after having debated whether to move the hospital or to divide its services, the commissioners recommended that an extension be built, but in the meantime that the number of patients in the Hôtel-Dieu be reduced. The institution was no longer to be obliged to accept the sick sent from the Hôpital-Général, and the latter institution was to acquire an infirmary to treat its own sick inmates. Smaller parish hospitals were also to be set up on the model of an institution established by Mme Necker in the parish of St-Sulpice-et-Gros-Caillou. It contained 120 beds with only one patient per bed. The wards were well aired and the service efficient; copper instruments were introduced to prevent the spread of germs; and a well-stocked pharmacy was set up. A doctor, surgeon general, apprentice surgeon, and twelve Sisters of Charity were attached to the institution; they served patients in their homes as well as in the hospital. A study of the functioning of the new institution between 1779 and 1785 revealed that its mortality rate was around 10 per cent, far below the 20 per cent recorded at the same period for the large Paris hospitals. At the same time, the cost of treatment never exceeded 17 sous 7 deniers per patient per day and more often it fluctuated around 16 sous 18 deniers, compared to about 20 sous per patient at the Hôtel-Dieu.[14] This approach, aimed at creating smaller hospitals to relieve the overcrowding at the large Paris institutions, became an integral part of the new crown rhetoric on welfare reform.

A second element in the hospital reform undertaken by Necker tried to address the financial problems of many of these institutions. He obtained the adoption of an edict in 1780 to treat hospital debts, which stipulated that institutions should reduce their services to correspond to their revenues. More important, it allowed indebted hospitals to sell real estate holdings in order to pay their debts, after which any surplus funds would be placed in the royal *caisse des domaines*, a national fund that would compensate poorer institutions with the surpluses of the richer ones and assure all of them a guaranteed annual revenue. In the original proposal for the edict, indebted hospitals would have been obliged to carry out the measures described, and this regulation would have given the crown a foothold in the management of hospital funds. Nevertheless, Bloch saw even the watered-down version of this edict as "the most important piece of older legislation concerning hospitals."[15]

Camille Bloch interpreted this series of interventions as constituting the basis of a crown policy in the field of welfare, but more recent historians are far more sceptical. Olwen Hufton, in a 1974 study of the poor in eighteenth-century France, was very critical of Bloch's approach. She admitted that his book was the "most powerful product" of a school of thought contending that social welfare was present even before the introduction of socialist approaches, but she accused Bloch and his contemporaries of producing work "of a decidedly partisan nature which fed on Enlightenment propaganda."[16] For her part, Hufton decided to concentrate upon the poor, the makeshift economy upon which they depended, and the totally inadequate social measures taken to alleviate their physical and financial difficulties. Reviewing the hôpitaux-généraux, the bureaux of charity, village poor relief, and the grants accorded by the central government, she demonstrated the huge gap between the needs of the poor and the modest aid that they received. She carried out her analysis using the periodic studies of local poor relief made under the controllers general of the Ancien Régime and by the Comité de Mendicité set up after the Revolution.

Based on these studies and on research into the internal workings of welfare institutions, Hufton showed the contradictions, inadequate conception, and functional difficulties of the major elements of what Bloch had seen as a policy of social assistance. Examining the dépôts de mendicité, she noted that the intendants' revenues, which were supposed to finance these institutions, were never sufficient and that coordination was often inadequate between the maréchaussée, who arrested vagabonds, and the curés, who were to certify their non-residence. The wrong people were frequently interned because of the difficulty of distinguishing between seasonal workers and vagabonds.[17] Illness and epidemics were rampant in the overcrowded, rundown facilities, and of the 71,760 vagabonds on record as having been arrested up to 1773, 13,899 died in the dépôts in the course of their three-to-six-month sentences.[18] Finally, as for organizing their internees into work detachments, the dépôts did not have a much better record than the hôpitaux-généraux. Because of errors in the initial arrests, the dépôts were full of sick and physically and mentally handicapped internees who should have been sent to hospitals and who were incapable of work. For those who could work, the results were not much better. In 1773 the task of providing employment and supplies for the dépôts was placed in the hands of a single company, Manie, Rimberge et Cie, which agreed to clothe and feed the internees at the daily rate of 6 sous per person and provide work for them. The company was rapidly disillusioned in its hopes of making money by selling the products of the internees' labour, and instead the directors turned to the idea of making profits by cutting back on services and care. Food was rationed, soap and clothing for the inmates became rare, and riots broke out in the dépôts.[19]

What Bloch had seen as Turgot's contributions fared no better under the critical eye of Olwen Hufton. Turgot attacked the large institutions such as the hôpitaux-généraux and the dépôts, arguing that local charitable initiatives organized around revitalized bureaux of charity provided more efficient services to the poor and cost considerably less to operate.

Table 7
Funds available for village poor relief in 1774 (in livres)

Diocese	Number of parishes reporting	Parishes, bureaux, or hospitals distributing relief				
		100+	50–99	1–49	0	unspecified
Rouen	343	55	24	46	215	3
Rennes	172	43	15	29	80	9
Mende	75	14	3	11	33	14
Clermont	86	1		3	57	25[1]
Montpellier	98	12	7	27	49	5

[1] Nineteen parishes of the diocese of Clermont possessed hospitals or bureaux of charity, but only one, Riom, specified its revenues.

Hufton noted, however, that in their replies to the commissioners appointed by him in 1774, towns and villages, including Caudebec, stated that they had only limited resources. In fact, the great majority of the villages and parishes that replied to the inquiries had absolutely no funds with which to distribute local aid (see Table 7).[20]

The bureaux of charity in which Turgot placed such confidence were unevenly distributed throughout the country. They had been founded in waves of charitable initiatives. Vincent de Paul and his successors had concentrated on the region around Paris and the northeastern part of the kingdom. The Jesuit fathers Chaurand, Dunod, and Guevarre had worked in the dioceses of Normandy, Brittany, Dauphiné, Provence, and Franche-Comté, and Bishop Pradel had encouraged local actions in his diocese of Montpellier. The locations of the bureaux existing in 1774 reflect these earlier initiatives since Rennes, Rouen, and Montpellier all distributed more aid than Clermont in the Massif Central, where there had been little missionary activity.

A second factor in explaining the existence of these bureaux was the presence in villages of benefactors affluent enough to make donations. Hufton noted that the combination of these factors explains the almost total absence of such bureaux in the poverty-stricken region of the Massif Central and the fact that few existed in the Comminges or the Alpine regions. For her, there is little to justify the faith that Turgot or Necker placed in bureaux of charity as the main source of relief for the deserving poor. It is true that these institutions corresponded to the government's encouragement of rural industry as a means of breaking the control of the urban guilds. The 1762 edict encouraging rural industry had been inspired by experiments in Normandy in which bureaux of charity had started up workshops (*manufactures des pauvres* or *écoles de filiature*) offering poor women and children a chance to work. However, the successes of these enterprises were spotty, and for Hufton, "revamped or otherwise, [they] could not support the burden of the eighteenth-century poor."[21]

As for Necker's attempt to abolish begging in 1777 and to reopen the dépôts, Olwen Hufton, citing the intendant of Brittany, saw the initiative as an "unqualified failure."[22] More promising, according to her, was the 1780 attempt to force hospitals to live within their means, to sell property to pay off their debts, and to transfer their remaining holdings over to a government caisse. Through this initiative, the crown could have made inroads into the previously reserved domain of the management of hospital resources; however, given the compromises that had to be made to obtain approval for the measure, she noted that the edict remained essentially "a dead letter."[23]

Olwen Hufton's severe judgment of the assistance "policy" described by Bloch certainly shows the limits and obstacles to royal intervention in the field of welfare and hospitals. Two more recent contributions to this debate have tempered her attack by emphasizing coherence and continuity in the logic developed by royal administrators from 1749 to the Revolution. Thomas M. Adams and Jean Imbert have both shown that there was a common line of argument by controllers general from Laverdy to Necker. Virtually every administration advocated three general changes to existing structures. First, they proposed the means to better identify the precise clientele to be treated in each institution and advocated creating special hospitals or services geared to their needs. Secondly, they questioned the efficiency and cost of the large urban institutions created to house the poor and the sick, urging instead the decentralization of aid and reinforcement of local relief services. Thirdly, they each proposed different means and objectives for reorganizing the existing hospital structure.[24]

While Olwen Hufton argued that there is no real evidence that any policy change improved the lives of the poor in France, these three proposals show that crown administrators agreed on the need for reform. However, all kinds of structural obstacles prevented the legislation to institute such reform. The inability of government agents to get their hands on the local hospitals and control their mandates and resources often resulted in alternative crown strategies, such as the creation of the dépôts de mendicité or the recourse to bureaux of charity. The defence of individual rights by the parlementaires made it impossible for the crown to obtain approval for the sentences prescribed for beggars or for the taxes needed to finance local bureaux of the poor. Many judges even refused to condemn beggars, arguing that they were merely doing what they could to survive in difficult times. Finally, rather than placing the accent on differences between Laverdy and Turgot over the dépôts, or between Turgot and Necker over how to best treat the poor, Adams and Imbert have emphasized the thread of continuity between the approaches of these men, who sought how best to reform health services and welfare. The problem was generally that the ideal solution was blocked by vested interests and power structures. As Turgot so astutely observed, the hospitals were defended by "powerful interests." These interests were responsible for blocking change, and they explain the apparent incoherence and inefficiency in crown initiatives observed by Olwen Hufton.

To move beyond this debate and the philosophy underlying the reports, proposals, and edicts brought forward between the 1760s and 1789, how did the hospitals at the local level react to the new suggestions for their decentralization, specialization, and participation with other institutions in dispensing their services? How did they deal with criticism that they had not sufficiently prepared the poor for the labour market? Among the eight institutions studied, there were obvious attempts to collaborate with the crown to reorient services. In many cases, the hospital directors had begun to offer such services long before they were recommended by royal officials, and in no case did an institution remain indifferent to suggestions, criticisms, and proposals for reform.

The hospitals had been regularly attacked for not promoting a work ethic by organizing their inmates into forced labour detachments. Of course, this was not true for Caudebec, which had installed a workshop to produce cotton cloth in 1727, shortly after being selected as a hôpital-général. By 1775 St-Vallier too had set up work facilities within its walls. The directors of the hospital at their meeting on 13 January proposed a workshop to spin wool. It was noted that Louis Jacquier of the Compagnie des Négociants of Lyon had offered to furnish the raw wool, the metal brushes for carding, and the spinning wheels necessary for the enterprise. The hospital, for its part, was to provide the workers, and two inmates were to be trained to oversee production. The hospital bureau recognized the "usefulness" of the proposed workshop, which would furnish employment for the children of the poor. It noted that the operation would be located in the large hall above the chapel, a room that had already been prepared to receive the workers.[25] In 1784 an inner staircase was constructed between the great hall of the hospital and the workshop in order to facilitate access to the installations without the need to go outside. A 1788 almanac noted that the workshop was still in existence and that it procured employment for the young people of the town and the poor.[26]

The schools set up by women's religious orders in the hospitals to teach poor girls were a type of innovation that closely resembled the St-Vallier workshop. These schools were established in the Grignan hospital in 1760 and in St-Vallier in 1784. At St-Vallier, the school was set up in the same large hall as the workshop, separated from it by pine boards. At both hospitals, the nuns taught knitting, carding, and spinning to poor girls.[27] Intended to instil work habits in the poor, these schools were attached to or grew out of many small hospitals. Kathryn Norberg has shown that in Grenoble the curé of St-Louis parish, Abbé Sadin, set up such a "little school" as a charitable gesture to accustom poor girls to work. "What could be more edifying," asked the curé, "than the spectacle of all these little children gathered together in two rooms, working in silence and with great industry and speed."[28] At the hospital in Buis-les-Baronnies, not far from Grignan, the Sisters of the Holy Sacrament established another of these schools, and in a 1777 deliberation it was noted that they taught handicrafts to the girls and sold the products of their work. In addition, they raised silkworms and marketed the cocoons. The revenues of these sales were then reinvested to buy raw materials for the school.[29]

A second innovation corresponding to the views of the crown and its agents can be found in the tendency of hospitals to spend more of their revenues helping the poor in their homes or stimulating community development. The distribution of grain to the poor and the needy was continued and expanded, particularly in the years of famine and unemployment so frequent in the 1770s and 1780s. At Savenay the hospital also distributed what were described as "remèdes" to the poor.[30] The distribution of these remedies refers to a project undertaken by Adrien Helvétius to combat epidemics in rural areas of the kingdom.[31] He oversaw the distribution of packages of medication, with instructions for their use, to trustworthy people in each area, who in turn would give out the appropriate medication to the sick. Helvétius, a Paris doctor whose father, a pharmacist, had been responsible for the introduction of ipecac in France, certainly did not play a disinterested role in coordinating the distribution. A plant imported from Brazil and used to induce vomiting, ipecac was promoted as a treatment for dysentery and was obviously one of the remedies included in the Helvétius packages. Among the other medications was anodyne coral powder, a derivative of opium that was to be taken with ipecac to combat dysentery. Alum powder was another of the favoured ingredients in the pills and syrup that Helvétius prepared; it was said to be particularly effective in controlling blood loss. Finally, reflecting the philosophy of supplying low-cost medication to the poor, a powder prepared from burned egg shells was promoted as a substitute for the more expensive quinine in the treatment of malaria. Small amounts of pure quinine were included in the packages, but they were ordered to be diluted and served as infusions. Jean-Pierre Goubert has argued that these efforts to obtain cheaper medication often invalidated the whole exercise, producing essentially worthless drugs.[32]

The widespread distribution of the packages was approved by Louis xiv, and Helvétius began to send them out to the intendants in 1706. Most of the généralités in France received the shipments, exceptions generally being in the south and southeast (Lyon, Grenoble, Aix, Languedoc, and Perpignan, as well as Caen, Alençon, Champagne, and Riom).[33] Between 47,000 and 60,000 dosages were distributed annually in the years from 1706 to 1709, costing 10,000 to 12,000 livres. Helvétius argued that the consignments should be doubled to meet the needs of the rural areas, and by royal arrêts of 1721 and 1722, Louis xv approved the increase for an annual cost of 30,000 livres.[34] From the instructions given for local distribution of the remedies at Belle-Île-en-Mer off the Brittany coast in 1735, two packages seem to have been sent to the community. The first contained two pounds of ipecac divided into five hundred doses, and the second was made up of twelve ounces of anodyne coral powder in four hundred doses.[35]

Considerable quantities of these remedies seem to have been sent to Brittany, especially during epidemic years, and the principal agents for their distribution were the nuns working in small parishes and hospitals or, in their absence, the curés of such parishes. Most small communities had no doctors or surgeons; even where they were present, provincial officials seem to have been sceptical of entrusting them with the distributions, fearing they might sell the medications.[36] On 25 September 1724 the controller general sent out a request to intendants asking for information concerning this program and the other "medical" facilities available in the kingdom. It noted the "positive results" obtained by the standardized packages of remedies prepared by the king's apothecary, Helvétius, and dispatched to the Sisters of Charity in the cities and towns of the kingdom. At the same time, it requested data on hospitals possessing proper equipment and staff: the number of beds, the financing, the buildings, and the personnel of each institution.[37] The replies to this inquiry were very limited, and up to the end of the Ancien Régime, the Helvétius packages continued to be one of the principal sources of medication for the rural population.

Outside relief, whether in the form of grain distribution or of medication, was not limited to Malestroit or Savenay. Other small hospitals, such as Grignan, Étoile, or Seyne, had always dedicated about 30 per cent of their budgets to such aid, handing out grain to the poor or small sums of money to formerly solvent residents who had fallen on hard times. Small institutions generally carried out this role, but the replies to the 1774 Turgot inquiry show that it was clearly limited since most villages and parishes in France possessed neither a hospital nor a foundation for poor relief.

A third example of innovation in hospital service comes from St-Antoine in Pontorson, the establishment that corresponds most clearly to a "medicalized" model. Directed by the Brothers of Charity, it was in the vanguard of such institutions, as was seen in the previous chapter. At the same time, it remained a small hospital: right up to 1792 there were only twelve beds available for the sick, and after 1730 the brothers used the crown rhetoric against vagabonds to eliminate the two or three places that it had maintained for itinerants.[38] Pontorson was also among the first hospitals to try to increase its revenues by taking in paying patients. There had always been a certain number of such residents, for it was an old monastic tradition to receive the aged and infirm as well as old soldiers. From 1666 to 1695, six men – four priests and two laymen, one of whom had been a tax collector in the town – had received "hospitality" in return for a certain sum of money.[39]

However, this type of voluntary resident disappeared after 1700, when the brothers began admitting a new and involuntary clientele: patients who were "mentally ill" or in need of "correction." In 1702 there were 6 of these *pensionnaires*, and by 1725 their number had risen to 22. To house them, the prior, Mathieu Gaillard, reinforced several dormitories in a wing that came to be known as the Exil. In 1750 there were 50 inmates crowded into the *maison de force*, and by 1757 the brothers had applied to begin the construction of a new building to house them.[40] Erected between 1758 and 1760, this new Exil was three storeys high with bars on its windows and thick, insulated walls. The prison aspect of the building was constantly reinforced, and in 1764 the ceiling below the attic had to be rebuilt and strengthened to prevent prisoners from escaping.[41] The number of inmates stabilized at around 50, with 42 in 1765 and 59 in 1779.[42]

The families of most of these new patients paid for their incarceration and their upkeep. The revenues received for their care came to represent a considerable proportion of the income of the institution. Most of the inmates were from well-placed families. Hélène Avisseau-Roussat has shown that of the 138 taken into the institution between 1745 and 1773, there were 110 civilians, 16 members of the clergy, and 12 military men. Among the 52 Normans interned, over half (28) were members of the nobility, 7 from merchant families, 5 priests, and 3 military men. Among the 56 Bretons placed, 25 were from noble families, 10 from merchant ranks, 9 priests, and 3 from the military.[43] The king paid for a few of the internees, but generally the families who brought their fathers or sons to be interned, with or without a *lettre de cachet* from the king, negotiated the cost of the services to be rendered. They paid sums ranging from 300 to 500 livres at the beginning of the seventeenth century, and by 1764 the hospital was signing agreements with families for 300, 400, 500, and 800 livres a year, depending upon the services and the quality of life to be accorded to the different inmates. From 1750 to 1779 the revenues from these pensions rose from 8,500 to more than 30,000 livres, and frequently this income constituted over half the annual revenue of the hospital.[44]

The harsh discipline and primitive conditions of detention for many of the inmates of this maison de force brought an atmosphere of increasing tension and latent violence to the establishment. Riots took place in 1767, 1774, and 1777 causing damage and injuries. In a letter to Minister Bertier just as Turgot was beginning his 1774 review of poor relief, M. de Fontette, the intendant at Caen, who was responsible for Pontorson, indicated the difficulties inherent in the system:

the administration of all the maisons de force in the kingdom is an area that appears to me to merit more attention. There are all sorts of subjects in these types of houses who are victims of hatred or self-interest. There are many others who, having been sufficiently punished, should be returned to society, but have been forgotten by their families. Finally, there are an infinite number who, without being able to recover their liberty, have daily needs that their families refuse because of indifference or greed. Humanity in general suffers from so many horrors that, although hidden away, are no less revolting. I do not know if I am wrong, but it seems to me that the administration of the maisons de force, in the sense that I see them, would benefit from the setting up in Paris of a commission that would report every six months on the condition and conduct of the pensionnaires, at least of those incarcerated at the request of their families.[45]

As Fontette suggested, controversy surrounded the procedures for internment in the maisons de force. The notorious lettres de cachet issued by the king and his representatives were generally at the origin of these detentions. Families who invoked mental illness or simply the antisocial behaviour of one of their members could easily obtain orders for internment. Thereafter the family paid for the incarceration and the "treatment" administered to the "patient."

The reasons for these internments varied, and of course, the real motives were never indicated. Glimpses of the accusations that led to internments can be obtained from the questioning carried out from time to time by the subdélégués who visited the patients at Pontorson. Among the clergy, lack of discipline or the inability to get along with colleagues seems to have played an important role. A Scottish priest, imprisoned in the Exil from 1753 to 1771, told Subdélégué Angot that he did not know the reasons for his confinement but that the other priests did not like him, had called him a schemer (*intriguant*), and had been pleased to see him taken away.[46] The cases of laymen varied even more. In 1762 the Sieur D—— told Angot that his brother had had him shut up to take control of his lands and holdings.[47] In some cases when the sons of noble families had broken the law, rather than standing trial, they were sent off to the Exil: according to the Subdélégué Mesle, the Sieur de R—— was supposed to have killed another man while hunting, but it had never been proved whether the death was accidental or not.[48] By the end of the Ancien Régime, institutions such as Pontorson were full of these types of inmates: alcoholic sons who had put their family fortune in jeopardy, others who were set on concluding what their families saw as dishonourable marriages, fathers whose gambling and drunkenness had placed their families at risk, military men considered deranged and a danger to their regiments, and priests whose bad habits posed problems for the church. The Brienne report submitted to Turgot in 1774 had noted the inadequacy of the procedures for obtaining the lettres de cachet that had filled institutions such as Pontorson with people who should not have been there.[49]

The creation of the maison de force fundamentally transformed the Pontorson hospital from a small twelve-bed institution for the sick and poor to a fifty-patient asylum for the mentally ill and those needing correction. Pontorson was not the only hospital that participated in this new direction. Most of the institutions run by the Brothers of Charity attached a maison de force to their traditional hospital; Charenton and Senlis became models for this new type of institution.[50] Near Rennes the small local hospital of St-Méen du Tertre de Joue underwent a transformation similar to that at Pontorson. Staffed by the Sisters of St-Thomas de Villeneuve, the institution embarked on a significant expansion after 1760, when the lettres de cachet became more frequent. There too the mentally ill, prodigal sons, debauched fathers, gamblers, prostitutes, and criminals were lumped together by order of their families. By 1777–79 the hospital was earning 72,279 livres annually from its pensionnaires.[51] It was precisely this movement that provided Michel Foucault with the great majority of his "horror stories." It is true that isolation cells, cages, ice-cold baths and showers, bleedings, and purgations were all associated with the treatments administered by these maisons de force.[52]

The additional revenues from the maison de force enabled Pontorson to double the number of beds allotted to sick patients, but at the same time this new "service" changed the institution. In contrast to the earlier confinement measures that grew out of societal concern and a certain vision of Christian charity, the asylums built around the lettres de cachet were clear manifestations of the new orientations of assistance. There were imperfect attempts to separate patients according to their illnesses as the government circulars recommended, but since the financial resources to undertake such changes were never approved, each institution had to do the best it could to carry out reform. The evolution of the hospital at Pontorson tends to demonstrate a certain breakdown in traditional notions of Christian charity in addition to a retreat from previous commitments to the sick and the poor, both of which concepts were present in crown efforts to "specialize" aid. But the creation of the maison de force was essentially a case of a traditional hospital trying to find new sources of financing.

These examples of the initiatives taken by the eight hospitals studied in this book show that, despite what Olwen Hufton saw as totally inadequate resources, at least some local institutions were able to evolve along the lines proposed by crown agents. In fact, the revenues of all eight of the institutions increased, in some cases dramatically, providing them with the means to implement some of the proposed changes (see Table 8).[53] When we look at the operating budgets and accounts of the

Table 8
Eighteenth-century operating budgets of the eight hospitals discussed in the text

Hospital	Years	Average annual budget for the sick and poor (in livres)	Average budget for outside aid (in livres)	Average patients admitted	No. of beds
Caudebec	1739–59	7,088		39	39 adults 28 children
Pontorson	1740–80	17,821		132	12 adults 40 maison de force
Malestroit	1740–80	735	503		4–6
Savenay	1746–60	1,814	487		6
Grignan	1747–77	2,437	1,156		4
Étoile	1764	1,923	723		13
Seyne	1740–59	3,430	987		
St-Vallier	1749–76	876			

eight hospitals, it becomes clear that, despite royal campaigns to cut back and restrict local institutions, all of them continued to receive the financial and moral support of their communities and the church. This support can be measured best by comparing Table 8 with Table 1 in chapter 1; it can be seen that the institutions had all improved their financial situations between the beginning of the seventeenth century and the middle of the eighteenth. Revenues had jumped almost thirty times at Pontorson, where the income from the maison de force accounted for an increase in the average annual budget from 635 livres taken in between 1612 and 1630 to the 17,821 livres received between 1740 and 1780. A tenfold increase can be observed at Caudebec, where the improved facilities created during the institution's years as an hôpital-général caused income to shoot up from an annual average of 671 livres between 1612 and 1630 to 7,088 livres between 1739 and 1759. Among the smaller institutions, Malestroit increased its intake over eight times, going from very limited yearly receipts of 173 livres between 1600 and 1630 to the more respectable 735 livres taken in between 1740 and 1780. In the same order, Seyne jumped from annual revenues of 130 livres between 1600 and 1630 to an average of 3,430 between 1740 and 1759. In most of the other institutions studied, budgets generally tripled. Étoile was the exception; there revenues only doubled, going from an average of 827 livres registered annually between 1604 and 1630 to the 1,923 received in 1764.

The budgets also show that five of the eight hospitals distributed outside aid to two categories of local inhabitants: those who had once been solvent before falling upon hard times (the pauvres honteux) and the poor and sick who could not earn a living for themselves or their families. The most evident example of outside aid was the weekly distribution of grain to town inhabitants who had been placed on the poor rolls. This aid varied considerably from year to year. At Malestroit during the period in question, the hospital consecrated an average of 68 per cent of its budget to such aid, but in years of crisis – crop failure, famine, unemployment – the assistance could reseach 80 per cent of the budget, while in normal years it dropped back to around 30 per cent. After the famine of 1668, the subdelegate evaluated the number of town poor at five hundred and asked for grain to be sent in. The intendant responded by dispatching 432 pounds of rice. In the subsequent economic crises of 1775 and 1785, with more stable revenues, the hospital increased its distribution of rye to the town poor. From 1773 to 1778, 70 per cent of the hospital revenues went to acquiring and distributing grain, and in 1780–85, over 80 per cent of the budget was spent on grain.[54]

The fact that four times more patients were treated at Pontorson than at Caudebec illustrates a fundamental difference between institutions primarily devoted to the sick and those that catered to the poor. At Caudebec, as in most of the other institutions, the sick and the injured always occupied a few places, but most of the hospital was left to the aged, the mentally or physically handicapped, and abandoned children. This latter category, the "poor," was primarily made up of long-term residents of the hospital who changed little from one year to another. This is the reason that an average of only 39 patients were treated each year. On the other hand, at Pontorson, in addition to the 40 beds reserved for the more permanent residents of the maison de force, there were 12 beds primarily reserved for sick patients. The turnover in these 12 beds was very high, explaining the average of 132 patients received annually in the hospital between 1739 and 1759. Injured patients were rarely kept for more than a month, and sick patients were often discharged after three or four days or as soon as their fever had abated. Such differences in the percentage of the sick and the poor admitted to each institution go a long way towards explaining the variations in the number of admissions. The fact that most small hospitals in France indiscriminately accepted the sick or the poor also helps to explain the difficulty in imposing a fundamental distinction between the type of care to be administered to each group. The essential advances in medical care to the sick that eventually changed the make-up of hospital inmates had only begun; it would be accelerated in the course of the nineteenth century.[55]

These institutions' capacity to help the local sick and poor should not be overestimated, however. Most of them could take in only the most afflicted members of their community during the last years of their lives, temporarily care for those injured in accidents, or look after abandoned children for a limited time. In their distribution of outside aid, they gave out grain to families placed on the town poor-relief rolls and money to the pauvres honteux. These actions maintained a level of local relief barely sufficient in years of average harvests, but totally insufficient in periods of crisis. After all, most of these hospitals did not deal with more than 300 to 500 people a year through outside aid and 40 to 50 patients a year who were treated within their walls.

As these budgets show, and as Olwen Hufton contended, there were severe limitations to hospital innovation. These limitations are illustrated by the reactions of the Caudebec hospital in the years after the crown suspended its grants to the hôpitaux-généraux. In 1733 Caudebec, like all the hospitals participating in the project, was advised that it would no longer be compensated for taking in arrested beggars and vagabonds.[56] However, royal officials asked the institutions to continue receiving those who were brought to their doors and to carry on the internment policy using their own funds. On 31 May 1734 the directors at Caudebec noted that their annual revenues now amounted to no more than 1,000 livres and that, with the suspension of grants, they had to cut services. They therefore decided that, in spite of crown appeals to continue internment, the hospital would no longer take in outsiders.[57] This decision eliminated the places set aside for the beggars and vagabonds arrested under the 1724 law, and it also ended aid given in the context of the passade, the traditional handouts and lodging given to itinerants in hospitals and hospices. With this change, the hospital directors abandoned the basic principles of traditional Christian charity; in accordance with the new Enlightenment rhetoric, it was presumed that aid and distributions to the undeserving poor increased their laziness and promoted vagabondage and vagrancy.

The change in policy, especially to the more traditional aid to itinerants, did not go unchallenged among Caudebec's local defenders of the poor. In 1746 several residents representing different social groups in the town complained that the administrators of the hospital no longer received "the poor outsiders who had come to live in the town and who subsequently fell ill."[58] They argued that this refusal prevented the hospital from doing the good for which it was created. The bureau replied that the administrators were only carrying out the policy that had been verbally adopted in 1734 and that they were convinced that if the outside poor knew that they would be received at the Caudebec hospital, they would flock to the town, depriving the town poor of the means to earn their livelihood. At this meeting in 1746, the policy of excluding outsiders was formally adopted.

The question was raised again in the late 1760s when it once more became clear that the directors were steadfastly refusing outsiders. On 30 January 1769 it was noted that the administrators had received a questionnaire from M. de Raltier, who was receveur and director of manufacturing for the poor of the town. He asked the directors for details on the employment of beggars and vagabonds in the hospital's workshops, and the assembly sent him a terse reply noting that the hospital received only the town poor and housed no vagabonds or beggars.[59] Eight months later, in the face of new problems with admissions and questions from the curé as to why outsiders were being refused, the directors repeated the criteria that had been officially adopted in 1746. The hospital was reserved for residents of the town; outsiders who were sick could be received by paying admission, but poor outsiders could not be admitted without a letter signed by at least three directors or submitting their cases to the assembly. Children placed in the institution and subsequently removed by their parents could not be readmitted. Caring for the town poor, the king's soldiers, and the sick were the priorities of the institution. The directors argued that difficulties were encountered when these criteria were not strictly applied, noting the case of a young boy who had entered the hospital with falsified papers and, after stealing food, had escaped under cover of night.[60]

This example from Caudebec demonstrates the importance of financial considerations for hospital directors. In contrast to Pontorson, which expanded its field of activity to take in new revenues, Caudebec cut back in order to balance its books, eliminating one of the traditional services of local hospitals. The constant preoccupation of the directors with balancing their accounts produced few debts or deficits at Caudebec, Pontorson, or the other institutions I have studied. These cases offer opposing evidence to the arguments of Camille Bloch that most hospitals were heavily indebted by 1789 or the judgment of Olwen Hufton that "by the end of the Ancien Régime a deficit was the norm."[61] Although they did not use quantitative analysis, both Léon Lallemand and Jean Imbert disputed these assessments, the first arguing that the source of Bloch's evaluations was incomplete and the second noting that judgments of hospital financial results for one or two years overlooked the way that these institutions functioned.[62] As Imbert noted, directors often allowed a deficit to be run up in a particularly difficult year, only to reduce expenses drastically during successive years so as to eliminate the accumulated deficit.[63]

In our examination of the case of Caudebec, it is clear that the directors of the hospital exposed themselves to regular criticism from the crown, the curé, and local residents by cutting back on traditional aid in order to balance the budget. The critics noted that the institution was not fulfilling its responsibilities to the poor, but in the eyes of hospital administrators, the problem was not so clear-cut. The passade and the internment of beggars were seen as encouraging bad habits by giving food and shelter to marginals who lived from handouts and thievery and as especially promoting the arrival of poor migrants from the countryside who competed with the local poor for seasonal jobs and charity.

Olwen Hufton, Jean Imbert, and Thomas Adams have argued persuasively that the royal welfare policy described by Camille Bloch was at best a series of proposals and projects regularly resisted by parlementaire elites and local notables. At its worst, it was a group of suggestions rendered incoherent by the fact that royal officials constantly tried to get around judicial resistance by reorienting their projects, replacing hospitals as centres of internment by dépôts de mendicité over which they had exclusive control, and reopening dépôts when the financial resources for meaningful local poor relief were refused. Although the major part of the policy was never given legal sanction, and its clauses with regard to the poor were regularly blocked in the parlements, hospitals were obviously affected by the proposals and criticism in royal reports and debates. They proceeded to transform and adapt their services to the new demands.[64] The workshops organized at Caudebec and St-Vallier, the pensionnaires housed at Pontorson, and the schools to teach skills and trades to poor girls at Grignan, St-Vallier, and Malestroit all corresponded to the types of welfare measures proposed in the reports and projects.[65] However, only in the distribution of medication sponsored by Helvétius can the crown be perceived as playing a direct role. At Pontorson there was an indirect crown responsibility for these innovations since the lettres de cachet created the conditions for the organization of the maison de force and the construction of the Exil. In the other cases, the new measures stemmed from the involvement of the community and from women's religious groups in teaching skills and organizing workshops.

The gap between the crown's inability to produce meaningful hospital legislation and the newer practices that evolved in the institutions brings us back to the theories of Foucault and his emphasis on practice. In effect, when we examine the innovations of most of the hospitals treated here, a real "policy" can be perceived that follows along the lines of most of the crown proposals. In effect, the attitudes of the directors of these institutions towards relief seem to have been strongly influenced both by the crown and Enlightenment rhetoric. As mentioned in chapter 3, even the supporters of traditional Christian relief had begun to incorporate a work-ethic philosophy into their ideas about aiding the poor.[66] Despite the obstacles to legislation, as Foucault noted, the practices of poor relief did change and came to constitute a relatively coherent approach. What modifies Foucault's analysis is the fact that the new practices represented both the movements for change, that is, the older Christian tradition that produced the religious orders, the "little schools" for poor girls, and the distribution of medication, and the more recent bourgeois-absolutist context that underlay the maisons de force and the workshops.

It has been argued that the local interventions of the absolute monarchy during the reign of Louis XIV were less oriented to contesting the traditional structures of town and village communities than had been previously thought. Hilton Root, using the case of Burgundy, contended that the crown actually reduced the weight of direct taxes and used its intendants to attack the power of arbitrary seigneurial justice and to side with local communities on such issues as the power and composition of town and village assemblies, the use of common lands, seigneurial dues, and grazing and gleaning rights.[67] Without arguing that the king's officials actually sided with the communities, Jean-Pierre Gutton and Yves-Marie Bercé both found that Louis XIV's reign brought a distinct reduction in friction with town and village representatives. Nevertheless, as they pointed out, an expanded maréchaussée, as well as crown attempts to transport grain out of certain regions to ensure a more equitable distribution throughout the kingdom, continued to provoke community discontent.[68] In the case of the offensive against local hospitals, there was certainly no turning point before Louis XIV's death in 1714. On this question, the change in crown attitudes came after the final series of reforms and closures of small hospitals between 1696 and 1700. It was only in the 1750s that royal officials really began to revise their perceptions of local hospitals and welfare institutions.

The Caudebec reply to the subdelegate in 1774 concerning the activities of its hospital was but one element in the eventual policy review begun by crown officials. From the 1750s to 1789, replies to similar inquiries were integrated into a series of reports, projects, and proposals that tried to reshape the structures of poor relief in the kingdom. They were directed at identifying and separating the clientele to be sent to increasingly specialized institutions as well as at suggesting the means to decentralize aid and reform the hospitals. The coherent implementation of these policies was regularly blocked in the parlements and the local courts of justice. Nevertheless, the visions for change behind these new orientations seem to have been adopted by the notables of the kingdom, who accepted the rhetoric for change that dominated Enlightenment discourse. Most important, the ideas were reflected in the innovations carried out by most of the hospitals studied. The crown policy of trying to shift relief efforts back to the communities was never adopted as such, but its elements came to be accepted in the outlook of the period, which in turn was transformed into individual interventions to reform aid to the poor.

During the eighteenth century, royal proposals to reform welfare certainly began to have an impact upon the eight hospitals studied. The institutions treated here take their place among the 1,034 other small-town hospitals that Muriel Jeorger has identified in the kingdom.[69] The limited number of these institutions, their uneven geographical distribution, and their lack of personnel and resources dramatically restricted the ability of the crown to use them to reform care for the poor and the sick. Institutional replies to the numerous inquiries carried out during the century only confirmed the existence of these problems. While specialists on the question such as Archbishop Loménie de Brienne argued in favour of two-, three-, or four-bed hospitals, he conceded the lack of such facilities, asking curés to assemble local notables to set up small hospitals and calling for a network of bureaux of charity and small institutions to distribute aid.[70] Necker, too, created a hospital and a bureau of charity as examples of how local welfare should be organized. After a century and a half of closing small institutions, expropriating their funds, and transferring their holdings to larger centralized hospitals, crown agents in the second half of the eighteenth century rediscovered the utility of locally distributed aid. The small hospitals were, in fact, slowly transforming their services to conform to the new demands of eighteenth-century society, but their numbers were far too limited to provide a base for the effective reform of either health or welfare relief.

Conclusion

The experiences of local hospitals in France from the sixteenth century to the Revolution can be seen as a long-term grass-roots effort to resist the forces of centralization and rationalization. They present us with a typical case in which the absolute monarchy tried to impose its diagnosis of inefficiency and its prescription of closure and expropriation upon institutions created and maintained by town and village communities. From the 1530s to the 1750s, crown officials were at work promoting different scenarios for expropriating the funds of local hospitals. They were convinced that in addition to being corrupt, these institutions held rich untapped sources of capital and land. Seeking ways to finance new initiatives and find new revenues to distribute as patronage, these officials tried directly and indirectly to get their hands on the hospitals' holdings.

From the 1530s to 1603, royal edicts encouraged local judges to inspect the poor-relief facilities in their districts and, on finding corruption or embezzlement, to close down the institutions and transfer their funds to better-organized establishments. By the early 1600s the monarchy's needs had changed, and under pressure to demobilize French armies after the Wars of Religion, the king sought to appease military officials by transferring revenues from the hospitals to old and injured officers. The majority of the appropriated funds came from the maladreries that had been founded as colonies for lepers or from the abbeys that had traditionally been responsible for receiving old soldiers. This project ran into difficulty when the institutions in question appealed the expropriations, arguing that they transferred private revenues to crown projects and that the operations went against the provisions of most of the institutions' charters.

By 1611, under the reign of Louis XIII, the monarchy, in response to this opposition, again changed priorities. Carrying out the mandate of the Chamber of the General Hospital Reform to inspect institutions founded to serve the poor and sick and to expropriate those that were judged corrupt or redundant, the crown stopped directing the confiscated revenues towards army officers and returned them to their original purpose, that is, to provide adequate treatment for the sick. By 1673 Louvois, minister of war to Louis XIV, proposed another method of diverting expropriated revenues from "corrupt" hospitals and "moribund" hospitaller orders to nobles and army officials. This time the state would not intervene directly but instead would turn over the task of inspection and closure to a hospitaller order, Notre-Dame of Mount Carmel and St-Lazare. The experiment lasted until Louvois's death in 1693, and it again ran into the problem of the crown's right to give a third party powers of expropriation over what were essentially private hospitals. Disputed in particular was the king's right to suppress a number of hospitaller orders without papal approval. Between 1693 and 1700 the last stage in royal attempts to close "inefficient" local hospitals brought direct crown intervention as a group of maîtres de requêtes and conseillers d'état revised the rulings on most of the hospitals that had been taken over by St-Lazare, integrating them into larger regional institutions.

Simultaneous with this effort at more or less direct crown intervention, a second movement, led by the urban hôpitaux-généraux, was also trying to obtain rights over the small, local hospitals. From 1663, the date of the edict ordering all major cities of the kingdom to set up hôpitaux-généraux, urban leaders and directors of the new institutions asked the crown for the right to expropriate the revenues of surrounding town and village hospitals. Louis XIV, through individual grants and a letter to the bishops in 1676, gave the hôpitaux-généraux permission to inspect and close down the small hospitals that had not already been granted to St-Lazare. Local hospitals, therefore, became one of the principal targets of the project to intern the poor and the beggars in the massive new urban institutions.

Despite the fact that these different initiatives were regularly opposed, they did have an impact. Thousands of local hospitals were inspected by commissioners from the different semi-judicial inquiries. They were accused of various evils and closed or partially expropriated. Over 4,078 hospitals were shut down or targeted for suppression by the Order of Notre-Dame of Mount Carmel and St-Lazare. After its operation ended, a review of the institutions to be re-established was undertaken by royal officials, who ordered that the holdings of 1,632 small hospitals be transferred to 608 regional institutions. Far from being repositories of the great wealth promised by the crown, the great majority of the suppressed institutions that were taken over between the 1530s and 1700 were found to be indebted, their buildings in ruins, and their landholdings non-existent. Given the number of local hospitals that were closed or expropriated by this movement, town and village hospitals can be placed among the "victims" of the early modern historical process in France.

It was true, as the crown argued, that many small hospitals were corrupt and inefficient. The problem was that the reform movements tried to shut down the well-managed, well-financed institutions along with those that were in ruins. Most of the communities that had possessed small hospitals lost them during the century and a half of inquiries, commissions, and judicial initiatives. A large percentage of local hospitals were effectively closed and expropriated in the period extending from 1530 to 1700. In addition, many other communities had never possessed such institutions; therefore, in a sense, the eight hospitals studied in this book are not exactly typical of town and village institutions. Despite all the efforts at reform and rationalization undertaken by the crown and the widespread resistance mounted by the institutions confronted with closure, the changes had not been very radical, as can be seen in the studies of hospital distribution carried out by the Comité de Mendicité after 1792. On the regional side, the pattern remained relatively similar to that of the seventeenth century at the beginning of the reforms. Provence continued to possess a relatively dense network of institutions; for every 10,000 inhabitants, it had almost two hospitals. For the same population, the Paris region had about one and a half, Dauphiné about one, and Brittany, Normandy and the Massif Central barely the equivalent of half a hospital.[1]

When we look at the hospitals' locations, however, the effects of all the reform movements are more evident, for the institutions had become far more concentrated in urban centers. The same analysis of the data gathered by the Comité de Mendicité shows that although only 18.8 per cent of the population lived in towns of 2,000 or more inhabitants, 57.27 per cent of the hôpitaux, hôtels-Dieux, and hôpitaux-généraux were located in such centers.[2] The departments containing a large city such as Paris, Grenoble, Marseille, Nantes, or Lyon were always among the best equipped because of the weight of their large urban institutions. The number of hospitals located in towns and villages of less than 2,000 inhabitants had certainly been reduced by the closures. There remained 1,034 hospitals in such centers, including the eight represented in this study. It is clear that these hospitals constitute cases where local efforts to support their institutions and resist rationalization had been more successful than in the majority of the towns and villages.

The Edict of Moulins in 1566 had recognized the responsibility of each community to care for its poor and sick, and the provisions of this edict were regularly repeated throughout the Ancien Régime. The eight hospitals studied in this book are representative of over a thousand cases in which local poor relief went beyond the efforts of the average community. They can be seen as model institutions, and their experiences in resisting closure and in expanding their services allow us to observe fundamental changes taking place in the community, the church, and the state. In other words, through the eyes of the local hospital operations we can analyse the fundamental forces responsible for most of the major changes in early modern French social history.

Traditional historiography has argued that from the end of the sixteenth century, town and village communities experienced economic and demographic stagnation leading to a long-term decline of their power and wealth. The attempts to close local hospitals reveal, on the one hand, the very real offensive represented by crown and urban initiatives to intervene in a recognized field of community responsibility and, on the other hand, attempts by local communities to preserve their institutions and renew their approach to welfare and to the treatment of the sick. It is clear that in the case of the hospitals, we are not in the presence of a long and inevitable decline of local power and institutions. Instead, the confrontations took place during periodic interventions, and expropriations and closures were followed by regular local protests and frequent reversals of policy. Many of the funds or holdings transferred from local hospitals were later returned to the institutions, the hospitals ordered to be closed down were frequently later reopened, and a large number of the establishments that received such orders simply ignored them.

The eight institutions studied here provide eloquent examples of the various survival strategies adopted by local hospitals in reaction to the new policies imposed by the absolute monarchy. Savenay and Malestroit were both ordered to be closed down in the reforms carried out between 1672 and 1693 by the Order of Notre-Dame of Mount Carmel and

St-Lazare, and Étoile had 100 livres expropriated in the same operation. Yet all three institutions continued to function, and their accounts reveal no concessions to the orders coming from above. At the same time, Pontorson was "asked" by the king to turn its hospital over to the Brothers of Charity in 1644. It complied, but for a century thereafter, town officials attempted to regain control over the institution. At Caudebec the administrators of the hospital were ordered by a 1724 edict to take in beggars from outside the town. They complied as long as the crown sent them subsidies for this new service, but as soon as the grants were eliminated, the hospital administrators decided to exclude poor outsiders from their institution despite demands from the crown to continue accepting them. It is clear that the crises confronting local hospitals were periodic and that frequently the community and the institution were able to return to the "normal" ways of functioning once the confrontation had passed.

In a rapidly evolving urban landscape, the possession of a hospital, along with a detachment of the royal constabulary and a seat of justice, became a criterion for determining which towns were to become regional centers. As hospitals were closed down and their revenues and holdings transferred to neighbouring institutions, it became important for a town not only to maintain its hospital, but to try to expand its services and benefit from the closure of nearby hospices and maladreries. For this reason, hospital directors vied with one another to obtain the lands and revenues of the institutions targeted for closure. The future position of their hospital, and indeed their town, often depended on their success in defending their institution.[3]

One of the reasons that the communities were so attached to their hospitals was the role played by the local elites in their operations. These groups were critical to the maintenance of the social patterns and value structures upon which small-town communities were based. Local notables had very close associations with the institutions for the sick and the poor. They were the principal contributors to the hospitals. Motivated perhaps by missionaries and the new church message in favour of helping the needy, notaries, lawyers, merchants, officials, and wealthy farmers gave through direct gifts or through their wills to support the local relief effort. These same men were the recteurs, councillors, and directors of the local hospitals, often serving as directors subsequent to having been mayors or consuls of their towns. Service on the hospital board became almost a litmus test of the town elite. At the same time, these men reaped benefits from their service. Enhancing their social prominence and their opportunities for building up a network of local clients, they could sign notes admitting townspeople or outsiders to the institution; they decided which individuals and families were to be placed on the poor rolls for the weekly distribution of grain; and they also determined in secret which formerly solvent families were to be given monetary aid to tide them over during hard times.

An even clearer benefit from their connections with the hospitals came from the decisions made by the directors concerning the use of the institutions' holdings and funds. The revenues received by the hospitals were to be loaned out and the landholdings rented, with the revenues from these operations going to the poor. The notables serving on individual hospital boards controlled considerable capital and landholdings, which almost constituted a local bank, and they could determine who should receive loans and at what interest rates. It is not surprising that a number of relatives of recteurs and board members figured among the beneficiaries of these operations. Finally, these men purchased most of the grain that was eventually distributed to those on the poor rolls. Again, the connections between the suppliers and the board members are clear: most of those who sold grain to the institution were former recteurs, councillors, or notables who had contributed regularly to support the hospitals. Furthermore, in the towns that possessed them, the hospitals were important elements in maintaining the internal coherence of the groups of local notables. The hospitals became bulwarks of community solidarity in the face of crown efforts to reduce local rights and centralize the administration of power.[4]

As to the poor, the sick, and the needy, obviously their connections with the institutions created to serve them were important. The two larger institutions under study had decidedly different orientations. At Pontorson the hospital primarily treated the medical problems of the sick and injured. It had a rapid turnover rate, and patients were sent home as soon as possible, although its attached maison de force was directed more towards the long-term internment of paying inmates. Caudebec, which was more oriented to receiving local poor and elderly residents, retained a large percentage of its inmates from year to year. For the other institutions, the most important aspect of their activity was outside relief. Few patients were actually interned in the small, local hospitals. Normally possessing between four and six beds, the majority of them took in patients who were approaching death and gave temporary care to victims of accidents and provisional shelter to unwed pregnant women and abandoned children. Far more substantial was the aid that they provided to poor townspeople through grain distributions, places in the hospital workshop, courses in the manual arts, or schools for the poor. All these activities became more valued in the course of the eighteenth century, and the problems of the poor and the needs of the local hospitals would be one of the major issues behind the creation of the Comité de Mendicité in 1790.[5]

Hospital records also allow us to observe the subtle manœuvring of the church on the question of charitable renewal. Trying to revise church doctrines and reach out to the faithful, the Catholic Reformation produced new types of initiatives by missionaries who went from town to town, carrying the church message in favour of aid to the poor and marginal groups. New religious orders were created to concentrate on serving the poor and the needy. Often they reluctantly became involved in the urban hôpital-général movement, but essentially they remained committed to traditional support for the sick and the poor wherever these individuals were to be found. St Vincent de Paul and his Lazarist missionaries travelled throughout the rural regions in central and eastern France asking every parish to set up bureaux of charity. Fathers Chaurand, Dunod, and Guevarre conducted missions from town to town in Brittany, Normandy, Languedoc, Provence, Dauphiné, and Franche-Comté, trying to convince communities to establish local hôpitaux-généraux or bureaux of the poor in order to stem migration towards the larger urban centers. Among the other new institutions proposed by the church to aid the poor and needy were monts de pitié, greniers d'abondance, and the distribution of packages of remedies and medicine sent to the provinces to combat epidemics. In each of the eight communities studied here, the impact of missions, sermons, and church teachings can be observed through the increased hospital donations and through the activity of the town elite in the field of poor relief.

An even more concrete result of seventeenth-century religious renewal was the foundation of women's religious orders to work in community hospitals as part of their service to the sick and the poor. These orders reinforced the organization and personnel of what had often been poorly equipped, understaffed local hospitals.[6] At the same time as they enlarged the opportunities for early modern women outside the household or the cloister, these nuns transformed the functioning of most of the hospitals of the kingdom. The new congregations were present in five of the eight hospitals under study, and they often had a major impact upon discipline, organization, and the services offered. Even in the communities without hospitals, the arrival of these congregations in local parishes led to the creation of convents, soup kitchens (*bouillons des pauvres*), and bureaux of charity that put women in public positions of authority and fundamentally changed the dynamic of local social services.

Finally, this study of local hospitals reveals a great deal about the obstacles confronted by the absolute monarchy in its attempts to influence and change the functioning of local power structures in the kingdom. First and foremost, the crown realized that the hospitals it sought to reform were essentially private institutions over which both it and the church shared certain rights. Because of his limited powers of direct intervention, the king always tried to have the reform agenda carried out by intermediaries: local judges, the commissioners of the Chamber of Christian Charity or its successor, the Chamber of the General Hospital Reform, or the members of the hospitaller Order of Notre-Dame of Mount Carmel and St-Lazare. Only in 1693 did royal commissioners become directly involved in deciding which hospitals, previously confiscated by St-Lazare, were to be re-established and which were to be merged with larger regional institutions.

Each of these interventions produced closures and expropriations, but in every case, hospitals appealed the decisions. They argued that the crown did not have the right, directly or indirectly, to ignore their charters or change the terms of the grants and legacies that had been left to them. Redirecting revenues and holdings that had been given to support lepers in order to provide care for old and injured soldiers or pensions for army officials was seen as untenable. Giving the right to confiscate the holdings of other "moribund" hospitaller orders to a new order, Notre-Dame of Mount Carmel and St-Lazare, without the pope's approval was argued to be illegal. The limits upon the powers of the absolute monarchy were evident in this resistance and in the fact that so many of the hospitals targeted for suppression continued to flourish.

In pursuing these types of confrontations with local communities, especially their elites, over the closing of hospitals and the expropriation of their holdings, the crown contributed to the tension and resistance that marked its relations with local communities until the eighteenth century. The disputes over local hospitals fit into a general pattern in which the absolute monarchy can be seen as questioning and trying to suppress or limit the powers of a number of local institutions in order to extend its own authority: the powers of *assemblées du pays*, town and village consulats, and *cours présidiales* were reduced or abolished, while new and heavier tailles and gabelles were imposed. In cases of local opposition, brigades of soldiers were lodged in the resisting communities.

Recently, many historians have argued that this type of confrontation between the central government and local communities ceased between 1660 and 1680 as direct taxes were replaced by more subtle, indirect impositions and as intendants began to defend the local communities against the exploitation of seigneurial courts and the exaggerated power of their elites.[7] Crown relations with the local hospitals demonstrate the same patterns of change, albeit not the same chronology. The attitude of the monarchy became less aggressive towards community hospitals, but only after the final rationalization of such institutions between 1693 and 1700. It was not until the 1750s that the full impact of the new policy became apparent.

By the 1760s the commissions and position papers prepared by crown officials had made a radical turnabout and begun to promote the very local relief efforts for the sick and the poor that their predecessors had denounced. This change came on the heels of interventions by Enlightenment writers and physiocrats who had produced scathing assessments of the cost and inefficiency of the hôpitaux-généraux and the other grandiose urban institutions created to intern the sick and the poor. Their critiques influenced royal policy. Local bureaux for the poor and hospitals with three to four beds were seen by the Turgot and Necker regimes to be more efficient and less expensive than the massive urban institutions created during the great confinement. The reversal in crown policy in favour of local charitable institutions followed the pattern established in the 1670s and 1680s of trying to harmonize relations between the central government and local communities. It was a significant change, but ironically, it was made after most local hospitals had been closed – victims of the previous century and a half of absolutist policy.

The eight institutions studied in this book resisted these closings and expropriations, remaining open and following the pattern of about a thousand other local hospitals in the kingdom. They perhaps do not constitute totally representative models of overall community treatment of the sick and the poor in early modern France, but in the route they decided to follow, they were profoundly influenced by a number of larger social forces. In this sense, they become vantage points from which we can observe the workings of these forces, be they urban efforts to push the absolute monarchy into the great confinement, the attempts by members of the second estate to obtain pensions for their services in the army, renewal in church approaches to charity, new women's activities in the field of welfare, or Enlightenment influences on social policy.

Although local hospitals in general may be seen as victims of the early modern historical process, they tell us a great deal about the wider evolution taking place in the social system and in Ancien Régime France as a whole.

All of the eight hospitals studied in this book survived the reorganizations imposed by the Revolution. During the nineteenth and twentieth centuries, their medical services and facilities were often expanded. However, all of them were affected by the renewed centralization of health services undertaken after World War II, particularly since the 1970s. St-Antoine in Pontorson was closed in 1955, and the hospitals in Grignan, Étoile, Caudebec, and Malestroit were transformed into homes for the elderly. Seyne took in the elderly while maintaining limited medical services. Savenay and St-Vallier continued relatively complete hospital services, although both of them are currently resisting new efforts to reform health services and cut back programs offered in small, local hospitals.

At first glance, these new attempts seem to confirm the thesis concerning the long-term, linear decline of small, local institutions in the face of centralization and urbanization.[8] This interpretation, however, loses sight of the fact that all eight hospitals had their facilities and services expanded at different periods between 1789 and the present, just as they did in the seventeenth and eighteenth centuries. The clinics and homes for the elderly and the presence of nurses in the towns in question all constitute a certain maintenance of community services, negotiated step by step with the central government. In the cases of the major hospitals of Savenay and St-Vallier, they constitute proof that communities, by solidly supporting the actions of their hospitals, could enable them to obtain increased services, personnel, and facilities. Through their protests, resistance, and demands for new services, they could even enable their institutions to obtain the status of regional hospitals and benefit from a certain degree of centralization. Just as in the seventeenth and eighteenth centuries, all of these movements were periodic, alternating in their tendency to centralize or regionalize. The experiences of local hospitals in France demonstrate the fact that what some see as the long, inexorable decline of small-town institutions has been marked by numerous halts, reversals in policy, and efforts at rebuilding brought about through local infrastructures and community elites.

Grignan Recteurs des Pauvres, 1661–1722

Date of mandate	Name	Occupation	Service as consul	Taille evaluations		
				1656	1681	1722
1661	Comte de Grignan					
1662	Comte de Grignan					
1663	Comte de Grignan					
1664	Comte de Grignan					
1665	Comte de Grignan					
1666	Comte de Grignan					
1667	Comte de Grignan					
1668	Firmin Salamon	notary	1668	3.72	25.20	
1669	Thomas Pascal	merchant	1673	25.25	22.50	
1670	Jean-Fr. Chambon	bourgeois	1676	54.08	58.35	
1671	Louis Gachon	lieutenant	1697		34.99	
1672	Anthoine Peyron		1671		20.48	
1673	Jacques Boyer	notary	1672		38.95	
1674	J.-P. Machabout		1671		5.55	
1675	Firmin Rivier				8.98	39.58
1676	Louis Fort		1675			
			1683		34.89	
			1691			
1677	Thomas Pascal	merchant	1673	25.25	22.50	
1678	Pierre Janvier				9.52	
1679	Pierre Rondil		1674	2.80	11.39	
1680	Anthoine Dufos		1682		21.74	119.90
1681	Anthoine Romanet	notary	1682		9.64	
1682	Joseph Rivier		1676		4.53	
1683	Louis Chaponton		1682			
1684	Anthoine Sauzet		1683		7.55	
1685	Guill. Poumeyer		1710			
			1719		3.18	

Date of mandate	Name	Occupation	Service as consul	Taille evaluations		
				1656	1681	1722
1686	Jean Sabol	blacksmith			7.50	
1687	Gab. Guintrandi	surgeon	1695			
1688	Anthoine Gourjon				2.75	
1689	Jean Basset				9.28	
1690	Joseph Dumas	notary	1717		2.98	
1691	August. Janvier		1697			
			1724		4.38	
1692	Jean Massot		1706			
1693	Pierre Rivier	blacksmith	1707		4.53	
1694	Pierre Rivier	blacksmith	1707		4.53	
1695	Fran. Bouttin		1728		5.26	
1696	Joseph Cazal	notary	1693		17.43	75.33
1697	Louis Bovery	notary	1694			168.56
1698	Pierre Gachon	doctor	1721			
			1722			96.01
1699	Guill. Poumeyer	notary	1710		7.85	96.75
1700	Joseph Dumas	notary	1717		10.60	57.81
1701	Gab. Guintrandi	surgeon	1695			
1702	Etienne Dubour		1688			25.33
1703	Nicolas Salomon		1706			
			1713			140.53
1704	Louis Fort		1675			
			1683		34.89	
			1691			
1705	Fran. Piallat					96.40
1706	Augustin Janvier	blacksmith	1724			41.69
1707	J.-B. Flachière		1713			
			1715			34.45
1708	Anthoine Martin	blacksmith	1725			13.93
1709	Jean Demar	wine merchant	1701			57.81
1710	Anthoine Jaubert		1692			
1711	Jean Rondil					51.47
1712	Jean Janvier		1716			86.90
1713	Pierre Rivier	blacksmith	1707			
1714	Jos. Meysonnasse	farmer	1717			21.04
1715	Étienne Piallat		1712			28.38
1716	Jean Demar	wine merchant	1701			57.81
1717	Jacques Conde				16.10	27.80
1718	Joseph Dumas	notary	1717		10.60	57.81
1719	Antoine Janvier		1718			115.47
1720	Jacques Boyer	notary			25.60	73.58
1721	Augustin Janvier	blacksmith	1724			41.69
1722	Jacques Rivier		1729			10.25

Note: This list has been drawn up using the Comptes des recteurs de l'Hôpital de Grignan, AD Drôme, 44 H 17, E9 (1656–79), E10 (1680–1700), and E11 (1701–26); the Deliberations of the Grignan consulate, AC Grignan, BB 19 (1668–72), BB 20 (1672–72), BB 21 (1674–1703), BB 22 (1706–17), and BB 23 (1721–40); and the taille rolls for Grignan, AC Grignan, CC 10 (1656), CC 12 (1681), and CC 15 (1722). It should be noted that the average evaluation differed considerably from one roll to another: in 1654 it was 6.71 livres, in 1681 it dropped back to 4.75 livres, and in 1722 it rose to 14.87 livres.

APPENDIX TWO

Seyne Recteurs of the Hospital, 1713–1750

Date of mandate	Name	Occupation	Previous mandates	Service as consul
1713	Antoine Laugier	notary		1695, 1702
1714	Alexandre Isoard	lawyer		1701
1715	Fr.-André Laugier		1721	1712
1716	René-Louis Remusat			1704, 1715
1717	Joseph Ebrard	notary		1716
1718	Gaspard Laugier	bourgeois		1717, 1723
1719	Joseph Rémusat	notary		1718
1720	Jacques Arnaud	doctor	1730	1698, 1719, 1730
1721	Fr.-André Laugier	notary	1715	1712, 1720
1722	Fr.-André Laugier	notary	1715	1712, 1720
1723	Jean-Bap. Salvat	procureur		1721, 1722, 1731
1724	Thérèse Isoard	veuve Lauger		
1725	Louis-And. Savorin	bourgeois		1724, 1738
1726	Pierre Rougon	bourgeois		1725
1728	Jean Juramy	merchant		
1729	Jean Juramy	merchant		
1730	Jacques Arnaud	doctor	1720	1698, 1719, 1730
1731	Jacques Arnaud	doctor	1720	1698, 1719, 1730
1732	Jean-Bap. Salvat	procureur	1723	1721, 1722, 1731
1733	Fr.-André Laugier	procureur	1715,1721	1712, 1720, 1732
1737	Ls.-And. Savournin	bourgeois	1725,1737	1712, 1738, 1747
1739	Jean-Bap. Salvat	procureur	1723,1732	1721, 1722, 1731
1740	Jean-Ant. Chauvet	notary		1739, 1740
1741	Jean-Ant. Chauvet	notary		1739, 1740
1742	Jean-Pierre Tiran	doctor		1726, 1733, 1741
1744	Jean-Pierre Turre	doctor		1742, 1743, 1760

Date of mandate	Name	Occupation	Previous mandates	Service as consul
1745	Jean-Pierre Turrel	doctor		1742, 1743, 1760
1747	Ls.-And. Savournin	bourgeois	1725,1737	1724, 1738, 1747
1748	Ls.-And. Savournin	bourgeois	1725,1737	1724, 1738, 1747
1749	Antoine Martin	merchant		
1750	Gaspard Savournin	notary		1749, 1762

Note: This list has been compiled from the appendix of consuls and mayors of Seyne in Allibert, *Histoire de Seyne*, 2–8, and from the Comptes des recteurs de l'Hôpital, 1713–51, AD Alpes-de-Haute-Provence, 54 H (Hôpital de Seyne), E7 (1713–14) and E8 (1715–50).

Notes

ABBREVIATIONS

AC Archives Communales
AD Archives Départementales
AGSSTV Archives générales des Sœurs de St-Thomas de Villeneuve
AN Archives Nationales, Paris
ASSJ Archives des Sœurs de St-Joseph, St-Vallier
ASSS Archives des Sœurs de St-Sacrement, Valence
BM Bibliothèque Municipale
BN Bibliothèque Nationale, Paris

INTRODUCTION

1 Mollat, "Les premiers hôpitaux," in Imbert, *Histoire des hôpitaux en France*, 15–30.
2 Foucault, *Folie et déraison*, 55–8.
3 Veyne, *Comment on écrit l'histoire*, 203–20.
4 Huppert, "*Divinatio et eruditio*"; Megill, "The Reception of Foucault by Historians."
5 Gutton, "À l'aube du XVIIe siècle"; Gutton, *La société et les pauvres*, 295–300.
6 Fairchilds, *Poverty and Charity in Aix-en-Provence*; Even, "L'assistance et la charité à La Rochelle"; Norberg, *Rich and Poor in Grenoble*; Cugnetti, "L'Hôpital de Grenoble."
7 Jones, *The Charitable Imperative*, 11.

8 Foucault, *Folie et déraison*, 13; Jeorger, "La structure hospitalière."

9 Jeorger, "La structure hospitalière," 1028–33.

10 Jacquart, "Immobilisme et catastrophes, 1560–1660"; Hickey, "Innovation and Obstacles to Growth."

11 Saint-Jacob, *Les paysans de la Bourgogne du Nord*; Poitrineau, *La vie rurale en Basse-Auvergne*.

12 Bouchard, *Le village immobile*, 338–44; Collomp, *La maison du père*, 277–320; Claverie and Lamaison, *L'impossible mariage*, 247–64.

13 Brémond, *Histoire littéraire du sentiment religieux*, vols. 1 and 2; Broutin, *La réforme pastorale en France*.

14 Delumeau, *Le Catholicisme entre Luther et Voltaire*, 256–92; Croix, *La Bretagne aux 16e et 17e siècles*, 2:1211–40.

15 Chill, "Religion and Mendicity in Seventeenth-Century France."

16 Allier, *La cabale des dévots*, chap. 4; Norberg, *Rich and Poor in Grenoble*, 27–64.

17 Châtellier, *La religion des pauvres*, 175–96.

18 Jones, *The Charitable Imperative*, 176.

19 On the question of education, see the contribution by Martine Sonnet in "Une fille à éduquer." This theme is also developed by Elizabeth Rapley in *The Dévotes*.

20 Jones, *The Charitable Imperative*, chaps. 3–5; Vacher, *Des "régulières" dans le siècle*.

21 Paultre, *De la répression de la mendicité*, part 3, chaps. 1 and 2. Léon Lallemand devotes a whole section of his *Histoire de la charité* to legislation concerning beggars and vagabonds and concerning the great confinement; see *Histoire de la charité*, vol. 4, *Les temps modernes*, 139–298.

22 Goubert, *L'Ancien Régime*, vol. 2, *Les pouvoirs*, 79–82 and 94–106.

23 Hufton, *The Poor of Eighteenth-Century France*, 131–76.

24 Imbert, *Le droit hospitalier de l'Ancien Régime*, 95–116.

25 Adams, *Bureaucrats and Beggars*, chap. 8.

26 Hickey, "Closing Down Local Hospitals."

27 M. de la Tour, intendant, to controller general, Marseilles, 4 mars 1777, AN, H 1417.

28 Intendant Bouchu, "Mémoire de la province de Dauphiné," 1698, BM Grenoble, U 908, f. 27.

29 "Révision des feux, 1699," AD Isère, 11 C 321, Étoile, f. 196 verso.

30 "Réponses à l'ordonnance de Le Bret, 1627," AC Grignan, CC 15.

31 Baratier, *La démographie provençale*, 163.

32 Gouhier, Vallez, and Vallez, *Atlas historique de Normandie*, vol. 2, *Institutions, économie, comportements*; see "Rolle des paroisses dont les élections

de la généralité d'Alençon." To translate the *feux* into population figures, I have used the multiple of 4.5 persons per *feux*, which is the generally accepted conversion rate for Normandy and Brittany.

33 État des maisons de l'élection d'Avranches, 1729, Pontorson, AD Calvados, C 293.

34 Gouhier, Vallez, and Vallez, *Atlas historique de Normandie*, vol. 2, *Almanach du département de la Manche pour l'an XI*.

35 Expilly, *Dictionnaire géographique, historique et politique*; cited in Guillemot, "L'Hôpital de Malestroit" (thesis), 1.

36 Hôpital de Savenay, "Historique", AD Loire-Atlantique, Savenay H, depôt 5, H 4.

37 Rôle de capitation, Savenay, 1741, AD Loire-Atlantique, B 3508; Capitation, l'an II, ibid., B 3511.

PART ONE

1 Versoris, *Journal d'un bourgeois de Paris*, 60.

2 "Déclaration portant commission au prévot de Paris de commettre un lieutenant pour visiter les rues, cabarets, lieux publics, et y saisir les vagabonds, gens sans aveu, mendians valides, blasphémateurs et gens surpris en flagrant délit, les conduire dans les prisons du Châtelet pour y en être fait justice," 7 mai 1526; "Édit sur les attributions et la juridiction des prévôts des maréchaux, et sur la punition des vagabonds et gens sans aveu," 25 janvier 1536; "Déclaration portant que les mendians valides seront employés par les prévôts des marchands et échevins de Paris à travailler aux ouvrages publics", 16 janvier 1545; in Isambert, *Recueil général des anciennes lois françaises*, 12:269–72, 531–3, 900–2.

CHAPTER ONE

1 Maître, *L'assistance publique dans la Loire-Inférieure*, 197.

2 Ibid.

3 Maître, *Histoire administrative des anciens hôpitaux de Nantes*, 72–3.

4 Natalie Davis, "Poor Relief, Humanism and Heresy," in N. Davis, *Society and Culture in Early Modern France*, 17–24, 38–9; Bataillon, "J.L. Vivès, réformateur de la bienfaisance."

5 Paultre, *De la répression de la mendicité*, 123–5, and Geremek, *La potence ou la pitié*, 203–6.

6 Panel, *Documents concernant les pauvres de Rouen*, 1:16.

7 Ibid., 1:41.

8 Among the numerous contributions to the history of changing perspectives on early modern poor relief, see Natalie Davis, "Poor Relief, Humanism and Heresy," in N. Davis, *Society and Culture in Early Modern France*, 42–8; Kingdon, "Social Welfare in Calvin's Geneva"; B.B. Davis, "Poverty and Poor Relief in Sixteenth-Century Toulouse"; Mentzer, "Organizational Endeavor and Charitable Impulse."

9 Acte de fondation, 1450, Hôpital de Savenay, AD Loire-Atlantique, Savenay H, dépôt 5, A 1. See the text of the act in Maître, *L'assistance publique dans la Loire-Inférieure*, 191–5.

10 Droguet, "La municipalisation des hôpitaux St. Nicolas."

11 X. Martin, "La part du corps de ville dans la gestion de l'Hôtel-Dieu d'Angers."

12 N. Davis, "Poor Relief, Humanism and Heresy," in N.Z. Davis, *Society and Culture in Early Modern France*, 19–20.

13 Imbert, "L'Église et l'État face au problème hospitalier."

14 "Édit attribuant aux baillis, sénéchaux et autres juges la surveillance de l'administration des hôpitaux et maladeries," Fontainebleau, 19 décembre 1543, in Isambert, *Recueil général des anciennes lois françaises*, 12:841–3.

15 Ibid., 842–3.

16 "Édit ordonnant que tous administrateurs d'hôpitaux seront tenus de rendre compte aux prochains juges des lieux ...," in Isambert, *Recueil général des anciennes lois françaises*, 12:897–900.

17 "Édit qui enjoint aux baillis, sénéchaux et autres juges d'établir dans les hôpitaux de leur ressort des commissaires administrateurs, et qui attribue à ceux-ci la connaissance des procès en cette matière," Rochefort, 26 février 1546, in Isambert, *Recueil général des anciennes lois françaises*, 12:920. Roger Doucet saw this edict, which was repeated in 1561, as resulting in the placement of all hospitals in France under the supervision of laymen; see Doucet, *Les institutions de la France au XVIe siècle*, 2:808.

18 The Edict of Fontainebleau was repeated on 19 May and 17 June 1544, 26 February 1546, 12 February 1553, 25 July 1560, December 1560, April 1561, July 1566, and in 1579. The Edict of St-Germain-en-Laye was modified in that of Rochefort on 26 February 1546, encouraging baillis and sénéchaux to establish commissioners in their jurisdictions to carry out the visits and reforms of the maladreries and hôpitaux.

19 Chalumeau, "L'assistance aux malades pauvres au XVIIe siècle," 81.

20 *Plaidoyez de Maître Claude Expilly, chevalier conseiller du roy en son Conseil d'État et président au Parlement de Grenoble* (Grenoble: Chez Laurent Durand, 1636); cited in Favier, "L'Église et l'assistance en Dauphiné sous l'Ancien Régime," 448.

21 Hickey, *Le Dauphiné devant la monarchie absolue*, and Gascon, "Immigration et croissance urbaine au XVIe siècle."

22 "Ordonnance sur la reforme de la justice," Moulins, février 1566, in Isambert, *Recueil général des anciennes lois françaises*, 14:209.

23 Ibid., 210–11.

24 Favier, "L'Église et l'assistance en Dauphiné sous l'Ancien Régime," 449.

25 Cloulas, "Les aliénations du temporel ecclésiastique sous Charles IX et Henri III."

26 AD Isère, B 2261, f. 62–9 et 76–7.

27 *Plaidoyez de Maître Claude Expilly, chevalier conseiller du roy au son Conseil d'État et président au Parlement de Grenoble*, 1636; cited in Favier, "L'Église et l'assistance en Dauphiné sous l'Ancien Régime," 448.

28 Basque, "L'assistance aux pauvres dans le Dauphiné rural," 44.

29 Le Grand, "Comment composer l'histoire d'un établissement hospitalier," 161–9.

30 "Testament de Guillaume de Poitiers, 1545," AC Étoile, AI.

31 "Historique de l'Hôpital la Charité" [seventeenth century], AC Étoile, B5–6, doc. B9.

32 "Contenu de la Charité, 29 décembre 1749," ibid., doc. B7.

33 Fillet, "Grignan religieux," 14:165–6.

34 Ibid., 14:166–9.

35 "Acte d'établissement d'un concierge à l'Hôpital de Grignan, 1664," AD Drôme, 44 H 23, FI.

36 "Comptes du rectorat de M. le Compte, 1664," AD Drôme, 44 H 17, E9/12, and "Comptes du rectorat de M. le Compte, 1645," ibid., E9/13.

37 "Règlements de l'hôpital de Grignan et additions aux règlements, 1676," AD Drôme, 44 H 11, E/2, and "Délibérations du Bureau de la charité," Grignan, 13 septembre 1676, ibid., E/1.

38 Allibert, *Histoire de Seyne*, 405–9.

39 Caise, *Histoire de Saint-Vallier*, 236.

40 Copy of the délibérations of 7 January 1683 of the Confrérie de la Charité; Délibérations of the Hotel-Dieu, Vienne, au sujet de la fondation de l'Hôpital de St-Vallier, 7 January 1683; MS. "Historique de l'Hôpital de St-Vallier," boîte "Hôpital de St. Vallier," ASSJ, 19–34.

41 Font-Reaulx, "L'Hôpital de Saint-Vallier," 319–21.

42 "Historique de l'Hôpital de Saint Vallier," boîte "Hôpital de St. Vallier," ASSJ, 22–3.

43 See Registre de la Confrérie de la Charité, 7 Janvier 1683; "Premier acte de fondation faict par Mr l'Abbé de St-Vallier, évêque de Québec en faveur des sœurs de St-Joseph servant les pauvres à l'hôpital établi à

St-Vallier, extrait des mémoires de Sœur Jeanne Burdier de l'Hôpital-Dieu de Vienne," ASSJ.

44 Registre des pièces les plus anciens de l'hôpital de Caudebec, no. 5, AD Seine-Maritime, 113 HP UI.

45 Compte des recettes et dépenses des chapelles St-Pierre, St-Maur, St-Julien et Ste-Anne, hôtel-Dieu et bureau des pauvres de Caudebec, 1612–44, AD Seine-Maritime, 113 HP E6.

46 Registre contenant l'analyse succincte des pièces les plus anciennes de l'hôpital (aujourd'hui égarés), AD Seine-Maritime, 113 HP UI.

47 Ibid.

48 Régime des hôpitaux, Caudebec, 1786, AD Seine-Maritime, 1 B 5514.

49 Ibid.

50 Cahier "ancienneté de l'hôpital," AD Manche, Hôpital de Pontorson, séries 2, 2.

51 Ibid. On St-Antoine of Pontorson, see the excellent thesis by Hélène Avisseau-Roussat, published under the title "L'Hôpital Saint-Antoine de la Charité de Pontorson (1644–1792)."

52 Cahier "ancienneté de l'hôpital," AD Manche, Hôpital de Pontorson, série 2, ff. 3–4.

53 Ibid.

54 Contrat entre frères de la charité et les habitants de Pontorson, 16 octobre 1644, AD Manche, Hôpital de Pontorson, A 1.

55 Procès-verbal faict de l'estat des lieux de l'hôpital, 25 October 1644, AD Manche, Hôpital de Pontorson, A 5.

56 Acte de fondation, 1450, Hôpital de Savenay, AD Loire-Atlantique, H Savenay, dépôt 5, A 1. See the text of the act in Maître, *L'assistance publique dans la Loire-Inférieure*, 191–5.

57 Ibid., article v, 192.

58 Historique de l'hôpital, 1439–1956, AD Loire-Atlantique, H Savenay, dépôt 5, H 4.

59 Maître, *L'assistance publique dans la Loire-Inférieure*, 197.

60 Rosenzweig, "L'Hôpital de Malestroit," 1–2.

61 Guillemot, "L'Hôpital de Malestroit" (thesis), 14.

62 Guillemot, "L'Hôpital de Malestroit," *Revue d'histoire économique et sociale*, 487.

63 Ibid., 508.

64 Ibid., 491–501.

65 Table 1 was created using data from Comptes des recettes et depenses, Chappelles Saint-Pierre, Saint-Maur, Saint-Julien et Sainte-Anne, Hôtel-Dieu et Bureau des pauvres de Caudebec, 1612–44, AD Seine-Maritime

113 HP E6; Avisseau-Roussat, "L'Hôpital Saint-Antoine de la Charité," 6, no 22:34; Comptes de l'Hôpital de Malestroit, AD Morbihan, 7 HS, E6, nos 29–36; Notes historiques sur l'Hôpital de Savenay, AD Loire-Atlantique, H Savenay, dépôt 5, H4; Comptes de l'Hôpital de Grignan, AD Drôme, 44 H 17, E4–6; Comptes de l'Hôpital de l'Étoile, 1600–30, AC Étoile, E7–21; Comptes de l'Hôpital de Seyne, AD Alpes-de-Haute-Provence, 54 H (Seyne), E1; also Croix, *La Bretagne aux 16e et 17e siècles*, 1:631.

66 Marchal, *Le droit d'oblat*, 72–77.

67 Bois, "Le vieillard dans la France moderne," 76–7.

68 Marchal, *Le droit d'oblat*, 59–61. For a more critical assessment of this practice, see Voitel-Grenon, "La Chambre de la generalle reformation des hopitaux," 150–1.

69 Marchal, *Le droit d'oblat*, 61–5.

70 Robert Chaboche has provided a very detailed study of handicapped soldiers during the Thirty Years War, and there is no reason to believe that the problem was less envident during the Wars of Religion; see Chaboche, "Les soldats français de la Guerre de Trente Ans."

71 Guérin, "Une tentative de reforme militaire et hospitalière, 1672–1693," 110.

72 Lot, *Recherches sur les effectifs des armées françaises*, 186 and 190.

73 Major, "Bellièvre, Sully, and the Assembly of Notables of 1596," 14–15.

74 Ibid., 15.

75 Chaboche, "Le sort des militaires invalides avant 1674," 130; Marchal, *Le droit d'oblat*, 74–9.

76 In his *Oeconomies*, Sully noted the reasons for this royal intervention: "le roy n'estimant pas que des capitaines mal payez, des soldats négligez … portassent jamais grande aimitié à ceux qui les emploieraient, … se résolut de préparer des moyens pour les souldoyer suffisament, et leur subvenir en leurs nécessitez, playes et maladies" (1604); in Sully, "Mémoires des sages et royales oeconomies," 1:4.

77 Édit du Roy pour la création de la Maison de la charité chrétienne, Paris, juillet 1604, AN, MM 233.

78 Edict du Roy faict en faveur des pauvres gentilhommes … Paris, juin 1606, AN, AD+ 141, pièce 4, pp. 7–8.

79 The names of the four *conseillers au Grand conseil* are not indicated in the edict, but they are listed on the first page of "Premier registre de la Chambre de la charité chrétienne," samedi, 5 août 1606, AN, V7 148. The increasingly important role of the grand aumônier in the organization of poor relief is underlined by Le Grand in "Comment composer l'histoire

d'un établissement hospitalier," 218–22, and by Portal in "Le grand aumônier de France."

80 "Premier registre de la Chambre de la charité chrétienne," AN, V7, 10–11.

81 Ibid., 12–13.

82 Minutes des enquêtes, 1607, AN, V7 126, 216 folios; 1609, AN, V7 127, 220 folios.

83 Registre d'audience de la Chambre de la charité, août 1606 à décembre 1607, AN, V7 148. This document was analysed by Marc Pître, who has prepared a thesis on the Chambre de la Charité Chretienne under my direction; see Pitre, "Henri IV et la Chambre de la Charité Chrétienne."

84 See François de la Barre vs l'Hôpital de Donzy, 19 novembre 1609, AN, V7 127; and Leonard Conault vs le prieur de Notre-Dame de Jorgny, 31 Mars 1609, AN, V7 127, f. 71

85 Corvisier, "Anciens soldats oblats, mortes-payés et mendiants," 13–14.

86 Ibid., 23.

87 Arrêt de Louis XIII, 1 septembre 1611, AN, AD+ 152.

88 Lettres patentes sur la réformation generalle des hôpitaux, hôtels-Dieu, maladreries et autres lieux pitoyables du Royaume, 24 octobre 1612, AN, AD 14, 1.

89 Chevalier, "Le diocèse de Die en l'année 1644," 83, 116–17, 138, 154, 156, 164, 170.

CHAPTER TWO

1 In the absence of Cachod's report, its principal findings can be reconstituted from the replies written by André Serret, *recteur moderne* of the Étoile hospital; see Sieur André Serret contre les chevaliers de St Jean de Jerusalem, 7 janvier 1681 and 17 juin 1681, AC Étoile, E 38.

2 Jean-Guy Basset, juge royal of Grenoble and subdélégué de la chambre royale, 13 mars 1681, AC Étoile, E 38.

3 Le Grand has noted that this inquiry produced some of the most critical archives for reconstituting the history of local hospitals in France; see Le Grand, "Comment composer l'histoire d'un établissement hospitalier," 192–200.

4 Petit, *L'Assemblée des notables de 1626–27*, 142.

5 Richet, *La France moderne*, 71–7 and 108–14.

6 Beik, *Absolutism and Society in Seventeenth-Century France*, esp. chaps. 10 and 11.

7 "Édit du roi en faveur de l'Ordre de Notre-Dame de Mont-Carmel et de St Lazare de Jérusalem," décembre 1672, AN, M 41, p. 5.

8 Dissard, *La réforme des hôpitaux et maladreries au XVIIe siècle*, 72–7. For the general context of this reform, see Jones, *The Charitable Imperative*, 41–2. This edict repeated an earlier one of 18 May 1669 in which Louis XIV confirmed the fusion of the two orders and ordered that a general chapter be held to draw up statutes and regulations for the new order. See "Extrait des registres du Grand conseil qui porte l'enregistrement des privilèges des chevaliers de l'Ordre Royal de Notre-Dame du Mont-Carmel et de St-Lazare," 18 mai 1669, AN, M 41, no 11, pp. 21–6. On the order in Normandy, see Mutel, "Recherches sur l'Ordre de Saint-Lazare de Jérusalem en Normandie."

9 Dissard, *La réforme des hôpitaux et maladreries au XVIIe siècle*, 6.

10 "Commissions … en exécution de l'Édit de décembre 1672," 7 février and 8 mars 1673, AN, M 41, no 12, 12–15. These directives named the members of a commission to oversee the transfer of the holdings of the Order of St-Esprit to the Order of St-Lazare.

11 Dissard, *La réforme des hôpitaux et maladreries au XVIIe siècle*, 72–4; R. Baillargeat, ed., *Les Invalides, trois siècles d'histoire*; Bois, "Les anciens soldats dans la société française au XVIIIe siècle"; Guérin, "Une tentative de réforme militaire et hospitalière, 1672–1693," 132–8 (I am indebted to Colin Jones for bringing the Guérin thesis to my attention).

12 Dissard, *La réforme des hôpitaux et maladreries au XVIIe siècle*, 76.

13 "Édit du Roi en faveur de l'Ordre de Notre-Dame du Mont-Carmel et de Saint Lazare de Jérusalem, décembre 1672," AN, MM 233, f. 6.

14 "Commission pour l'établissement de la Chambre Royale," 8 février 1673, AN, M 41, no 12, 10–12.

15 Norberg, *Rich and Poor in Grenoble*, 65–80.

16 "Mémoires servant de réponse à Mrs les Commissaires du Conseil concernant l'Ordre de St Lazare," AN, MM 223.

17 "Edict du Roi en faveur de l'Ordre de Notre-Dame du Mont-Carmel et de St-Lazare," décembre 1672, AN, M 41, no 12, 4.

18 "Édit du Parlement de Grenoble ordonnant que tous les hôpitaux, leproseries et maladreries de la Commanderie de Valence de l'Ordre de Saint-Esprit soient réunis à l'Ordre de Notre Dame de Mont-Carmel et de St Lazare, 1 mars 1678," in *Recueil des édits et déclarations du roy*, 2, doc. 98.

19 "Ordre de St Lazare, Pouille ou Recueil Général de toutes les maladreries du Royaume, hôpitaux, hôtels-dieu, aumôneries et avec leurs prix, 1682," AN, MM 219.

20 Dissard, *La réforme des hôpitaux et maladreries au XVIIe siècle*, 75.

21 Dupâquier, *Histoire de la population française*, 2:75–80.

22 Guérin, "Une tentative de réforme militaire et hospitalière," 406–8 and 524.

23 The close links between the *dévots* and the Company of the Holy Sacrament in the founding of the general hospitals is clearly demonstrated in the case of the Grenoble hospital; see Kathryn Norberg, *Rich and Poor in Grenoble*, 27–64.

24 Foucault, *Folie et déraison*, 57–63 and 76–81; Gutton, "À l'aube du xviie siècle," 87–97, and *La société et les pauvres*, 85–122.

25 Gutton, *La société et les pauvres*, 295–302 and 326–50.

26 On the debate over the change to more practically oriented welfare, see Callahan, "Corporate Charity in Spain"; N. Davis, "Poor Relief, Humanism and Heresy," in N. Davis, *Society and Culture*, 39–52; Gutton, *La société et les pauvres*, 215–46.

27 Chill, "Religion and Mendicity in Seventeenth-Century France."

28 Norberg, *Rich and Poor in Grenoble*, 170–1.

29 Édit, 12 juin 1662, in Isambert, *Recueil général des anciennes lois françaises*, 18:18–23.

30 Lettre aux évêques pour l'établissement d'un hôpital-général en chaque ville, 1676, AN, MM 227.

31 Déclaration du Roi en faveur des hôpitaux généraux et hôtels-Dieu du Royaume, Versailles, 24 mars 1674, AN, M 41, no 14, 1 and 2.

32 Imbert, *Le droit hospitalier de l'Ancien Régime*, 99.

33 Gutton, *La société et les pauvres*, 394–5.

34 Joret, "Le P. Guévarre et les bureaux de charité au xviie siècle."

35 Ibid., 356.

36 Ibid.

37 Ibid., 357.

38 Ibid.

39 Chaurand to Calloët-Querbrat, secrétaire de l'Assemblée charitable de Paris, Morlaix, 22 avril 1678, BN, Coll. Morel de Thoisy, mss. 319, ff. 58–66.

40 See the justification of the Franciscan method in "Avis ... ces confréries et hôpitaux ne doivent rien demander ...," 1670, in BN, Coll. Morel de Thoisy, mss. 319, ff. 52–4.

41 In fact, during Chaurand's missionary activities in the years 1677–82, 38 hôpitaux or bureaux de charité were founded, of which 24 obtained letters patent. By the end of the seventeenth century, 44 hôpitaux-généraux had been set up in the province. This information comes from meetings with Jean-Luc and Guylène Bruzulier, who are completing theses on the general-hospital movement in Brittany; see the forthcoming

thesis by Jean-Luc Bruzulier, "Les pauvres, les pouvoirs et l'assistance: Les hôpitaux-généraux en Bretagne, 1676–1724."

42 *Reglemens des assemblées politiques de charité des paroisses, suivant les ordonnances de nos Rois ... lesquelles assemblées ont esté établies dans toutes les paroisses de Bretagne ...*, AN, AD 14, 2, p. I. (I am indebted to Jean-Luc Bruzulier for sending me a photocopy of this document.)

43 Ibid., 5–16.

44 Ibid., 16–31.

45 *La mendicité abolie dans le diocèse d'Aix par l'établissement d'un hôpital général ou d'une maison de charité en chaque ville et gros bourg et par un bureau de charité en chaque lieu ou l'on ne pouvait pas enfermer les pauvres. Avec la response aux principales objections que l'on peut faire contre ces établissements* (Aix, n.d. [1687]), Bibliothèque Ingebertine, Carpentras, 13 024.

46 Ibid., 51–62.

47 Dissard, *La réforme des hôpitaux et maladreries au XVIIe siècle*, 79–82.

48 Hôpital de l'Étoile, Comptes, 1682, AC Étoile C 44.

49 "Ordre de St. Lazare, Poullie, 1682,: AN, MM 219, Grenoble, f. 224, Die, f. 226, Valence, f. 253, and Senez, f. 256.

50 Sieur André Serret, recteur moderne de l'Hôpital de l'Étoile contre l'Ordre de St-Lazare, 7 janvier 1681, AC Étoile, E 38.

51 Sieur André Serret, recteur moderne de l'hôpital de l'Étoile contre Monseigneurs le Grand Vicaire-général, Commandeurs et Chevaliers de l'Ordre de Notre Dame de Mont Carmel et de St Lazare de Jérusalem, 17 juin 1681, ibid.

52 See the report on the case by Sieur Rouillé du Coudray, delivered before the Chamber of the Arsenal, 17 March 1683, AN, Z I N 24, and the report on a second hearing, which maintained the initial judgment, 28 March 1685, AN, Z I N 26. A third hearing was accorded on 19 August 1686, which again upheld the initial judgment; see AN, Z I N 27.

53 Accounts by Jean-Antoine Point, Hôpital de l'Étoile, AC Étoile, E 44, f. 104.

54 "Ordre de St. Lazare, Poullie, 1682," AN, M 46 Grand prieuré de Bretagne, ff. 142–9.

55 Pouille des biens, hôpitaux, maisons et revenus de l'Ordre régulier du Saint-Esprit de Montpellier [Paris, n.d.], AN, M 46, ff. 30–59.

56 Judgement on Savenay, 19 June 1674, AN, Z 7607; cited in Maître, *L'assistance publique dans la Loire-Inférieure*, 199.

57 Arrêt de la Chambre de la réformation des hôpitaux, 26 janvier 1677, AN, S 4857.

58 Hôpital de Malestroit, comptes de Julien Garson, 1672–75, AD Morbihan, 7 HS6 (Malestroit), E6, no 48.

59 Guillemot, "L'Hôpital de Malestroit," *Revue d'histoire économique et sociale*, 438 and 496.

60 Dissard, *La réforme des hôpitaux et maladreries au XVIIe siècle*, 109–11.

61 From the very beginning of the "reform," the Vatican had opposed the transfer of foundations belonging to the traditional hospitaller orders. Father Coquelin had been sent to Rome in 1672 and 1673 to try to negotiate this question with the pope, but the mission was a failure. The Vatican insisted that the issue be addressed in negotiating the Régale, and again in 1687 the Marquis de Chamlay tried to negotiate a settlement with the new pope, Innocent XII, under which the 1672 edict could be maintained. This second failure seems to have led Louis XIV to envisage rescending the edict. On this question, see Guérin, "Une tentative de réforme militaire et hospitalière," 352–78, 489–502, and 513.

62 Ibid., 485–507. Guérin notes that among the twelve commissioners, Louis XIV appointed his chancellor, two ministers of state, and eminent jurists, but he also named partisans of Louvois, such as Boucherat and Pelletier, as well as his ennemies, including du Pussort.

63 Mémoire pour résoudre les difficultés des commissaires préposés à l'examen de l'édit de 1672, BN, MS. 20332, f. 232.

64 Claire Guérin has analysed in detail the arguments of each of the Chamlay reports; see Guérin, "Une tentative de réforme militaire et hospitalière," 489–99.

65 "Édit de désunion de l'Ordre de Mont Carmel et de St Lazare," mars 1693, AN, F 15.

66 "Déclaration du 24 août 1693," AN, AD 14, 2. See the explanations of this document in Dissard, *La réforme des hôpitaux et maladreries au XVIIe siècle*, 127–30.

67 Even as the St-Lazare reform was proceeding, the activity of the dévots was evident. Huguenot consistories and their holdings, including a certain number of rural hospitals in such places as Nyons, were suppressed and their revenues transferred to the new urban general hospitals such as Grenoble; see Norberg, *Rich and Poor in Grenoble*, 79. In addition, in 1676 the king ordered that French bishops aid the new hôpitaux-généraux by suppressing and expropriating the funds of poorly managed rural poor-relief institutions in the cases where their holdings has not already been given over to another organization; see Dissard, *La réforme des hôpitaux et maladreries au XVIIe siècle*, 119–20.

68 Jones, *The Charitable Imperative*, 41.

CHAPTER THREE

1 The maladreries in question were Fécamp, Contremoulins de Marolles, Mesmoulins, St-Nicolas d'Etretat, Senneville, Bec-de-Mortagne, and Froberville.

2 Réunion des administrateurs des hôpitaux de Coudebec, Fécamp, Saint Romain de Colbuse et Montivilliers, 23–25 mai, 3 and 10 octobre 1697, AD Seine-Maritime, 113 HP, A3 cahier 5.

3 Déclaration du Roy en interprétation de l'édit du mois de mars 1693, Versailles, 15 avril 1693, AD Ille-et-Vilaine, C 1265.

4 Déclaration du Roy en interprétation de l'Édit de mars 1693 et de la déclaration du 15 avril suivant, Versailles, 24 août 1693, AD Ille-et-Vilaine, C 1265.

5 Mémoire pour messieurs les Archevêques & Évesques, Intendans & Commissaires départis dans les provinces ... concernant l'exécution de l'Édit du mois de mars 1693 & des déclarations du 15 avril & 24 aoust 1693, AD Ille-et-Vilaine, C 1265; Édit du Roi portant nomination des commissaires par sa majesté pour l'exécution de l'Édit du mois de mars & de la déclaration du 15 avril 1693, dans *Estat général des unions faites des biens et revenus des maladreries, léproseries, aumôneries*, annexe 4.

6 This map has been drawn up from data presented in the *Estat général des unions faites des biens et revenus des maladreries, léproseries, aumôneries*.

7 Ibid. No information is given in that source for the dioceses of Digne and Sénez.

8 Dénombrement des hôpitaux, maladreries et aumôneries de Dauphiné ... avec leurs revenues dressé par diocèse, février 1692, BM Grenoble, R80, p. 532.

9 The names of the maîtres de requêtes or conseillers d'État are noted for each act adopted in the Conseil d'État. The acts for thirty-three hospitals in Dauphiné are contained in the correspondance of the Parlement of Grenoble, all dated October 1696; see AD Isère, B 2363, f. 90–126.

10 This map has been reproduced from Favier, "Enfermement et assistance aux villages en Dauphiné au XVIIIe siècle," 2.

11 Vaganet, "Pouvoir et notabilité à Nyons, 1692–1768," 91–3.

12 Assignations données pour le paiement à l'hôpital de Valence, 1705, Archives de l'Hôpital de Valence, III B 3.

13 "État des biens et revenus de l'hôpital de l'Étoile ... pour satisfaire la déclaration du 11 février 1764," AD Drôme, C293.

14 For the généralité of Rouen, d'Ormesson is mentioned in an act concerning the Hôtel-Dieu of Rouen; see AN, St-Lazare, Z 1 N/33. For Caen,

see Le Cacheux, *Essai historique sur l'Hôtel-Dieu de Coutances*, 1st section, *L'Hôtel-Dieu 1209–1789*, 193.

15 Vaudreuil, 4 mars 1700, AD Seine-Maritime, 1 B 5513.

16 This map has been drawn up from data obtained from several sources: "Suppressions et réunions d'hospices après l'Édit de 1693," 22 octobre 1694, AD Seine-Maritime, 1 B 5513; "Hôpitaux et maladreries," AD Calvados, 1 B 5513–16; "Intendance: villes avec fondations qui pourraient être réuni aux hôpitaux," 1724–25, AD Ille-et-Vilaine, C 1285; Léchaudé-d'Anisy, "Recherches sur les léproseries et maladreries," 149–212; Le Cacheux, *Essai historique sur l'Hôtel-Dieu de Coutances*, 193 and 211; Lecanu, *Histoire du diocèse de Coutances et d'Avranches*, 2:16–19 and 27.

17 Intendance, Lettres patentes de réunions, Fécamp, 1697, AD Seine-Maritime, 113 HP A3. See also A. Martin, *L'Hôtel-Dieu de Fécamp*, 9–10.

18 Transactions concernant la réunion de diverses maladreries, 1695–1705, Archives de l'Hôpital de Caudebec, AD Seine-Maritime, 113 HP A3.

19 Procès de l'Hôpital de Bernay contre l'Hôpital d'Orbec, 1708–1710, AD Calvados, H Supp 1321 (Hôpital d'Orbec), A4.

20 Jones, *The Charitable Imperative*, 42.

21 On the creation of these hôpitaux-généraux, see Croix, *La Bretagne aux 16e et 17e siècles*, 2:672–84; Gutton, *L'État et la mendicité*, 87–103; Schwartz, *Policing the Poor*, 34–92; Norberg, *Rich and Poor in Grenoble*, 86–92; Fairchilds, *Poverty and Charity in Aix-en-Provence*, 101–15.

22 "Déclaration du 18 juillet 1724 concernant les mendiants et vagabonds," Chantilly, 18 juillet 1724; see text in Gutton, *L'État et la mendicité*, 225–30.

23 Gutton, *L'État et la mendicité*, 29.

24 Ibid., 26. See also "Édit du Roi portant suppression de tous les officiers archers des maréchaussées et établissement de nouvelles compagnies de maréchaussée dans toute l'étendue du royaume," mars 1720, AD Loire-Atlantique, B 402.

25 Schwartz, *Policing the Poor*, 59.

26 Gutton, *L'État et la mendicité*, 87–103.

27 Gutton, *La société et les pauvres*, 489.

28 Schwartz, *Policing the poor*, 209–22.

29 Cameron, *Crime and Repression in the Auvergne and the Guyenne*. A number of historians have questioned the efficiency of the constabulary, an "outside" force, in dealing with local communities, but it must be remembered that its work in incarcerating the poor was more clearly defined, and as Schwartz argues, it was frequently in the interest of the rural communities. For those who debate the incapacity of the constabulary, see N. Castan, *Justice et répression en Languedoc* and *Les criminels de*

Languedoc; Y. Castan, "Mentalités rurales et urbaines à la fin de l'Ancien Régime"; and LeGoff and Sutherland, "The Revolution and the Rural Community in Eighteenth Century Brittany."

30 These inquiries seem to have been translated into questionnaires distributed to the hospitals in 1721 and 1723. The first round asked each intendant to supply information on the institutions of his généralité, indicating (1) the number of hospitals and beds, (2) the characteristics of each institution and the restrictions placed upon it, such as receiving only local inhabitants, only soldiers, or only one sex, and (3) the financing of the hospital. Under Dodun the questionaire of 21 August 1723 was simpler, probably because the replies from the earlier inquiry had already supplied most of the required information. The new questionaire sought only to know the number of hospitals in each province and their responsibilities and revenues, seemingly with the goal of establishing three classes of institutions. See Jeorger, "Les enquêtes hospitalières au xviiie siècle," 52–3.

31 Gutton, *L'État et la mendicité*, 50.

32 Ibid. Muriel Jeorger has noted that this request for information was limited strictly to evaluating the capacity of each hospital to intern the beggars and vagabonds to be arrested under the new law; see Jeorger, "Les enquêtes hospitalières au xviiie siècle," 53.

33 "Mémoire sur les établissements faits dans la province de Dauphiné pour le renfermer les mendiants," 18 juillet 1724, BN, Ms.fr. 8468, ff. 114–18.

34 Schwartz, *Policing the Poor*, 63.

35 Richer, Intendant, à Monsieur le Régent, 12 mai 1720, AD Calvados, c 596.

36 "Augmentations proposés pour les bâtiments des Hôpitaux de Caen ...," 1720, AD Calvados, c 596.

37 De la Granville to Dodun, 7 août 1724, AD Puy-de-Dôme, c 1046; cited in Gutton, *L'État et la mendicité*, 51.

38 Dodun to de la Granville, 2 septembre 1724, AD Puy-de-Dôme, c 1047; cited in Gutton, *L'État et la mendicité*, 51.

39 Gutton, *L'État et la mendicité*, 54.

40 "Instruction concernant l'exécution de la déclaration des mendiants," 24 juillet 1724; cited in Gutton, *L'État et la Mendicité*, appendix.

41 Gutton, *L'État et la mendicité*, 72.

42 Délibérations, Consulate of Grignan, 18 avril 1724, AC Grignan, BB 23, f. 63.

43 Ibid., 27 décembre 1724.

44 Ibid., 23 août 1726, f. 91.

45 Gutton, *L'État et la mendicité*, 75.

46 Jeorger, "Les enquêtes hospitalières," 53.

47 Mémoire concernant la vingt-quatrième partie due aux pauvres des paroisses sur toutes les dixmes, n.d. [1724], AD Isère, II c 1001; cited in Favier, "L'Église et l'assistance en Dauphiné sous l'Ancien Régime," 460.

48 Favier, "L'Église et l'assistance en Dauphiné sous l'Ancien Régime," 461.

49 Mémoire concernant la vingt-quatrième partie due aux pauvres, n.d. [1724], AD Isère, II c 1001.

50 Mémoire sur les établissements faits dans la province de Dauphiné pour renfermer les mendiants, 1724, BN, Ms.fr. 8468, ff. 137–46.

51 Favier, "L'Église et l'assistance en Dauphiné sous l'Ancien Régime," 461–2.

52 Subdélégué à l'Intendant, Quimperlé, 1724, AD Ille-et-Vilaine, c 1289.

53 Intendance; villes avec fondations qu'on pourrait réunir aux hôpitaux, 1724–25, AD Ille-et-Vilaine, c 1285.

54 Fondations qui peuvent être réuni, 1724–25, AD Ille-et-Vilaine, c 1285.

55 Hôpitaux de Bretagne avec gages et augmentations, juillet 1727, AD Ille-et-Vilaine, c 1285.

56 Gutton, *L'État et la mendicité*, 72–3.

57 Chapalain-Nougaret, *Misère et assistance dans le pays de Rennes au XVIIIe siècle*, 201.

58 Ibid.

59 Ibid., 202–7, and Poulet, "Pauvreté, mendicité et assistance de l'État en Bretagne au XVIIIe siècle," 40–8.

60 Chapalain-Nougaret, *Misère et assistance dans le pays de Rennes au XVIIIe siècle*, 206.

61 Registre des dépenses pour la restauration de l'hospice de Caudebec (1685) and lettres patentes pour la transfert de l'hôpital, mois d'octobre 1693, AD Seine-Maritime, 113 HP, E23.

62 Registres d'entrées, sorties et morts commençant le 15 septembre 1705 et finissant le 21 septembre 1717, ibid., F1.

63 Hôpital de Caudebec, Registre des admissions, 1 janvier 1724–30 août 1724, ibid.

64 Registre des entrées et sorties, Hôpital de Caudebec, 17 février 1716, ibid.

65 Registre des entrées et sorties, Hôpital de Caudebec, 28 avril 1717, ibid.

66 Registre des entrées et sorties, Hôpital de Caudebec, 1718, ibid.

67 Registre des entrées et sorties, Hôpital de Caudebec, février et avril 1724, ibid.

68 Hôpital général de Caudebec, Registre des entrées, 1 septembre–30 décembre 1724, ibid., F2.

69 Hôpital de Caudebec, comptes de Narin Barin, 1 mars 1700–31 décembre 1708, ibid., E9; comptes de Guillaume Née, 1709–20, ibid., E11; comptes de 1721–23, ibid., E11.

70 Hôpital de Caudebec, comptes de Vivien Nicollet, maréchal, 1724–28, ibid., E11; comptes de Louis Pascal Falloppe, 1728, 1729, 1730, ibid., E16.

71 Hôpital de Caudebec, comptes de Vivien Nicollet, 1724–28, ibid., E11.

72 These statistics are derived from comparisons between the statistics on inmates in the Caudebec hospital admissions and the budgets of the hospital in the accounts; see Registres d'entrée, Hôpital de Caudebec, 1724, ibid., F2, and 1728 and 1730, ibid., F3; see also Comptes, Hôpital de Caudebec, 1724 par Vivien Nicollet, ibid., E11, and 1728 and 1730 par Louis Pascal Falloppe, ibid., E16.

73 Registres d'entrée, Hôpital de Caudebec, 1732, ibid., F3; Comptes, Hôpital de Caudebec, 1732 par Louis Pascal Falloppe, ibid., E16.

74 Robert Schwartz shows that Avranches received 3,306 livres in 1727, 5,426 in 1728, and 2,750 in 1732, compared to Carentan with 2,937 in 1727, 5,426 in 1728, and 2,200 in 1732; see Schwartz, *Policing the Poor*, 75.

75 Comptes, Hôpital de Caudebec, 1724–27 par Vivien Nicollet, AD Seine-Maritime, 113 HP E11.

76 Délibération, Hôpital de Caudebec, 1 septembre 1775, ibid., E3.

77 Comptes, Hôpital de Caudebec, 1724–27 par Vivien Nicollet, ibid., E11, and 1734, ibid., E16.

78 Favier, *Les villes du Dauphiné aux XVIIe et XVIIIe siècles*, 101–16.

CHAPTER FOUR

1 Cahier des délibérations du Bureau des pauvres, Grignan, 1736–72, octobre 1736, AD Drôme, 44 H 11 E1/6.

2 Ibid., 17 mai 1736.

3 Norberg, *Rich and Poor in Grenoble*, 175–82.

4 Hufton, *The Poor of Eighteenth-Century France*, 173–6. Among specific treatments of English institutions is Roy Porter, "The Gift Relation: Philanthropy and Provincial Hospitals in Eighteenth Century England," in Granshaw and Porter, *The Hospital in History*, 149–77. The historic "rights" of the English poor were reflected in the debate over the introduction of the 1834 Poor Law; see Apfel and Dunkley, "English Rural Society and the New Poor Law," 54–6; and Blaug, "The Myth of the Old Poor Law and the Making of the New."

5 Gutton, *La société et les pauvres*, 215–24.

6 Imbert, "Les prescriptions hospitalières du Concile de Trente," 10.

7 Ibid., 11–12.

8 "Conseil sur le fait du Concile de Trente par Messire Charles du Moulin," in *Caroli Molinaeri … omnia quae extant opera* (Paris, 1681), 5:356; cited in Imbert, "Les prescriptions hospitalières du Concile de Trente," 19.

9 Imbert, "Les prescriptions hospitalières du Concile de Trente," 20–1.

10 Ibid., 12–14.

11 Brémond, *Histoire littéraire du sentiment réligieux en France*, 5:260–74.

12 Delumeau, *Le Catholicisme entre Luther et Voltaire*, 135–54; Pérouas, *La diocèse de La Rochelle de 1648 à 1724*, 309–52; Croix, *La Bretagne aux 16e et 17e siècles*, 2:1211–40.

13 Croix, *La Bretagne aux 16e et 17e siècles*, 2:1212–33.

14 Coste, *Le grand saint du grand siècle*, 1:312.

15 Châtellier, *La religion des pauvres*, 177.

16 Ibid., 178.

17 Ibid., 179.

18 Délibérations de la Confrérie de la Charité de St Vallier, 1637, ASSJ, ff. 19–20.

19 Recettes, 1681–83 and 1689–92, Archives de l'Hôpital de Saint-Vallier, 2E1; 1706–09, ibid., 2E4.

20 Hôpital de Caudebec, Recettes, 1612–14, AD Seine-Maritime, 113 HP E6.

21 Avisseau-Roussat, "L'Hôpital Saint-Antoine de la Charité," *Revue du département de la Manche* 6, no 22:108.

22 Venard, "Catholicisme et usure au XVIIe siècle," 59–74.

23 Venard, "Les œuvres de charité en Avignon," 138; De Vourric, *Traité de l'usure et les vrais moyens de l'esviter*; Salomon, *Public Welfare, Science, and Propaganda*, 52.

24 Venard, "Les œuvres de charité en Avignon," 136.

25 Mandon, *Histoire du prêt-gratuit de Montpellier*, 2:234–8. It should be noted as well that it was not just the church that was favourable to the monts de piété. One of the earliest supporters was Théophraste Renaudot, a Huguenot who was behind the founding of the mont de piété in Paris in 1638. See Salomon, *Public Welfare, Science, and Propaganda*, 45–52.

26 Assemblée du Bureau de l'hôpital de Grignan, 25 mars 1709, AD Drôme, 44 H 23, G1/1.

27 Bureau de l'Hôpital de Grignan, État et rolle de ceux qui doivent du grain au mont de pitié, 26 août 1761, ibid., G1/3, and Organisation du mont de piété, 14 avril 1770, ibid., G1/4.

28 Mont de pitié, 14 avril 1770, ibid., G1/3.

29 Ordonnance du recteur, AC Rousset, HHI, in Lacroix, *Inventaire sommaire*, 4:277.

30 Délibérations du bureau, 1 octobre 1737, AC Remuzat, GG 2, and "Livre de compte de mont frumentaire," 1754–83, ibid., GG 3, in Lacroix, *Inventaire sommaire*, 4:101.

31 Délibérations consulaires, Marsanne, 29 juin 1727, AC Marsanne, BB 10, and Délibérations consulaires, Vinsobres, 2 août 1782, AC Vinsobres, BB 25; both published in Lacroix, *Inventaire sommaire*, 4:370 and 63–4.

32 Ordonnance de l'évêque de Vaison pour un mont de grains, 16 juin 1721, AC Vinsobres, BB 13, in Lacroix, *Inventaire sommaire*, 4:60.

33 "Histoire horrible," BN, Coll. Morel de Thoisy, mss. 319, f. 62.

34 "Mandament de Mgr de Lescar pour établir des Confréries de St-Charles dans ses paroisses," 1677, ibid., f. 50.

35 "Pour l'examen des pauvres," ibid., ff. 93–4.

36 Chaurand, "Hôpital de Tréguier," ibid. 319, ff. 58–9; "Hôpital de Lannion," 19 février 1678, ibid., f. 60; "Hôpital de Guingamp," 26 mars 1678, ibid., f. 60; "Hôpital de Morlaix," 22 avril 1678, ibid., f. 61.

37 Objections and replies in "Avis," ibid., ff. 53–4.

38 "La manière d'établir le confrérie de charité," ibid., ff. 113–14.

39 See the forthcoming thesis by Jean-Luc Bruzulier entitled "Les pauvres, les pouvoirs et l'assistance: Les hôpitaux-généraux en Bretagne, 1676–1724."

40 Mémoire sur la Bretagne, 1705, AN, KK 1104, ff. 3–6.

41 Croix, *La Bretagne aux 16e et 17e siècles*, 2:1216–17.

42 Hoffman, *Church and Community*, 98–138, and Luria, *Territories of Grace*, 126.

43 Basque, "L'assistance aux pauvres," 47–8.

44 Chevalier, "Le diocèse de Die en l'année 1644," 84.

45 Tackett, *Priest and Parish in Eighteenth-Century France*, 151–69; Croix, *La Bretagne aux 16e et 17e siècles*, 2:1234.

46 Gutton, *La sociabilité villageoise dans l'ancienne France*, 185–205.

47 Ibid., 192–6; Luria, *Territories of Grace*, 168.

48 Bouchard, *Le village immobile*, 329–37; Luria, "Conflict and the Constitution of Moral Order in Old Regime Rural Society," 139–44.

49 Norberg, Fairchilds, Gutton, and Vovelle have all noted that charitable bequests increased regularly in size and frequency after 1630, peaking at different points in the first half of the eighteenth century. At the same time, studies of urban testaments have demonstrated that the social groups responsible for the charitable bequests differed markedly from one region and century to another. Norberg argues that magistrates were

the principal initiators in Grenoble, followed by nobles and bourgeois *rentiers*, while in seventeenth-century Paris, Chaunu contends that noble families set the pattern. See Norberg, *Rich and Poor in Grenoble*, 117–37; Vovelle, *Piété baroque et déchristianisation en Provence*, 229–64; Fairchilds, *Poverty and Charity in Aix-en-Provence*, 18–37; Gutton, *La société et les pauvres*, 419–37; Chaunu, *La mort à Paris*, 392–427; Croix, *La Bretagne aux 16e et 17e siècles*, 1:685–709.

50 Berger, "Rural Charity in Late Seventeenth Century-France.

51 Vovelle, *Piété baroque et déchristianisation*, 253–4.

52 Ibid., 254–5.

53 Basque, "L'assistance aux pauvres," 47–52.

54 "Comptes des recteurs de l'hôpital," AD Drôme, 1656–79, 44 H 17, E/9, and 1680–1700, 44 H 17, E/10

55 Délibérations, 26 septembre 1723, Consulat of Grignan, AC Grignan, BB 23.

56 Délibérations, 17 mars 1723, ibid.

57 The archival holdings of almost every hospital in the Valentinois and Diois contain extensive legal proceedings showing the regular contestation of these deathbed grants to institutions of charity; see the H series under each town and village in Lacroix, *Inventaire sommaire*. It should also be noted that Maurice Basque observed the refusal of many heirs to honor the monetary clauses of wills made out to local hospitals; see Basque, "L'assistance aux pauvres," 84–5.

58 Vovelle, *Piété baroque et déchristianisation*, 109–26; Vovelle, *Mourir autrefois*, 46–53; Chaunu, *La mort à Paris*, 249–60.

59 Figure 2 is based on annual accounts of the eight hospitals: Étoile, AC Étoile, E7–9, E20, E32, E35, E37, E40, E42, E44–5, E48–50, E54–5; Grignan, AD Drôme, 44 H 12–18; Saint-Vallier, Archives hospitalières de St-Vallier, 2E1–5; Seyne, AD Alpes-de-Haute-Provence, 54 H E1–2, E7–8; Caudebec, AD Seine-Maritime, 113 HP E6–14; Pontorson, Avisseau-Roussat, "L'Hôpital Saint-Antoine," *Revue du département de la Manche* 6, no 22 91–112; Savenay, Archives de l'Hôpital de Savenay, E3–4; Malestroit, AD Morbihan, 7 HS 6, E6, no 29–69. The revenues were calculated in livres and then deflated by dividing them by the price of wheat on the Grenoble market using the data collected by Robert Latouche and published in Hauser, *Recherches et documents sur l'histoire des prix en France de 1500 à 1800*, 365–70. I would like to thank Professor Albert Hamscher for suggesting this method of compensating for devaluations and inflation.

60 Bloch, *L'assistance et l'État*, 282.

61 At Pontorson the Brothers of Charity often had to call upon the father provincial or other houses of the order (Grenoble and Paris) to aid them in operating the hospital; see Avisseau-Roussat, "L'Hôpital Saint-Antoine de la Charité," 6, no 22; 108. At Caudebec in 1733, the hospital administrators immediately cut back aid to "outsiders" when the intendant suspended grants for their internment. In 1746 they defended this action and refused to readmit "outsiders," arguing that the hospital did not have sufficient funds; see Délibérations, Hôpital de Caudebec, 8 janvier 1746, AD Seine-Maritime, 113 HP, E4, f. 2.

62 Avisseau-Roussat, "L'Hôpital Saint-Antoine de la Charité," 6, no 22: 73–9.

63 Délibérations, Hôpital de Caudebec, 16 septembre et 7 décembre 1765, AD Seine-Maritime, 113 HP E4. This question has been further explored by Marc Robichaud, "L'Hôpital de Caudebec," 75–80.

64 Ibid., 3 avril 1766.

65 Ibid., 18 février 1769.

66 Vovelle, *Piété baroque et déchristianisation*, 257–64; Norberg, *Rich and Poor in Grenoble*, 239–66; Chaunu, *La mort à Paris*, 392–427.

67 Registre des entrées, Hôpital de Caudebec, AD Seine-Maritime 113 HP F4.

68 Délibérations, Hôpital de Caudebec, 15 décembre 1759, ibid.

69 Registre des entrées, Hôpital de Caudebec, ibid.

70 Avisseau-Roussat, "L'Hôpital Saint-Antoine de la Charité," (thesis), plate 19.

71 Avisseau-Roussat, "L'Hôpital Saint-Antoine de la Charité," 6, no 22:106–7.

72 Délibérations, Hôpital de Seyne, registre 1753–80, AD Alpes-de-Haute-Provence, 22 J 4.

73 Ibid. and Arnaud-Duc, "L'entretien des enfants abandonnés en Provence sous l'Ancien Régime," 57. Arnaud-Duc notes that the 120 livres was judged insufficient by most hospitals, for which it cost 300 livres to raise a child. The approved amounts did increase under the pressure of hospital directors, rising to 150 livres in 1765 and to 175 in 1778, but the experience of Seyne seems to indicate that children were frequently paid for with individual, short-term grants.

74 Avisseau-Roussat, "L'Hôpital Saint-Antoine de la Charité," 6, no 23:155.

75 Ibid., 156–7.

76 Pierre Bourdieu has argued that this type of initiative was an integral part of the "strategy" for social reproduction, that families of notables or those desiring to enter the local elite consciously or unconsciously imitated the gestures (such as donations) that would gain them respectability

and consolidate their place as members of the elite; see the discussion of his article "Les stratégies matrimoniales dans le système de reproduction," in Bourdieu, *Choses dites*, 78–93.

77 Their domination of charitable agencies gave them much the same power as in urban areas; see Trexler, "Charity and the Defense of the Urban Elites in the Italian Communes"; Norberg, *Rich and Poor in Grenoble*, 297–304; Fairchilds, *Poverty and Charity in Aix-en-Provence*, 147–58; Cavallo, *Charity and Power in Early Modern Italy*, chap. 3; Cavallo, "Charity, Power, Patronage in Eighteenth-Century Italian hospitals," 107–10; Cavallo, "The Motivations of Benefactors."

78 Marco H.D. Van Leeuwen has argued the theoretical aspects of this question in an article discussing what the poor and the rich respectively had to gain from charity; see "Logic of Charity." Pierre Bourdieu has underlined the position of force that capital contributions assured to local donors: in a pre-capitalist economy, their symbolic role was inevitably recognized by the community, which associated them with other prestigeous families, trusted them with community decisions, and accorded them places of honour in local ceremonies; see Bourdieu, *Le sens pratique*, 191–207.

79 See in particular the accounts of Louis Tesserand, 1603–04, Hôpital de l'Étoile, AC Étoile, E7.

80 The question of their trustworthiness was frequently brought to the attention of the town consulate, which followed closely the financial reports of the outgoing recteur of the poor. In Grignan the report, or *reliquat*, of the previous recteur was brought up for scrutiny, or the councillors called for him to reimbourse additional amounts in August 1669, April and August 1670, March 1672, July 1673, December 1707, January 1712, December 1713, November 1718, July 1721, September 1722, March 1723, September 1723, and September 1732; see Deliberations, Consulat de Grignan, AC Grignan, BB 19–23.

81 Sandra Cavallo, examining the complicity between the elite of Turin and the San Giovanni hospital, argues that the "reforms" proposed by the central government created a new local elite dependant upon royal structures. These new notables replaced the more traditional city elite; see Cavallo, "Charity, Power, Patronage," 109.

82 "Délibération du Bureau des pauvres de Seyne," 15 mars 1625, AD Alpes-de-Haute-Provence, 54 H, Seyne, E 1.

83 "Délibérations, établissement du bureau des distributions, 1676," AD Drôme, 44 H II, EI/1.

84 "Ordonnance de Mgr. le Compte, 1686," ibid., EI/2.

85 For Grignan, see "Comptes," 1600–01, AD Drôme, 44 H 12, E4, and "Comptes," 1680, ibid., 44 H 17, E10/1. For Étoile, see "Journal que tient Loys Tosserand, procureur de l'hôpital, 1603–04," AC Étoile, E7, and Comptes de Charles Point, 1666–67, ibid.

86 "Journal que tient Loys Tosserand, procureur de l'hôpital, 1603–04," AC Étoile, E7.

87 Comptes de Charles Point, Hôpital d'Étoile, 1667–69, ibid., E37.

88 Allibert, *Histoire de Seyne*, 405–9.

89 Bruzullier, "Les tentatives de reformes d'un petit hôpital général à la fin du XVIIIeme siècle."

90 Hôpital de Malestroit, Comptes, AD Morbihan, 7 HS 6 (Malestroit), E6, Comptes, 1601–1704.

91 Guillemot, "L'Hôpital de Malestroit," 485–8.

92 Ibid., 490.

93 Ibid., 491.

94 Ibid., 492–3.

95 Gutton, *L'État et la mendicité*, 121–3 and 231–40.

96 Avisseau-Roussat, "L'Hôpital Saint-Antoine de la Charité," 6, no 22: 91–2.

97 Délibérations, Hôpital de Meursault, Archives de l'Hôtel-Dieu de Beaune, 1 G15 1904; cited in Guyob, "Pauvreté et assistance dans le monde rural," 118–19.

98 Croix, "Les notables ruraux dans la France du XVIIIe siècle."

99 Gutton, *La sociabilité villageoise*, 136–54.

100 Root, *Peasants and King in Burgundy*, 208–33.

CHAPTER FIVE

1 Contrat entre la ville de Malestroit et la Communauté de St-Thomas de Villeneuve, 17 October 1666, AGSSTV, CO 34, f. 13vo.

2 Lallemand, *Histoire de la charité*, 4:32–54.

3 Bournafous-Sérieux, *Une maison d'aliénés et de correctionnaires*, 18, and Avisseau-Roussat, "L'Hôpital Saint-Antoine de la Charité," 6, no 22:58.

4 Délibérations, Bureau de l'Hôpital de Caudebec, 3 janvier 1690 and 6 mars 1695, AD Seine-Maritime 113 HP E1.

5 Ibid., 6 novembre 1699.

6 Ibid., 6 novembre 1699, 30 décembre 1699, and 26 janvier 1700.

7 Ibid., 26 janvier 1700.

8 Délibérations, Bureau de direction de l'Hôpital Saint-Armal de Savenay, 1 août 1760, Archives de l'Hôpital de Savenay, B2.

9 Rapley, *The Dévotes*, 10–22; Vacher, *Des "régulières" dans le siècle*, 13–43; Jones, *The Charitable Imperative*, esp. chap. 3.

10 Council of Trent, session 25:5; cited in Schroeder, *Canons and Decrees of the Council of Trent*, 220–1.

11 Vacher, *Des "régulières" dans le siècle*, 16.

12 Rapley, *The Dévotes*, 28–34.

13 St Vincent de Paul, *Correspondance*, 14:125; cited in Rapley, *The Dévotes*, 81.

14 St Vincent de Paul, *Correspondance*, 9:209; cited in Rapley, *The Dévotes*, 82.

15 Rapley, *The Dévotes*, 82–3.

16 Règlement de la charité mixte de Joigny, in St Vincent de Paul, *Correspondance*, 447; cited in Rapley, *The Dévotes*, 83.

17 Jones, *The Charitable Imperative*, 98.

18 Ibid., 84.

19 Rapley, *The Dévotes*, 82.

20 Ibid., 85–6.

21 Ibid., 87.

22 Jones, *The Charitable Imperative*, 40, 112, 163.

23 Ibid., 176.

24 Délibérations, 24 décembre 1764, Hôpital de Grignan, AD Drôme, 44 H II, EI/6

25 Délibérations, Hôpital de Caudebec, 2 novembre 1725, AD Seine-Maritime, 113 HP E5.

26 Délibérations, 1 août 1760, Bureau de direction de l'Hôpital St-Armal de Savenay, Archives de l'Hôpital de Savenay, B2.

27 Vacher, *Des "régulières" dans le siècle*, 79–96.

28 Ibid., 58–74. See also Bois, *Les Sœurs de Saint-Joseph*, 33–50.

29 Vacher, *Des "régulières" dans le siècle*, 82.

30 Ibid., 133–4.

31 Anon., "À Lamballe, au XVIIe siècle," 4.

32 Laplume, "Un Augustin français du XVIIe siècle," 344–5.

33 Nécrologie pour père Ange Le Proust, AGSSTV, Père Ange/34.

34 Contrat qui unit la Confrérie de la Charité avec l'Hôpital de Lamballe, 6 February 1661, AGSSTV, LAM/1.

35 Anon., "À Lamballe, au XVIIe siècle," 11.

36 Hickey, "Preaching and Teaching," 30–1.

37 Vernet, *La Congrégation des religieuses du Très-Saint-Sacrement*, 48.

38 See manuscript by Antoinette Ponthier (niece of Pierre Vigne and third superior of the order), "Premièrement le temps que cette congrégation a commencé," 1724, ASSS, 2.

39 See *mémoire* by Pierre Vigne in Vernet, *La Congrégation des religieuses du Très-Saint-Sacrament*, 57.

40 Ponthier,"Premièrement le temps que cette congrégation a commencé," 1724, ASSS, 3.

41 Vacher, *Des "régulières" dans le siècle*, 46–58.

42 Ibid., 162. It should be noted that another woman from Le Puy, Marguerite de Saint-Laurans, was associated with the six founding sisters. Although not mentioned in the 1650 document, she was identified in 1654 as "supérieure" of the community. She too was literate.

43 Professions des sœurs de St Joseph de Vienne, 1681–1792, AD Isère, 21 H 1.

44 Bernaville, *Dans le sillage de Monsieur Vincent*, 33–5. Anon., "À Lamballe, au XVIIe siècle," 8–13.

45 Copies des extraits mortuaires des sœurs décédées de 1668 à 1933, documents établis en 1924 et 1933, AGSSTV.

46 It should be noted that for the religious communities, the profession date of their nuns was far more important than their birth date, for with their vows they entered into a new spiritual life and the date of this event took on the greatest chronological importance. That is why the profession date is almost always given in death notices. On these death notices, see Rapley, "Women and the Religious Vocation in Seventeenth-Century France," 614–17; Drillat, "Les Visitandines françaises (1667–1767)," 189–205; Houdaille, "La mortalité des Carmélites en France de 1736 à 1792"; Dinet, "Mourir en religion aux 17e et 18e siècles."

47 Copies des extraits mortuaires des sœurs décédées de 1668 à 1933, documents établis en 1924 et 1933, AGSSTV.

48 Croix, *La Bretagne aux 16e et 17e siècles*, 2:325.

49 Ponthier, "Premièrement le temps que cette congrégation a commencé," 1724, ASSS, 2. It is noted by Abbé Veyrenc that the house was, in fact, purchased by Father Vigne in 1715 and turned over to the three sisters.

50 Vernet, *La Congrégation des religieuses du Très-Saint-Sacrement*, 49, and Veyrenc, *Essai sur la vie du Père Vigne*, 296.

51 Ponthier, "Premièrement le temps que cette congrégation a commencé," 1724, ASSS, 5.

52 Vernet, *La Congrégation des religieuses du Très-Saint-Sacrement*, 56, and Veyrenc, *Essai sur la vie du Père Vigne*, 323–5.

53 Veyrenc, *Essai sur la vie du Père Vigne*, 303–4.

54 "Tableau des sœurs reçues à la profession dans notre communauté de Boucieu-le-Roi en Vivarais, de 1722 à 1789," ASSS, 1.

55 Rapley, "Women and the Religious Vocation."

56 Ibid., 619.

57 Ibid., 620–1.

58 Note from Sister Dunoyer to hospital administration, St-Vallier, n.d. [mid-seventeenth century]; copy in ASSJ.

59 Rapley, "Women and the Religious Vocation," 624–6.

60 Ibid., 627–31.

61 Châtellier, *La religion des pauvres*, 175–96.

62 Laslett, *The World We Have Lost: Further Explored*, 113–16.

63 Dupâquier, *La population française*, 60–1.

64 Hufton, "Women without Men," 368–71. The positions that the women held in the hospitals were important, but as Colin Jones has argued, "they [the nuns] were offered a new scope for action – on condition that they renounce any participation in the exercise of power – in the more private sphere of gratuity and compassion." Within this context, they always remained hierarchically subordinant to men, either the directors of the hospital, the "father founder" of the order, or the bishop; see Jones, *The Charitable Imperative*, 112. See also Claverie and Lamaison, *L'impossible mariage*, 181–6.

65 The choice of Mme Rouxel de Thierry as procuratrice was intended to maintain a secular opening for the order. She could represent the sisters before the courts and in the face of any legal problems with the hospitals. The importance of this position can be seen in the fact that the procuratrice was one of the three general superiors of the order along with the "spiritual father" and the mother superior; see Bernaville, *Dans le sillage de Monsieur Vincent*, 60–1.

66 Supplique à sa Majesté et son conseil de confirmer l'ordonnance de M. l'Archevêque de Paris approvant le déménagement de la maison-mère de la Société de St Thomas de Villeneuve à Paris, 30 mars 1697, AGSSTV.

67 Langlois, *Le Catholicisme au féminin*, 418.

68 Bernaville, *Dans le sillage de Monsieur Vincent*, 33–4.

69 Langlois, *Le Catholicisme au féminin*, 418.

70 Marguerite Walsh de Valois, supérieure générale, "Liste des noms et des ages des hospitalières de St Thomas de Villeneuve dans les maisons du diocèse de Paris," 29 mars 1790, AN, D XIX 7, ch 103, no 10.

71 Vacher, *Des "régulières" dans le siècle*, 217–8.

72 Ibid., 135–40.

73 Ibid., 237.

74 Ibid., 145–6.

75 Langlois, *Le Catholicisme au féminin*, 74–5 and 103.

76 Ponthier, "Premièrement, le temps que cette congrégation a commencé," 1724, ASSS, 5.

77 Mgr Jean de Catellan, bishop of Valence, to Louise Bouveyron, superior, Valence, 13 août 1721; cited in Veyrenc, *Essai sur la vie du Père Vigne*, 288–9.

78 Veyrenc, *Essai sur la vie du Père Vigne*, 299.

79 Vernet, *La Congrégation des religieuses du Très-Saint-Sacrement*, 58–9.

80 Veyrenc, *Essai sur la vie de Père Vigne*, 396.

81 Vernet, *La Congrégation des religieuses du Très-Saint-Sacrement*, 57.

82 Ibid., 57.

83 Langlois, *Le Catholicisme au féminin*, 99.

84 "État de l'Hôpital en 1656"; cited in Avisseau-Roussat, "L'Hôpital Saint-Antoine de la Charité," 6, no 23:131.

85 Mémoire des religieux, 25 février 1739; cited in ibid., 131.

86 1er registre des inventaires, 1693, and 2e registre des inventaires, 1720; cited in ibid., 131.

87 Registres d'entrée des malades, 1665–83, 1701–22, and 1747–81, AD St-Lô, Archives de l'Hôpital de Pontorson, fonds découvert par M. Nédélec, reg. 43, 44, 45.

88 Diderot, "Hôtel-Dieu," in *L'Encyclopédie ou dictionnaire raisonné des sciences, des arts et des métiers*, 8:319–20. The differences within physiocratic circles over public assistance is reflected in the different entries in the *Encyclopédie*; see Roland Mortier, who discusses the debate over the extent to which Diderot actually wrote the entry, in his article "Diderot et l'assistance publique, ou la source et les variations de l'article *hôpital* de l'*Encyclopédie*," published in Bingham and Topazio, *Enlightenment Studies in Honour of Lester G. Crocker*, 175–85.

89 Foucault, *Folie et déraison*, 54–81 and 90–1. It should be noted that several historians have contested Foucault's account both in terms of its methodology and of its accuracy. His methodology has been treated in Huppert, "*Divinatio et eruditio*," and Megill, "The Reception of Foucault by Historians." As to Foucault's accuracy in the case of hospitals, see Jones, *The Charitable Imperative*, chap. 2.

90 Meuvret, "Les crises de subsistance et la démographie de la France d'Ancien Régime," 277–8.

91 Registre des entrées, 1724–60, Hôpital de Caudebec, AD Seine-Maritime, 113 HP, F2–4, and Registre des sorties, 1724–60, ibid., F9–10. The death rates have been calculated according to the method suggested by Colin Jones: the number of deaths noted in the registers is divided by the number of entries plus the number of poor residents in the institution; see Jones, *Charity and Bienfaisance*, 222, note 89. (These calculations have been carried out by my assistant, Marc Robichaud.)

92 Registres d'entrées, Hôpital de Pontorson, 1676, AD Manche; AD St-Lô, Archives de l'Hôpital de Pontorson, fonds découvert par M. Nédélec, reg. 43.

93 "État au vray," 1649, Hôpital de Pontorson, AD St-Lô, A 20; cited in Avisseau-Roussat, "L'Hôpital Saint-Antoine de la Charité," 6, no 22:67–8.

94 Fosseyeux, "Le service médical à l'Hôpital de la Charité," 3, no 5:119; also Avisseau-Roussat, who notes that sixteen apprentices in pharmacy and surgery were sent to Pontorson between 1662 and 1691; see "L'Hôpital Saint-Antoine de la Charité de Pontorson," 6, no 23:122.

95 Fosseyeux, "Le service médical à l'hôpital de la Charité," 3, no 5:118.

96 Avisseau-Roussat, "L'Hôpital Saint-Antoine de la Charité," 6, no 23:122.

97 Fosseyeux, "Le service médical à l'hôpital de la Charité," 3, no 5:118. On the larger repercussions of this case see Gelfand, *Professionalizing Modern Medicine*, 106–7.

98 Fosseyeux, "Le service médical à l'hôpital de la Charité," 3, no 5:119.

99 Avisseau-Roussat, "L'Hôpital Saint-Antoine de la Charité," 6, no 23:122.

100 Herault, "Soigner en montmorillonnais au début du XVIIIe siècle." See also Herault, "Les pauvres et l'amputation à la Maison-Dieu de Montmorillon aux XVIIe et XVIIIe siècles," and *Dieu, la maladie et les Montmorillonnais*.

101 Délibérations, Hôpital de Caudebec, 9 janvier 1719, AD Seine-Maritime, 113 HP E2.

102 Ibid., 25 décembre 1724.

103 Ibid., 2 novembre 1725.

104 Ibid., 29 juillet 1772, ff. 4–5.

105 Beyland, *Le Père Le Valois, Elisabeth de St-Simon, Marie Barbe de Coudraye*, 37.

106 Délibérations, Hôpital de Caudebec, 25 novembre 1724, AD Seine-Maritime, 113 HP E2, ff. 27–8. In the accounts for 1772, the nun was still receiving 50 livres; see Comptes, 1772–89, ibid., E20.

107 Délibérations, Hôpital de Grignan, 30 décembre 1764, AC Grignan, 44 H 11, E1/6.

108 Délibérations, 11 mars 1778, Hôpital de Savenay, Archives de l'Hôpital de Savenay, B2.

109 Comptes, 1768–69, Hôpital de l'Étoile, AC Étoile, E55.

110 Délibérations, 1753–80, Hôpital de Seyne, AD Alpes-de-Hautes-Provence, 22 J 4.

111 Jones, *The Charitable Imperative*, 170–200.

112 Ibid., 174.

113 Contracts d'engagement, AGSSTV, CO.

114 Jones, *The Charitable Imperative*, 172.

115 Ibid., 177.

116 Contrat de Malestroit, 17 octobre 1666, AGSSTV, CO 34, f. 13.

117 Colin Jones, *The Charitable Imperative*, 178.

118 Contrat d'établissement, Hôpital de Malestroit, 17 octobre 1666, AGSSTV, CO 34, f. 13.

119 Contrat d'engagement, Hôpital de Moncontour, 26 février 1661, ibid., CO 20, f. 15.

120 Contrat d'établissement, Hôpital de Lamballe, 16 février 1661, ibid., CO 23.

121 Délibérations, Hôpital de Caudebec, 17 juin 1725, AD Seine-Maritime, 113 HP E3.

122 Délibérations, Bureau de l'Hôpital de Caudebec, 28 avril 1719, ibid.

123 Ibid., 29 juillet 1719, ff. 27–8. Nine years later, in 1728, the same problem was again brought before a general assembly of the hospital. Sieur Falloppe again complained that Le Brunent, the surgeon, was furnishing "médicaments" to his patients. This time the board did not just leave the conflict to the nuns; it was more directivist. Noting that Falloppe paid 200 livres to the crown for the right to practice his "art" and that he prepared free "remedies" for the town poor, it gave him the exclusive right to dispense "drogues" to the inmates of the hospital at the same time that Le Brunent's right to treat inmates and to "heal their wounds" was confirmed; ibid., 12 février 1728, f. 45.

124 Délibérations, Hôpital de Caudebec, 29 avril 1729, ibid., f. 50.

125 Historique de l'Hôpital de Saint-Vallier, boîte "Hôpital de St Vallier," ASSJ, 27–8.

126 Comptes de Hyacinthe Fleury, trésorier, Hôpital de St-Vallier, 6 juillet 1731, Archives de l'Hôpital de St-Vallier, 2E5. For the nuns' version, see Historique de l'Hôpital de St Vallier, boîte "Hôpital de St Vallier," ASSJ, 28.

127 Guillemot, "L'Hôpital de Malestroit," 492–3.

128 Rosenzweig, "L'Hôpital de Malestroit," 11–12.

129 Ibid., 12–13.

130 Gutton, "La mise en place du personnel soignant dans les hôpitaux français," 16–18.

131 The interest in herb gardens on the part of the nuns was not really new in hospital terms since the men's nursing orders had almost always used herb medicines; on the Augustinians, see Herault, "Soigner en montmorillonnais au début du XVIIIe siècle," 65–71 and 99–109, and on the Brothers of Charity, see Avisseau-Roussat, "L'Hôpital Saint-Antoine de la Charité," 6, no 23:124–5.

132 Lebrun, *Se soigner autrefois*, 18–25, 79–85.

133 Contrat d'engagement entre l'Hôpital de Dol et les Sœurs de St-Thomas, 24 July 1673, AGSSTV, CO 55a.

134 Délibérations, Confrérie de la Charité, St-Vallier, 1697, ASSJ.

135 Jones, *The Charitable Imperative*, 196.

136 Ibid.

CHAPTER SIX

1 Délibérations, Hôpital de Caudebec, 23 décembre 1774, AD Seine-Maritime, 113 HP E5, f. 26.

2 État général des hôpitaux et établissements de charité de la généralité de Rouen, 1775, AD Seine-Maritime, C 995, f. 127.

3 Jeorger, "Les enquêtes hospitalières."

4 Ibid., 56–7.

5 Ibid., 58.

6 Bloch, *L'assistance et l'État*, 450.

7 Ibid., 138.

8 Ibid., 164–78. There have been several recent contributions to the history of the dépôts de méndicité. The most important has come from Thomas McStay Adams; see his thesis "An Approach to the Problem of Beggary in Eighteenth-Century France." Much of the information in that study has been incorporated into his book *Bureaucrats and Beggars* and an article, "Mœurs et hygiène publique au XVIIIe siècle." See also Schwartz, *Policing the Poor*, 158–78; Norberg, *Rich and Poor in Grenoble*, 216–26; Fairchilds, *Poverty and Charity in Aix-en-Provence*, 149–54.

9 Bloch, *L'assistance et l'État*, 181.

10 Ibid., 193–4.

11 Ibid., 196–205.

12 Ibid., 218–20.

13 Ibid., 222–4.

14 Ibid., 229–31.

15 Ibid., 311.

16 Hufton, *The Poor of Eighteenth-Century France*, 4.

17 Ibid., 226–9.

18 Ibid., 232.

19 Ibid., 232–7.

20 This table has been drawn up using the information included in appendix 1 of Hufton, *The Poor of Eighteenth-Century France*, 369–81.

21 Ibid., 173.

22 Ibid., 244.

23 Ibid., 159.

24 Adams, *Bureaucrats and Beggars*, and Imbert, *Le droit hospitalier de l'Ancien Régime*. It should be noted that I have chosen these three themes to illustrate the much larger concepts developed in each of these books.

25 Délibérations, 13 janvier 1775, Registre de l'hospice de St-Vallier, 1692–1784, Archives de l'Hôpital de Saint-Vallier, 1 EZ, f. 167.

26 Almanac of 1788; cited in Caise, *Histoire de Saint-Vallier*, 237–8.

27 Fillet, "Grignan religieux," 234. In the case of St-Vallier, besides manual arts, the nuns taught reading and writing; see Caise, *Histoire de Saint-Vallier*, 238.

28 Norberg, *Rich and Poor in Grenoble*, 164–6.

29 Viale, "L'Hôpital de Buis au XVIIIe siècle," 34.

30 Délibérations, Hôpital de Savenay, "Confirmation à faire sur le compte de Mlle Genodeau, sœur hospitalière de Savenay," 5 juin 1769, Archives de l'Hôpital de Savenay, B2.

31 This initiative followed upon similar efforts by Paul Pellison, administrator of the *caisse des conversions*, to pay Huguenots to adopt the Catholic faith. He operated within the charitable initiatives taken by Calloët-Querbrat and Chaurand to distribute pills and ointments to the countryside. Prepared with the collaboration of Dr Chomel, Pellison's packages contained little true scientific medication; rather, they resembled more the empirical types of remedies; see Gutton, *La société et les pauvres*, 394–6, and BN, MS fr. 6.801, D'Aguesseau, "Mémoire concernant la distribution des remèdes faitte depuis 1680," f. 325.

32 Lafond, *La dynastie des Hélvetius*, 70–124 and chap. 10; Nicolle, *Apothicaires et pharmaciens de Morbiha*, 141–2. Jean-Pierre Goubert has argued that the limits placed by Helvétius on the distribution of quinine and the attempt to find a substitute for it certainly did nothing to combat the ever-present malaria in Brittany; see *Malades et médecins en Bretagne*, 316–17.

33 Lafond, *La dynastie des Helvétius*, 126–7.

34 Ibid., 145.

35 Nicolle, *Apothicaires et pharmaciens de Morbihan*, 141.

36 Lafond, *La dynastie des Helvétius*, chap. 10. The absence of doctors and surgeons in rural Brittany is documented in Goubert, *Maladies et médecins en Bretagne*, 52–118.

37 Jeorger, "Les enquêtes hospitalières," 53.

38 Avisseau-Roussat, "L'Hôpital Saint-Antoine de la Charité," 6, no 23:115–16, 131–2.

39 Ibid., 132.

40 Ibid., no 22:74–5.

41 Ibid., 78–9.

42 Avisseau-Roussat, "L'Hôpital Saint-Antoine de la Charité" (thesis), plate 19.

43 Avisseau-Roussat, "L'Hôpital Saint-Antoine de la Charité," 6, no 23:134.

44 Ibid., no 22:106–7.

45 M. de Fontette to Bertier, ministre d'État, 29 mai 1774; cited in ibid., no 23:165.

46 Avisseau-Roussat, "L'Hôpital Saint-Antoine de la Charité," 6, no 22:136.

47 Ibid., 136.

48 Ibid., 137.

49 Mémoire sur la mendicité, 1774, BN, Ms.fr. 8129, f. 271 v.

50 Bonnafous-Sérieux, *Une maison d'aliénés et de correctionnaires*, 36–65.

51 Guillochon, "L'Hôpital et Aumônerie de Saint-Méen," 70–116 and 152.

52 Foucault, *Folie et déraison*, chap. 5.

53 This table has been composed using the following sources: Comptes, Hôpital de Caudebec, AD Seine-Maritime, 113 HP, E17–18 and F4; Comptes, Hôpital de Pontorson, AD Manche, Fonds découverts par M. Nédélec, Registres de dépenses, nos 23–37, and Registres des entrées des malades, 1747–81, no. 45; Comptes, Hôpital de Malestroit, AD Morbihan, 7 HS 6 (Malestroit), E6, nos 68–73; Étoile, Enquête Laverty, 1764, AD Isère, 11 C 1004; Comptes, Hôpital de Seyne, AD Alpes-des-Haute-Provence, 54 H E8; Comptes, Archives de l'Hôpital de Saint-Vallier, 2E7–9; Comptes, 1745–60, Distribution aux pauvres, 1745–60, Archives de l'Hôpital de Savenay; Comptes, Hôpital de Grignan (1746–79), AD Drôme, 44 H 19, E 13.

54 Guillemot, "L'Hôpital de Malestroit," 519–21.

55 Ramsey, *Professional and Popular Medicine in France*, chap. 2; Léonard, "Les médecins de l'Ouest au XIXe siècle," esp. 1: part 1, "Situation initial."

56 Intendant de la Bourdonnaye aux administrateurs de l'hôpital de Caudebec, 5 November 1733, AD Seine-Maritime, Hôpital de Caudebec, 113 HP E6.

57 These deliberations are resumed during a 1770 meeting, see Délibérations, Hôpital de Caudebec, 17 août 1770, ibid., E4, ff. 122–3.

58 Ibid., 8 janvier 1746, f. 2.

59 Ibid., 30 janvier 1769, ff. 108–9.

60 Ibid., 30 septembre 1769, ff. 112–13.

61 Bloch, *L'assistance et l'État*, 281–315; Hufton, *The Poor of Eighteenth-Century France*, 154.

62 Lallemand, *Histoire de la charité*, 4:387–92.

63 Imbert, *Le droit hospitalier de l'Ancien Régime*, 256–62.

64 An exception can be noted in the field of medicalization. If Pontorson remained in the vanguard of medical treatment, most of the other hospitals dragged their feet. The Caudebec hospital possessed a pharmacy only in 1771 after initially refusing to appropriate the money for its establishment in 1725. However, all the other six institutions continued to have their remedies and treaments furnished by the local apothecary, doctor, or surgeon.

65 Gutton, *La société et les pauvres*, 467–77. These changes in hospital services to the poor and the sick were not limited to the eight institutions studied in this book. Jean-Pierre Gutton has traced the same tendency of the hospitals in the Lyonnais to follow the general lines of Enlightenment thought and crown proposals for reform. Even if the monarchy failed in its attempts to force a new conception of poor relief upon the hospitals, institutions in the Lyonnais installed workshops, often directed by the textile companies. The experience seems to have worked so well that after 1761 Abbé Pupil, recteur of the poor in Lyon, even imported poor girls from other hospitals to work in the Lyon shops. "Work schools" to teach knitting, weaving, and handicrafts to children were also set up in most of the smaller hospitals of the region. Schools to instruct the poor in the rudiments of reading and writing were established as annexes to the hospitals by the Sisters of St-Joseph.

66 Robert Schwartz has noted increased acceptation of the idea of incarcerating the dangerous poor and trying the reform and teach work habits to the others, see *Policing the Poor*, 209–17.

67 Root, *Peasants and King in Burgundy*, 77–86, 109–50.

68 Gutton, *La sociabilité villageoise*, 141–154; Bercé, *Histoire des croquants*, 1:257–93.

69 Jeorger, "La structure hospitalier," 1031.

70 "Mémoire sur la mendicité," BN, MS fr. 8129, ff. 266–72.

CONCLUSION

1 Jeorger, "La structure hospitalière," 1050–1.

2 Ibid., 1034–7.

3 Favier, *Les villes du Dauphiné aux XVIIe et XVIIIe siècles*, 349–430.

4 Bercé, *Croquants et nu-pieds*, 82–4; Gutton, *La sociabilité villageoise*, 141–54.

5 Forrest, *La Révolution française et les pauvres*, 52–3.

6 They prepared the hospitals to become the centres for the experiments that were to be carried out in dissection, anatomy, and medical training in the course of the nineteenth century; see Ramsey, *Professional and Popular Medicine in France*, 72–102; Foucault, *Naissance de la clinique*, 38–86.

7 Root, *Peasants and King in Burgundy*, chap. 2; Bercé, *Croquants et nupieds*, 82–118.

8 Weber, *Peasants into Frenchmen*, and Mendras, *Sociétés paysannes*, chap. 8.

Bibliography

ARCHIVAL SOURCES

ARCHIVES NATIONALES, PARIS

AD+ 14, 141, 152 Édits et déclarations royaux

AD 14, 2 *Règlements des assemblées politiques de charité des paroisses, suivant les ordonnances de nos Rois ... lesquelles assemblées ont esté établies dans nos paroisses de Bretagne ...* Rennes et Paris, n.d. [1681]

D XIX 7, ch 103, no 10 "Liste des noms et des ages des hospitalières de St Thomas de Villeneuve dans les maisons du diocèse de Paris," 29 mars 1790

F 15 "Édit de désunion de l'Ordre de Mont Carmel et Saint-Lazare, 1693"

F 15, 138 Mémoires sur la mendicité, conférence de Montigny, 1764

H 1417 Lettres et mémoires sur la mendicité, 1776–77

KK 1104 Mémoire sur la Bretagne, 1705

M 30–64 Documents et relevés permettant l'Ordre de Mont Carmel et St-Lazare d'acquérir maladreries et hôpitaux, et surtout d'exproprier les biens des ordres hospitaliers supprimés, 1673–92

MM 199–237 Édits, papiers et documents concernant l'Ordre de Mont Carmel et St-Lazare, y compris des relevés de leurs biens, 14e–17e siècles

S 4812–915 Relevés des titres de biens et propriétés, organisés par diocèse, qui ont passé sous l'emprise de l'Ordre de Mont Carmel et St-Lazare, 1673–93

V 7 126–47 Documents et procédures légales initiés par la Chambre de la Charité Chrétienne et la Chambre de la Réformation générale des hôpitaux, 1607–73

V 7 148–52 Registres des jugements de la Chambre de la Charité Chrétienne, 1606–11 z 1 n 1–33 Papiers, correspondances et décisions des commissions extraordinaires du Conseil du Roi pour les officiers concernant hôpitaux et maladreries (Chambre de la Réformation générale, 1612–72; la Chambre de l'Arsenal, 1673–92; Commission, 1693)

z 7607 Décisions rendues par la Chambre de l'Arsenal

BIBLIOTHÈQUE NATIONALE, PARIS

Ms.fr. 6.801, f. 325–46 D'Aguesseau, "Mémoire concernant la distribution des remèdes faitte depuis 1680 aux pauvres malades des provinces par ordre du roi sous la direction de Mons Pellison," 1680–1768

Ms.fr. 8129 "Mémoires sur la mendicité," 1774

Ms.fr. 8468 "Mémoire sur les établissements faits dans la province de Dauphiné pour le renfermer les mandians," 1724

Coll. Morel de Thoisy, mss. 319 Imprimés provenants de Calloët Querbrat et de Père Chaurand sur l'établissement des hôpitaux-généraux dans le royaume

ARCHIVES DÉPARTEMENTALES DES ALPES-DE-HAUTE-PROVENCE, DIGNE

54 h Fonds de l'Hôpital de Seyne (anciens papiers, comptes), 1616–1789

22 j Délibérations des directors, Hôpital de Seyne

ARCHIVES DÉPARTEMENTALES DU CALVADOS, CAEN

1 b 5513–16 Intendance, documents traitant des hôpitaux

h Supp 1321 (Hôpital d'Orbec), a4 "Defense contre les protestations des administrateurs de l'Hôpital de Bernay"

c 293 "État des maisons de l'Election d'Avranches," 1729

c 995 "État général des hôpitaux et établissements de charité de la généralité de Rouen," 1775

c 596 Intendance, correspondance et papiers traitant la mise en œuvre de la loi de 1724

ARCHIVES DÉPARTEMENTALES DE LA DRÔME, VALENCE

44 h 11–23 Fonds de l'Hôpital de Grignan (anciens documents, quelques délibérations et comptes), 1610–1789

c 293 "État des biens et revenus de l'Hôpital de l'Étoile … pour satisfaire la déclaration du 11 février 1764"

ARCHIVES DÉPARTEMENTALES DE L'ILLE-ET-VILAINE, RENNES

c 1265 Édicts et déclarations royaux

c 1265–310 Intendance, documents traitant des hôpitaux, 1672–1771

ARCHIVES DÉPARTEMENTALES DE L'ISÈRE, GRENOBLE

II C 321 Revision des feux, 1699

II C 1001 "Mémoire concernant la vingt-quatrième partie des tailles due aux pauvres," 1724

II C 1002–5 Enquête Laverty sur les hôpitaux de Dauphiné, 1764

B 2363, fol. 90–126 Actes constituants les 33 hôpitaux, 1792

21 H 1 Professions des sœurs de St-Joseph de Vienne, 1681–1792

ARCHIVES DÉPARTEMENTALES DE LA LOIRE-ATLANTIQUE, NANTES

Savenay H, dépôt 5 Fonds de l'Hôpital de Savenay, déliberations, comptes 1450–1793

B 3508 Rôle de capitation, Savenay, 1741

B 3511 Capitation, 1793

ARCHIVES DÉPARTEMENTALES DE LA MANCHE, ST-LÔ

Fonds de l'Hôpital de Pontorson (séries anciennes et nouvelles), anciens papiers, délibérations, comptes, quelques registres d'entrées et de sorties, 1644–1789

ARCHIVES DÉPARTEMENTALES DU MORBIHAN, VANNES

7 HS 6 Fonds de l'Hôpital de Malestroit (anciens papiers, délibérations et comptes), 1450–1789

ARCHIVES DÉPARTEMENTALES DE LA SEINE-MARITIME, ROUEN

I B 5513–14 Suppressions et fusionnement des hôpitaux, 1694

113 HP Fonds de l'Hôpital de Caudebec-en-Caux (anciens papiers, délibérations, comptes, registres d'entrées et de sorties), 1538–1789

ARCHIVES COMMUNALES DE L'ÉTOILE

Fonds de l'Hôpital de l'Étoile (séries A, B, C and E), 1582–1789

ARCHIVES COMMUNALES DE GRIGNAN

BB 19–23 Délibérations du conseil municipale, 1668–1732

CC 10, 12, 15 Rôles de taille de Grignan, 1654, 1681, 1722

BIBLIOTHÈQUE MUNICIPALE DE GRENOBLE

U 908 Intendant Bouchu, "Mémoire de la province de Dauphiné," 1698

R 80 "Dénombrement des hôpitaux, maladreries et aumôneries de Dauphiné … avec leurs revenus," fév. 1692

ARCHIVES DE L'HÔPITAL DE ST-VALLIER

1E2 Registre de l'hospice, avec copie des actes depuis 1637 et 1670

2E1–2E9 Comptes et documents financières, 1681–1809
2H6 Réunion des revenus et bénéfices, 1772–79

ARCHIVES DE L'HÔPITAL DE SAVENAY
Délibérations du bureau, 1745–1790; lettres et comptes, 1731–93

ARCHIVES DE L'HÔPITAL DE VALENCE
III B 3 Assignations données pour le paiement à l'Hôpital de Valence, 1705

ARCHIVES DES SŒURS DE ST-JOSEPH DE ST-VALLIER, ST-VALLIER
"Historique de l'Hôpital," dans boîte "Hôpital de Saint Vallier"
Registre de la Confrérie de la Charité, 1662–93
Sœur Dunoyer à l'administration de l'Hôpital de St-Vallier, vers 1750

ARCHIVES DES SŒURS DE SAINT-SACREMENT, VALENCE
"Premièrement, le temps que cette congrégation a commencé," 1724
"Tableau des sœurs reçues à la profession dans notre communauté de Boucieu-le-Roi en Vivarais, de 1772 à 1789"

ARCHIVES GÉNÉRALES DES SŒURS DE ST-THOMAS DE VILLENEUVE, NEUILLY
Père Ange/34 Nécrologie pour père Le Proust
LAM/1 Contrat de la Confrérie de charité avec l'Hôpital de Lamballe
Copies des extraits mortuaires des sœurs décédées de 1668 à 1933
"Supplique à sa Majesté ... de confirmer l'ordonnance ... approuvant le déménagement de la maison-mère de la Société ... à Paris," 30 mars 1697
CO Séries de contrats entre la congrégation et les hôpitaux

PUBLISHED BOOKS AND ARTICLES

Anonymous. "À Lamballe, au XVIIe siècle: La formation de la Société de Saint-Thomas de Villeneuve." *Mémoires de la Société d'Émulation des Côtes-du-Nord* 115 (1977): 1–21
Adams, Thomas McStay. "An Approach to the Problem of Beggary in Eighteenth-Century France: The *Dépôts de Mendicité*." PhD dissertation, University of Wisconsin 1972
– *Bureaucrats and Beggars: French Social Policy in the Age of the Enlightenment.* New York: Oxford University Press 1990
– "Mœurs et hygiène publique au XVIIIe siècle: Quelques aspects des dépôts de mendicité." *Annales de démographie historique*, 1975, 93–105

- "Turgot, mendicité et réforme hospitalière: L'apport d'un mémoire inédit." *Actes du 99e Congrès national des Sociétés Savantes*, Besançon, 1974, Section d'histoire moderne, vol. 2. Paris: Bibliothèque Nationale 1976

Allibert, C. *Histoire de Seyne, de son baillage et de sa viguerie.* Barcelonnette, 1904; reprint, Marseille: Jeanne Lafitte 1972

Allier, Raoul. *La cabale des dévots, 1627–1666.* Paris: Armand Colin 1902

Almanach du département de la Manche pour l'An x. Cherbourg 1804

Apfel, William, and Dunkley, Peter. "English Rural Society and the New Poor Law: Bedfordshire, 1834–47." *Social History* 10 (1985)

Ariès, Philippe. *L'homme devant la mort.* Paris: Seuil 1977

Arnaud-Duc, Nicole. "L'entretien des enfants abandonnés en Provence sous l'Ancien Régime." *Revue historique de droit français et étranger* 1 (1969): 29–65

Asselin, Henri-Georges. "Les conceptions hospitalières de Piarron de Chamousset (1717–1773)." *Bulletin de la Société française de l'histoire des hôpitaux* 29 (1974): 69–79

Avisseau-Roussat, Hélène. "L'Hôpital Saint-Antoine de la Charité de Pontorson (1644–1792)." Thèse pour l'École des Chartes 1963

- "L'Hôpital Saint-Antoine de la Charité de Pontorson (1644–1792)." *Revue du département de la Manche* 6, no 22 (avril 1964): 43–112; 6, no 23 (juillet 1964): 115–200

Baillargeat, R., ed. *Les Invalides, trois siècles d'histoire.* Paris: le Musée de l'Armée 1974

Baratier, Édouard. *La démographie provençale du xiiie au xvie siècle avec des chiffres de comparaison pour le xviiie siècle.* Paris: sevpen 1961

Basque, Maurice. "L'assistance aux pauvres dans le Dauphiné rural du xviie siècle: L'exemple du diocèse de Die." Thèse de maîtrise, Université de Moncton 1986

Bataillon, Marcel. "J.L. Vivès, réformateur de la bienfaisance." *Bibliothèque d'humanisme et de la Renaissance* 14 (1952): 141–58

Beik, William. *Absolutism and Society in Seventeenth-Century France: State Power and Provincial Aristocracy in Languedoc.* Cambridge: Cambridge University Press 1985

Bercé, Yves-Marie. *Croquants et nu-pieds: Les soulèvements paysans en France du xvie au xixe siècle.* Paris: Gallimard/Julliard 1974

- *Histoire des croquants: Étude des soulèvements populaires au xviie siècle dans le sud-ouest de la France.* 2 vols. Genève: Droz 1974

Berger, Patrice. "Rural Charity in Late Seventeenth-Century France: The Pontchartrain Case." *French Historical Studies* 10 (Spring 1979): 393–415

Bernaville, Gaétan. *Dans le sillage de Monsieurs Vincent: Les religieuses de St-Thomas de Villeneuve (1661–1953).* Collection "Les grands ordres monastiques et instituts religieux," no 44. Paris: Grasset 1953

Beyland, Hugues. *Le Père Le Valois, Elisabeth de St-Simon, Marie Barbe de Coudraye et les hôpitaux de Rouen et Lisieux.* Lille: Établissements et Archives 1975

Bingham, Alfred J., and Topazio, Virgil W. *Enlightenment Studies in Honour of Lester G. Crocker.* Oxford: Oxford University Press 1979

Blaug, Mark. "The Myth of the Old Poor Law and the Making of the New." *Journal of Economic History* 24 (1964): 229–45

Bloch, Camille. *L'assistance et l'état en France à la veille de la Révolution: Généralités de Paris, Rouen, Alençon, Orléans, Châlons, Soissons, Amiens (1764–1790).* Paris, 1908; reprint, Genève: Slatkine 1974

Bois, A. *Les Sœurs de Saint-Joseph: Filles du petit dessein de 1648–1949.* St-Vallier 1949

Bois, Jean-Pierre. "Les anciens soldats dans la société française au XVIIIe siècle." Thèse de doctorat d'état, Université de Paris IV 1986

– "Le vieillard dans la France moderne, XVIIème-XVIIIème siècles: Essai de problématique pour une histoire de la vieillesse." *Histoire, économie et société* 1 (1984): 67–94

Bonnafous-Sérieux, Hélène. *Une maison d'aliénés et de correctionnaires au XVIIIe siècle: La charité de Senlis.* Paris: Presses Universitaires de France 1936

Bouchard, Gérard. *Le village immobile: Sennely-en-Sologne au XVIIIe siècle.* Paris: Plon 1972

Bourdieu, Pierre. *Choses dites.* Paris: Editions de minuit 1987

– *Le sens pratique.* Paris: Éditions de minuit 1980

– "Les stratégies matrimoniales dans le système de reproduction." *Annales (ESC)* 27 (1972): 1105–27.

Bourgeois, Roy. "Les visites pastorales et le visage religieux du diocèse de Die au XVIIe siècle." Thèse de maîtrise, Université de Moncton 1987

Brémond, Henri. *Histoire littéraire du sentiment religieux en France depuis la fin des guerres de religion jusqu'à nos jours.* 11 vols. Paris: Bloud et Gay 1916–36

Broutin, Paul. *La réforme pastorale en France au XVIIe siècle.* 2 vols. Paris: Desclée et Cie 1956

Bruzulier, Jean-Luc. "Les pauvres, les pouvoirs et l'assistance: Les hôpitaux-généraux en Bretagne, 1676–1724." Forthcoming thesis, Université de la Haute Bretagne, Rennes

– "Les tentatives de réformes d'un petit hôpital général à la fin du XVIIIème siècle: L'hôpital général d'Auray." To appear in *Bulletin de la Société française d'histoire des hôpitaux*

Caise, Albert. *Histoire de Saint-Vallier, de son abbaye, de ses seigneurs et de ses habitants.* Valence, 1876; reprint, Roanne: Éditions Horvath 1988

Callahan, William J. "Corporate Charity in Spain: The Hernaudad del Refugio of Madrid, 1618–1814." *Social History* 9 (1976): 159–86

Cameron, Iain A. *Crime and Repression in the Auvergne and the Guyenne, 1720–1790.* Cambridge: Cambridge University Press 1981

Castan, Nicole. *Les criminels de Languedoc, 1750–1790.* Toulouse: Privat 1980

– *Justice et répression en Languedoc à l'époque des Lumières.* Paris: Flammarion 1980

Castan, Yves. "Mentalités rurales et urbaines à la fin de l'Ancien Régime dans le ressort du Parlement de Toulouse d'après les sacs à procès criminels (1730–1790)." *Cahiers des Annales* 33 (1971): 109–86

Cavallo, Sandra. *Charity and Power in Early Modern Italy: Benefactors and Their Motives in Turin, 1541–1789.* Cambridge: Cambridge University Press 1995

– "Charity, Power, Patronage in Eighteenth-Century Italian Hospitals: The Case of Turin." *The Hospital in History.* Edited by Lindsay Granshaw and Roy Porter. London: Routledge 1989. 93–122

– "The Motivations of Benefactors: An Overview of Approaches to the Study of Charity." *Medicine and Charity Before the Welfare State.* Edited by Jonathan Barry and Colin Jones. London: Routledge, 1991. 46–62

Chaboche, Robert. "Les soldats français de la Guerre de Trente Ans, une tentative d'approche." *Revue d'histoire moderne et contemporaine* 20 (janvier–mars 1973): 10–24

– "Le sort des militaires invalides avant 1674." *Les Invalides, trois siècles d'histoire.* Edited by R. Baillargeat. Paris: le Musée de l'Armée, 1974. 127–46

Chalumeau, R.P., "L'assistance aux malades pauvres au xviie siècle." *xviie siècle* 90–1 (1971): 75–86

Chapalain-Nougaret, Christine. *Misère et assistance dans le pays de Rennes au xviiie siècle.* Nantes: cid Éditions 1989

Châtellier, Louis. *La religion des pauvres: Les sources du Christianisme moderne, xvie–xxe siècles.* Paris: Aubier 1993

Chaunu, Pierre. *La mort à Paris aux xvie, xviie et xviiie siècles.* Paris: Fayard 1978

Chevalier, Jules, ed. "Le diocèse de Die en l'année 1644: Procès-verbal d'une visite pastorale." *Bulletin de la Société d'archéologie et de statistique de la Drôme* 47 (1913): 1–110

Chill, Emmanuel. "Religion and Mendicity in Seventeenth-Century France." *International Review of Social History* 7 (1962): 400–25

Claverie, Elisabeth, and Lamaison, Pierre. *L'impossible mariage: Violence et parenté en Gévaudan, xviie, xviiie, xixe siècles.* Paris: Hachette 1982

Cloulas, Ivan. "Les aliénations du temporel ecclésiastique sous Charles ix et Henri iii (1563–1587)." *Revue d'histoire de l'Église de France* 44 (1958): 5–56

Collomp, Alain. *La maison du père: Famille et village en Haute-Provence aux xviie et xviiie siècles.* Paris: Presses Universitaires de France 1983

Les Confréries de Pénitents (Dauphiné – Provence). Actes du Colloque de Buis-les-Baronnies, October 1982. Valence: Gregoire 1988

Corvisier, André. "Anciens soldats oblats, mortes-payes et mendiants dans la première moitié du XVIIe siècle." *97e Congrès national des sociétés savantes, histoire moderne* 2 vols. Paris: Bibliotheque Nationale 1972. 1: 7–29

Coste, Pierre. *Le grand saint du grand siècle: Monsieur Vincent.* 3 vols. Paris: Desclée de Brouwer 1931

Croix, Alain. *La Bretagne aux 16e et 17e siècles: La vie, la mort, la foi.* 2 vols. Paris: Maloine 1981

– "Les notables ruraux dans le France du XVIIIe siècle: Une clé de la sociabilité." *De la sociabilité, spécificité et mutations.* Edited by Roger Levasseur. Montréal: Boréal, 1990. 39–58

Cugnetti, Patrice. "L'évolution du patrimoine hospitalier de Valence du XIe au XVIIIe siècle." *Liber amicorum. Hommage au Doyen Gérard Chauvet.* Valence: Faculté libre de droit 1990. 69–74

– "L'Hôpital de Grenoble des origines à la fin du Second Empire." 2 vols. Thèse de doctorat, Université de Grenoble II, 1980

Davis, Barbara Beckerman. "Poverty and Poor Relief in Sixteenth-Century Toulouse." *Historical Reflections* 17 (1991): 267–96

Davis, Natalie Zemon. "Assistance, humanisme et hérésie: Le cas de Lyon." *Études sur l'histoire de la pauvrété (Moyen Âge–XVIe siècle).* Edited by Michel Mollat. 2 vols. Paris: Publications de la Sorbonne, 1974. 2: 761–824

– *Society and Culture in Early Modern France.* Stanford: Stanford University Press 1975

De Font-Reaulx, J. "L'Hôpital de Saint-Vallier." *Bulletin de la Société d'archéologie et de statistique de la Drôme* 65 (1935–36): 319–21

Delumeau, Jean. *Le Catholicisme entre Luther et Voltaire.* Paris: Presses Universitaires de France 1971

Delumeau, Jean, ed. *La mort des pays de Cocagne: Comportements collectifs de la Renaissance à l'âge classique.* Paris: Université de Paris Sorbonne, Centre de recherches d'histoire moderne 1976

Depauw, Jacques. "Pauvres, pauvres mendiants, mendiants valides ou vagabonds? Les hésitations de la législation royale." *Revue d'histoire moderne et contemporaine* 21 (1974): 401–18

De Vourric. *Traité de l'usure et les vrais moyens de l'esviter par l'usage de divers contrats licites, etc., avec un règlement pour les Monts-de-Piété gratuits.* Avignon: L. Lemolt 1687

Dinet, Domonique. "Mourir en religion au 17e et 18e siècles: La mort dans quelques couvents des diocèses d'Auxerre, Langres et Dijon." *Revue historique* 259 (1978): 30–54

Dissard, Françoise. *La réforme des hôpitaux et maladreries au XVIIe siècle.* Paris: Éditions internationales 1938

Doucet, Roger. *Les institutions de la France au XVIe siècle*. 2 vols. Paris: J. Picard et Cie 1948

Drillat, Geneviève. "Les Visitandines françaises (1667–1767)." *La Mort des pays de Cocagne*. Edited by Jean Delumeau. Paris: Publications de la Sorbonne 1976. 189–205.

Droguet, Alain. "La municipalisation des hôpitaux St Nicolas et St Yves de Vitré (1549–1578)." *Bulletin et mémoires de la Société archéologique du Département de l'Ile-et-Vilaine* 71, no. 9 (1976): 53–5

Dupâquier, Jacques. *Histoire de la population française*. 4 vols. Paris: Presses Universitaires de France 1989

– *La population française aux XVIIe et XVIIIe siècles*. Paris: Presses Universitaires de France 1979

L'Encyclopédie ou dictionnaire raisonné des sciences, des arts et des métiers par une société de gens de lettres. Edited by Diderot et d'Alembert. 17 vols. Paris, 1751–65; Neufchastel: S. Faulche 1765

Estat général des unions faites des biens et revenus des maladreries, léproseries, aumôneries et autres lieux pieux aux hopitaux des pauvres malades. Paris 1705

Even, Pascal. "L'Assistance et la charité à La Rochelle." 3 vols. Thèse pour l'École des Chartes 1985

Expilly, Jean Joseph d'. *Dictionnaire géographique, historique et politique des Gaules et de la France*. 6 vols. Paris: Dessaint et Saillant 1762–70

Fairchilds, Cissie C. *Poverty and Charity in Aix-en-Provence, 1640–1789*. Baltimore: Johns Hopkins University Press 1976

Favier, René. "Les activités rurales des villes dauphinoises au XVIIIe siècle." *Des économies traditionnelles aux sociétés industrielles*. Edited by P. Bairoch and A.M. Piuz. Genève: Droz 1985. 59–80

– "L'Église et l'assistance en Dauphiné sous l'Ancien Régime: Le vingt-quatrième des pauvres." *Revue d'histoire moderne et contemporaine* 21 (1984): 448–64

– "Enfermement et assistance aux villages en Dauphiné au XVIIIe siècle." Unpublished paper presented at Montpellier, February 1986

– "Les petites villes dauphinoises face à leur environnement rural au XVIIIe siècle: Emprise foncière, financière, humaine." *Petites villes du Moyen Âge à nos jours*. Edited by J.-P. Poissou et Philippe Lours. Paris: CNRS 1987. 323–34

– *Les villes du Dauphiné aux XVIIe et XVIIIe siècles*. Grenoble: Presses Universitaires de Grenoble 1993

Favreau, Robert. "La pauvreté en Poitou et en Anjou à la fin du Moyen Âge." *Études sur l'histoire de la pauvreté (Moyen Âge–XVIe siècle)*. Edited by Michel Mollat. 2 vols. Paris: Publications de la Sorbonne 1974. 1: 589–620

Fillet, L. "Grignan religieux." *Bulletin de la Société d'archéologie et de statistique de la Drôme* 14 (1880): 165–6; 13 (1879): 175–93; 14 (1880): 5–20, 150–70, 225–34

Font-Reaulx, Jacques de. "L'Hôpital de Saint-Vallier." *Bulletin de la Société d'Archéologie et de Statistique de la Drôme* 55 (1935–36): 318–28

Forrest, Alan. *La Révolution française et les pauvres*. Paris: Perrin, 1986

Fosseyeux, Marcel. "Les premiers budgets municipaux d'assistance: La taxe des pauvres au XVIe siècle." *Revue d'histoire de l'Église de France* (1934): 20 407–32

– "Le service médical à l'Hôpital de la Charité aux XVIIe et XVIIIe siècles." *Aesculape* 3, no. 5 (mai 1913): 117–21 and no. 6 (juin 1913): 150–4

Foucault, Michel. *Folie et déraison: Histoire de la folie à l'âge classique*. Paris: 10/18 1961

– *Naissance de la clinique: Une archéologie du regard médical*. 2d ed., rev. Paris: Presses universitaires de France 1972

– et al. *Les machines à guérir (aux origines de l'hôpital moderne)*. Paris: Institut de l'environment 1976

Gallot-Lavallée, Pierre. *Un hygiéniste au XVIIIe siècle: Jean Colombier, rapporteur du Conseil de santé des hôpitaux militaires, inspecteur général des hôpitaux et prisons du royaume (1736–1789)*. Paris, 1913

Gascon, Richard. "Immigration et croissance urbaine au XVIe siècle: L'exemple de Lyon." *Annales ESC* 25 (1970): 988–1001

Gelfand, Toby. *Professionalizing Modern Medicine: Paris Surgeons and Medical Science and Institutions in the 18th Century*. Westport Conn.: Greenwood Press 1980

Geremek, Bronislaw. *La potence ou la pitié: L'Europe et les pauvres du Moyen Age à nos jours*. Paris: Gallimard 1987

Goubert, Jean-Pierre. *Malades et médecins en Bretagne, 1770–1790*. Paris: Klincksieck 1974

Goubert, Pierre. *L'Ancien Régime*. Vol. 2, *Les pouvoirs*. Paris: Armand Colin 1973

Gouhier, Pierre, Vallez, Anne, and Vallez, Jean-Marie, eds. *Atlas historique de Normandie*. Vol. 2, *Institutions, économies, comportements*. Caen: Université de Caen, Centre de recherche de l'histoire quantitative 1972

Granshaw, Lindsay, and Porter, Roy, eds. *The Hospital in History*. London: Routledge 1989

Guérin, Claire. "Une tentative de réforme militaire et hospitalière, 1672–1693: Son application en Normandie." Thèse pour l'École des Chartes 1975

Guevarre, André. *La mendicité abolie dans le diocèse d'Aix par l'établissement d'un hôpital général ou d'une maison de charité en chaque ville et gros bourg et par un bureau de charité en chaque lieu où l'on ne pouvait pas enfermer les pauvres. Avec la response aux principales objections que l'on peut faire contre ces établissements*. Aix, n.d. [1687]

Guillemot, André. "L'Hôpital de Malestroit du milieu du XVIIe siècle à la Révolution." Thèse de DES, Université de Rennes 1967

– "L'Hôpital de Malestroit du milieu du XVIIe siècle à la Révolution." *Revue d'histoire économique et sociale* 48 (1970): 483–524

Guillochon, Marc. "L'Hôpital et Aumônerie de Saint-Méen du Terte de Joué près de Rennes, 1627–1789: Naissance et évolution d'une institution à vocation hospitalière sous l'Ancien Régime." Thèse, École nationale de la santé, Rennes 1979

Gutton, Jean-Pierre. "À l'aube du XVIIe siècle: Idées nouvelles sur les pauvres." *Cahiers d'histoire* 10 (1965): 87–97

– *L'état et la mendicité dans la première moitié du XVIIIe siècle: Auvergne, Beaujolais, Forez, Lyonnais.* Saint-Étienne: Centre d'études foreziennes 1973

– *Guide du chercheur en histoire de la protection sociale.* Vol. 1, *Fin du Moyen Age – 1789.* Paris: Association pour l'étude de l'histoire de la securité sociale 1994

– "La mise en place du personnel soignant dans les hôpitaux français (XVIe–XVIIIe siècles)." *Bulletin de la Société française d'histoire des hôpitaux* 54 (1987): 11–19

– *La sociabilité villageoise dans l'ancienne France: Solidarités et voisinages du XVIe au XVIIIe siècle.* Paris: Hachette 1979

– *La société et les pauvres: L'exemple de la généralité de Lyon, 1534–1789.* Paris: Les Belles-Lettres 1971

Guyob, L. "Pauvreté et assistance dans le monde rural: L'exemple de Meursault, 1500–1760." Thèse de maîtrise, Université de Paris 1 1987

Hauser, Henri. *Recherches et documents sur l'histoire des prix en France de 1500 à 1800.* Paris: Presses modernes 1936

Herault, Pascal. *Dieu, la maladie et les Montmorillonnais: Quand la Maison-Dieu soignait l'âme et le corps aux XVIIe et XVIIIe siècles.* Guide to an exhibition presented 13 July–2 October 1994 at the Maison-Dieu, Montmorillon

– "Les pauvres et l'amputation à la Maison-Dieu de Montmorillon aux XVIIe et XVIIIe siècles: Contribution à l'histoire de la chirurgie hospitalière." *Bulletin de la Société française d'histoire des hôpitaux* 69 (1993): 23–33

– "Soigner en montmorillonnais au début du XVIIIe siècle (d'après le *Livre des remèdes et voyages* de l'Augustinian Jean Rozet)." *Annales de Bretagne* 100, no. 1 (1993): 61–120

Hickey, Daniel. "Closing Down Local Hospitals in Seventeenth-Century France: The Mount Carmel and St. Lazare Reform Movement." *Social History/Histoire sociale* 25, no. 49 (May 1992): 9–33

– *Le Dauphiné devant la monarchie absolue.* Grenoble; Moncton: Presses Universitaires de Grenoble/Éditions d'Acadie 1993

– "Innovation and Obstacles to Growth in the Agriculture of Early Modern France: The Example of Dauphiné." *French Historical Studies* 15 (1987): 208–40

– "Preaching and Teaching: Pierre Vigne and the Sisters of the Holy Sacrament; The Grass Roots of the Catholic Reformation." *Proceedings of the*

Annual Meeting of the Western Society for French History 19:29–38 Riverside, Calif. 1992

Hoffman, Philip. *Church and Community in the Diocese of Lyon, 1500–1789.* New Haven: Yale University Press 1984

Houdaille, J. "La mortalité des Carmélites en France de 1736 à 1792." *Population* 26 (1971): 745–8

Hufton, Olwen. *The Poor of Eighteenth-Century France, 1750–1789.* Oxford: Oxford University Press 1974

– "Women without Men: Widows and Spinsters in Britain and France in the Eighteenth Century." *Journal of Family History* 9 (1984): 355–76

Huppert, George. "*Divinatio et eruditio*: Thoughts on Foucault." *History and Theory* 13 (1974): 191–207

Imbert, Jean. *Le droit hospitalier de l'Ancien Régime.* Paris: Presses Universitaires de France 1993

– "L'Église et l'État face au problème hospitalier au xvie siècle." *Études d'histoire du droit canonique dédiées à Gabriel Le Bras.* Paris: Sirey 1965. 577–92

– ed. *Histoire des hôpitaux en France.* Toulouse: Privat 1982

– "Les prescriptions hospitalières du Concile de Trente et leur diffusion en France." *Revue d'histoire de l'Église de France* 42 (1956): 5–28

Isambert, François André, et al., eds. *Recueil général des anciennes lois françaises depuis l'an 420 jusqu'à la Révolution de 1789.* 26 vols. Paris: Belin-Leprieur 1822–33

Jacquart, Jean. "Immobilisme et catastrophes, 1560–1660." G. Duby and A. Wallon, eds., *Histoire de la France rurale*, sec. 2, vol. 2, *L'Age Classique des paysans.* Paris: Seuil 1975. 185–259

Jaher, Frederic C., ed. *The Rich, the Well Born, and the Powerful: Elites and Upper Classes in History.* Urbana: University of Illinois Press 1973

Jenny, J. "Les œuvres de charité et les institutions hospitalières dans le diocèse de Bourges (xviie–xviiie siècles)." *Trente-deuxième congrès de la Fédération des sociétés savantes du Centre.* Guéret 1973. 66–80

Jeorger, Muriel. "Les enquêtes hospitalières au xviiie siècle." *Bulletin de la Société française d'histoire des hôpitaux* 31 (1975): 51–60

– "La structure hospitalière de la France sous l'Ancien Régime." *Annales ESC* 32 (1977): 1025–51

Jones, Colin. *The Charitable Imperative: Hospitals and Nursing in Ancien Régime and Revolutionary France.* London: Routledge 1989

– *Charity and Bienfaisance: The Treatment of the Poor in the Montpellier Region, 1740–1815.* Cambridge: Cambridge University Press 1983

Joret, Charles. "Le P. Guevarre et les bureaux de charité au xviie siècle." *Annales du Midi* 3 (1889): 340–93

Kingdon, Robert M. "Social Welfare in Calvin's Geneva." *American Historical Review* 76 (1971): 50–70

Lacroix, André. *Inventaire sommaire des Archives départementales antérieures à 1790, Drôme.* 8 vols. Valence: Chenevier et Pessieux 1865–1910

Lafond, Louis. *La dynastie des Helvétius: Les remèdes du roi.* Paris: Occitania 1926

Lallemand, Léon. *Histoire de la charité.* Vol. 4, *Les temps modernes (du XVIe au XIXe siècle).* Paris: Alphonse Picard et fils 1910

Langlois, Claude. *Le Catholicisme au féminin: Les congrégations françaises à supérieur général au XIXe siècle.* Paris: CERF 1984

Laplume, Stanislas-Kostka. "Un Augustin français du XVIIe siècle: Le Père Ange Le Proust (1624–1697)." *Sonderdruck aus Homo Spiritalis: Festgabe für Luc Verheijen OSA.* Würzburg: Augustinus-Verlag 1987: 340–52

Laslett, Peter. *The World We Have Lost: Further Explored.* London: Scribners 1984

Lebrun, François, ed. *Histoire des Catholiques en France du XVe siècle à nos jours.* Toulouse: Privat 1980

– *Les hommes et la mort en Anjou aux XVIIe et XVIIIe siècles: Essai de démographie et de psychologie historiques.* Paris: Flammarion Science 1971

– *Se soigner autrefois: Médecins, saints et sorciers aux 17e et 18e siècles.* Paris: Temps Actuels 1983

Le Cacheux, Paul. *Essai historique sur l'Hôtel-Dieu de Coutances, depuis l'origine jusqu'à la Révolution, avec cartulaire général – l'Hôpital Général et les Augustines hospitalières.* 2 vols. Paris: A. Picard et fils 1895–99

Lecanu, Auguste-François. *Histoire du diocèse de Coutances et d'Avranches depuis les temps les plus reculés jusqu'à nos jours, suivie des actes des saints et d'un tableau historique des paroisses du diocèse.* 2 vols. Coutances: Salettes, 1877–78

Léchaudé-d'Anisy, M.A. "Recherches sur les léproseries et maladreries dites vulgairement maladreries qui existent en Normandie." *Mémoires de la Société des antiquaires de Normandie,* 17 (1847): 149–212

Le Goff, Jacques, and René Raymond, eds. *Histoire de la France religieuse.* Vol. 2, *XIV–XVIIIe siècles.* Paris: Seuil 1988

Le Goff, T.J.A., and D.M.G. Sutherland. "The Revolution and the Rural Community in Eighteenth-Century Brittany." *Past and Present* 62 (1974): 96–119

Le Grand, Léon. "Comment composer l'histoire d'un établissement hospitalier: Sources et méthode." *Revue d'histoire de l'Église de France* 16 (1930): 161–239

Léonard, Jacques. "Les médecins de l'Ouest au 19e siècle." 3 vols. Lille: Université de Lille, Atelier des thèses 1979

Le Roy Ladurie, Emmanuel, Jean Jacquart, and Hugues Neveux. *L'âge classique des paysans, 1340–1789.* Vol. 2 of *Histoire de la France rurale.* Edited by George Duby and Armand Wallon. 4 vols. Paris: Seuil 1975

Le Roy Ladurie, Emmanuel, and Michel Morineau. *Paysannerie et croissance*. Vol. 1, Pt. 2 of *Histoire économique et sociale de la France*. Edited by Fernand Braudel and Ernest Labrousse. 4 vols. Paris: Presses Universitaires de France 1977

Levasseur, Roger, ed. *De la sociabilité: Spécificité et mutations*. Montréal: Boréal 1990

Lot, Ferdinand. *Recherches sur les effectifs des armées françaises des Guerres d'Italie aux Guerres de religion, 1492–1562*. Paris: SEVPEN 1962

Luria, Keith P. "Conflict and the Constitution of Moral Order in Old Regime Rural Society." *Proceedings of the Annual Meeting of the Western Society for French History* 16: 139–44 Auburn, Alabama 1989

– *Territories of Grace: Cultural Change in the Seventeenth-Century Diocese of Grenoble*. Berkeley: University of California Press 1991

Maître, Léon. *L'assistance publique dans la Loire-Inférieure avant 1789: Étude sur les léproseries, aumôneries, hôpitaux-généraux et bureaux de charité*. Nantes: Société académique 1879

– *Histoire administrative des anciens hôpitaux de Nantes*. Nantes, 1879; reprint Marseille: Jeanne Lafitte 1981

Major, J. Russell. "Bellièvre, Sully, and the Assembly of Notables of 1596." *Transactions of the American Philosophical Society*, new series, 64, pt. 2 (1974): 1–34

Mandon, L. *Histoire du prêt-gratuit de Montpellier, 1684–1891*. 2 vols. Montpellier: J. Martel Ainé 1892

Marchal, Jean. *Le droit d'oblat: Essai sur une variété de pensionnés monastiques*. Paris: Abbaye Saint-Martin 1955

Martin, Alphonse. *L'Hôtel-Dieu de Fécamp*. Le Havre: Imprimerie Lepelletier 1883

Martin, Xavier. "La part du corps de ville dans la gestion de l'Hôtel-Dieu d'Angers à la fin du XVIe siècle." *Annales de Bretagne et des pays de l'Ouest* 82 (1975): 149–62

Massevile, Louis Levasseur de. *État géographique de la province de Normandie*. Rouen: J.B. Besongne le fils 1722

Megill, Allan. "The Reception of Foucault by Historians." *Journal of the History of Ideas* 48 (1987): 117–41.

Mendras, Henri. *Sociétés paysannes*. Paris: Armand Colin 1976

Mentzer, Raymond A., Jr. "Organizational Endeavor and Charitable Impulse in Sixteenth-Century France: The Case of Protestant Nîmes." *French History* 5 (1991): 1–29

Merle, L. *L'Hôpital du Saint-Esprit de Niort (1665–1790): Contribution à l'histoire de la lutte contre la mendicité sous l'Ancien Régime*. Fontenay-le-Comte: Lussaud 1966

Meuvret, Jean. "Les crises de subsistance et la démographie de la France d'Ancien Régime." *Cahiers des Annales* 32 (1971): 271–80

Mezzadri, Luigi. *Vincent de Paul (1581–1660)*. Paris: Desclée et Brouwer 1985

Mitchell, Harvey. "Politics in the Service of Knowledge: The Debate over the Administration of Medicine and Welfare in the Late Eighteenth Century." *Social History* 6 (1981): 185–207

Molette, Charles. *Guide des sources de l'histoire des congrégations féminines françaises de vie active*. Paris: Éditions de Paris 1974

Mollat, Michel. *Les pauvres au Moyen Âge: Étude sociale*. Paris: Complexe 1978

Mutel, André. "Recherches sur l'Ordre de Saint-Lazare de Jerusalem en Normandie." *Annales de Normandie* 33 (1983): 121–42

Nicolle, Louis. *Apothicaires et pharmaciens de Morbihan: Contribution à l'histoire de la pharmacie dans le Morbihan des origines au début du xxe siècle*. Paris: Oberthur 1962

Norberg, Kathryn. *Rich and Poor in Grenoble, 1600–1814*. Berkeley: University of California Press 1985

Olejniczak, William John. "The Royal Campaign against Beggary and Vagrancy in France during the Eighteenth Century as Implemented in the *Généralité* of Champagne." PHD dissertation, Duke University 1983

– "Working the Body of the Poor: The *Ateliers de Charité* in Late Eighteenth Century France." *Journal of Social History* 24 (1990): 87–107

Panel, Gustave, ed. *Documents concernant les pauvres de Rouen*. 3 vols. Rouen: Lestringant; Paris: Picard 1917–19

Paultre, Christian. *De la répression de la mendicité et du vagabondage en France sous l'Ancien Régime*. Paris 1906; reprint Genève: Slatkine-Megariotis 1975

Pérouas, Louis. *Le diocèse de La Rochelle de 1648 à 1724: Sociologie et pastorale*. Paris: SEVPEN 1964

– *Grignon de Montfort: Un aventurier de l'Évangile*. Paris: Éditions ouvrières 1990

Petit, Jeanne. *L'Assemblée des notables de 1626–27*. Paris: École pratique des hautes études 1937

Pitre, Marc R. "Henri IV et la Chambre de la Charité Chrétienne 1606–1611: L'assistance aux anciens militaires invalides et une tentative de réforme hospitalière au début du 17e siècle." MA thesis, Université de Moncton 1996

Poitrineau, Abel. *La vie rurale en Basse-Auvergne au XVIIIe siècle (1726–1789)*. 2 vols. Paris 1965; reprint Marseille: Lafitte 1979

Portal, Michel. "Le grand aumônier de France jusqu'à la fin du XVIIe siècle." *Revue de l'assistance publique à Paris* 29 (1954): 291–306

Poulet, Catherine. "Pauvreté, mendicité et assistance de l'état en Bretagne au XVIIIe siècle." Mémoire de maîtrise, Université de la Haute-Bretagne 1975

Pullan, Brian. *Rich and Poor in Renaissance Venice: The Social Institutions of a Catholic State to 1620.* Cambridge, Mass.: Harvard University Press 1971

Ramsey, Matthew. *Professional and Popular Medicine in France, 1770–1830: The Social World of Medical Practice.* Cambridge: Cambridge University Press 1988

Rapley, Elizabeth. *The Dévotes: Women and the Church in Seventeenth-Century France.* Montreal-Kingston: McGill-Queen's University Press 1990

– "Women and the Religious Vocation in Seventeenth-Century France." *French Historical Studies* 18 (1994): 613–31

Recueil des édits et déclarations du roy: Lettres patentes et ordonnances de sa majesté, arrests et règlements de ses conseils et du Parlement de Grenoble. 26 vols. Grenoble: Chez Gaspard Giroud et André Giroud 1690–1783

Richet, Denis. *La France moderne: L'esprit des institutions.* Paris: Flammarion Science 1973

Robichaud, Marc. "L'Hôpital de Caudebec, 1693–1789: Un exemple de l'assistance locale en France à l'époque des Lumières." MA thesis, Université de Moncton 1996

Root, Hilton. *Peasants and King in Burgundy: Agrarian Foundations of French Absolutism.* Berkeley: University of California Press 1987

Rosenzweig, Louis. "L'Hôpital de Malestroit." *Annuaire statistique, historique et administratif de Morbihan.* Part 2. Vannes 1864. 1–52

Salomon, Howard M. *Public Welfare, Science, and Propaganda in Seventeenth-Century France: The Innovations of Théophraste Renaudot.* Princeton: Princeton University Press 1972

Saint Jacob, Pierre de. "Mutations économiques et sociales dans les campagnes bourguigonnes à la fin du XVIe siècle." *Études rurales* 1 (1961): 34–49

– *Les paysans de la Bourgogne du Nord au dernier siècle de l'Ancien Régime.* Toulouse: Privat 1960

Schmitt, Thérèse-Jean. *L'organisation ecclésiastique et la pratique religieuse dans l'archidiaconé d'Autun de 1650 à 1750.* Autun: Marcelin 1957

Schroeder, H.J. *Canons and Decrees of the Council of Trent.* St Louis: Herder 1941

Schwartz, Robert M. *Policing the Poor in Eighteenth-Century France.* Chapel Hill: University of North Carolina Press 1988

Sonnet, Martine. "Une fille à éduquer." *Histoire des femmes.* Edited by N. Davis and A. Farge. Vol. 3, *XVI–XVIII siècles.* Paris: Plon 1991. III–40

Sully, Duc de. "Mémoire des sages et royales œconomies d'estat de Henri le Grand." Vol. 1. *Collection des mémoires relatifs à l'histoire de la France, depuis l'avènement de Henri IV, jusqu'à la paix de Paris, conclu en 1763; avec des notices sur chaque auteur, et des observations sur chaque ouvrage.* Edited by Claude Bernard Petitot, Alexandre Petitot, and Louis Monmerqué. Second series. 76 vols. Paris: Foucault 1820–29

Tackett, Timothy. *Priest and Parish in Eighteenth-Century France: A Social and Political Study of Curés in a Diocese of Dauphiné, 1750–1791.* Princeton: Princeton University Press 1977

Trexler, Richard C. "Charity and the Defense of the Urban Elites in the Italian Communes." *The Rich, the Well Born, and the Powerful: Elites and Upper Classes in History.* Edited by Frederic C Jaher. Urbana: University of Illinois Press 1973. 64–109

Vacher, Marguerite. *Des "régulières" dans le siècle: Les sœurs de Saint-Joseph du Père Médaille aux xviie et xviiie siècles.* Clermont-Ferrand: Adosa 1991

Vacher, Thérèse. *Les archives des congrégations françaises de Saint-Joseph.* Lyon: Publications du DEA d'histoire religieuse 1991

Vaganet, Fabienne. "Pouvoir et notabilité à Nyons, 1692–1768." Thèse de maîtrise, Université de Lyons II 1987

Van Leeuwen, Marco H.D. "The Logic of Charity: Poor Relief in Preindustrial Europe." *Journal of Interdisciplinary History* 24 (1994): 589–613

Venard, Marc. "Catholicisme et usure au xviie siècle." *Revue d'Histoire de l'Église de France* 52 (1966): 59–74

– "Les œuvres de la charité en Avignon à l'aube du xviie siècle." *xviie siècle* 90–1 (1971): 127–46

Vernet, Félix. *La Congrégation des religieuses du Très-Saint-Sacrement de Valence (1715–1940).* Lyon: Lescuyer 1941

Versoris, Nicolas. *Journal d'un bourgeois de Paris sous François Ier.* Edited by Philippe Joutard. Paris: 10/18 1963

Veyne, Paul. *Comment on écrit l'histoire augmenté de Foucault révolutionne l'histoire.* Paris: Seuil-histoire 1978

Veyrenc, Jean-Baptiste. *Essai sur la vie du Père Vigne, missionnaire apostolique, fondateur de la Congrégation des religieuses du Saint-Sacrement dont la maison-mère est actuellement à Romans (1868).* Valence: Jules Céas 1868

Viale, Annick. "L'Hôpital du Buis au xviiie siècle: Structures diverses et rôle des femmes." *Bulletin de l'Association "Les Amis du Buis des Baronnies"* 40 (1982): 11–35

Voitel-Grenon, Geneviève. "La Chambre de la généralle réformation des hôpitaux, hôtels-Dieu et maladreries de France (1612–1672)." Thèse pour l'École des Chartes 1973

Vovelle, Michel. *Mourir autrefois: Attitudes collectives devant la mort aux xviie et xviiie siècles.* Paris: Gallimard/Archives 1974

– *Piété baroque et déchristianisation en Provence au xviiie siècle.* Paris: Seuil-histoire 1973

Weber, Eugen. *Peasants into Frenchmen: The Modernization of Rural France, 1870–1914.* Stanford: Stanford University Press 1976

Index

absolutism and the hospitals: thesis, 9–10; crown perception of hospital mismanagement, 36–7, 43; difficulties in trying to intervene, 43–4; new intervention through Notre-Dame of Mount Carmel and St-Lazare, 45–6; opposition of the hospitaller orders, 64–5; dispute with pope over crown rights, 64; holdings restored, 66; royal officials redistribute hospitals, 79; setting up the hôpitaux-généraux to intern beggars, 79–86; Turgot and Necker attempt to reorient hospital activities. *See also* Chamber of Christian Charity; Chamber of the Arsenal; Chamber of the General Hospital Reform; Notre-Dame of Mount Carmel and St-Lazare; royal edicts, declarations, and ordinances
Adams, Thomas M., 183, 184, 195

Adhémar, Louis d', Comte de Grignan, 27, 116–17
Adrets, Baron des, 23
Aguesseau, Sieur d', *conseiller d'état*, 71
Aiguillon, Duchesse d', 139
Aix-en-Provence: city, 5, 55, 59, 116, 186; diocese, 11, 59–60, 74; *La mendicité abolie*, 60
Alembert, Jean le Rond d', 178
Alençon: généralité, 52; intendant, 78
Alezeron, Rose-Marie, 167
Allain, Jeanne, 167
Allard, Guy, 74
Allex: hospital of, 76
almshouses, 15, 25, 47, 75
Ambray, Madame d', 165
Amiens: diocese of, 50, 52, 73
Angers, 20, 41, 107, 168
Anne of Austria (queen mother), 152
Ardèche, 9, 144, 159
Arles, 116
army: size of standing army (sixteenth century), 38; injuries and amputations, 38; budget of and 1596

Assembly of Notables, 38–9; Louvois and Notre-Dame of Mount Carmel and St-Lazare, 48; construction of Invalides, 48; king's justification of new aid for officers and soldiers, 49; goal of St-Lazare experiment, 67
Arnaud, Dr Jacques, 124
Arouel, Denis, 30
Arras: hospital, 72; town, 52
Assemblies of Notables: 1596, 38; 1626, 46
Aumône Générale of Lyon, 18, 19, 20, 110
Aunay, 81
Auray: Chartreuse d'Auray, 89; hospital of, 128
Aurillac: hospital of, 84
Auriol, Alix, Dame d', 27
Auvergne: généralité of, 83, 84, 85; hospital at Issoire, 56
Avignon: mont de piété, 107; town, 146
Avisseau-Roussat, Hélène, 188
Avranches: bishop of, 122; diocese of, 83, 94

St-Nicolas: maladrerie of, 20, 78, 88
St-Paul-de-Léon: diocese of, 62
St-Père-en-Retz: hospital of, 18
St-Romain-de-Colbusc: hospital of, 69
St-Ruf: priory of, 28
St-Sauveur: hospital of, 58
St-Sauveur-le-Vicomte: hospital of, 83
St-Sulpice-et-Gros-Callou: parish of, 180
St-Vallier, Mgr de. See Lacroix-Chevrières, Jean-Baptiste de
St-Vallier, hospital of, 29, 105, 146, 155–6, 195, 207; previous charitable foundations, 28; organization of a charitable confraternity by Abbé Gernus (1639), 281; donation by Abbé Jean-Antoine de Bret, 28; donations by Jean-Baptiste de la Croix- Chevrières, 28–9; bringing in Sisters of St-Joseph, 141; organization of a workshop, 184–5
St-Vallier, town of, 12, 28–9, 155
Salers, 84
Salpêtrière. See Paris, hospitals of
Santiago de Compostela: pilgrimage of, 13
Savenay, Hôpital St-Armal of, 13, 17–18, 21, 32, 36, 66, 117, 130, 136, 141, 167, 187, 201, 207; origins, 33; attempt by Hôtel-Dieu of Nantes to take over, 33–4; attempts by Notre-Dame of Mount Carmel and St-Lazare to suppress, 62–3; distribution of packages of medication, 185–6
Savenay, town of, 13, 17–18
Savournin, Louis-André, 124
Schwartz, Robert, 81

Senlis: hospital of, 190
Sens: archbishop, 40; town, 52, 73
Serre, Janine, 117
Serret, André, 45, 61–2
Servant, Madelaine, 150
Seyne, hospital of, 61, 121–4, 128, 167, 187, 207; origins, 27; fusion of Hôpital St-Jacques and the Hôtel-Dieu in 1656, 27; new building approved in 1680, 27; taking in paying clients, 122; service of local elites, 124
Seyne, town of, 12, 27, 35–6, 118, 121, 124–5, 141, 167, 191
Sinard, 44
Sisteron, 74, 146, 155
Sisters of Calvary, 145
Sisters of Charity (Ladies or Daughters of Charity), 8, 138–41, 147–51, 154, 155, 167–9, 173, 180, 186; beginnings, 138–41; struggle against cloister, 137–41. See also Marillac, Louise de; Vincent de Paul, St
Sisters of Providence, 141, 171
Sisters of St-Joseph, 8, 28, 148, 150, 161, 165, 173; beginnings, 141–3; founding sisters, 145–6; decentralized structures, 154–8
Sisters of St-Thomas de Villeneuve, 8, 134–5, 141, 143–4, 146–8, 150, 154, 165, 171–2, 173, 190; beginnings, 143–4; founding sisters, 146–8; role of a lay director, 152–3; contracts negotiated with hospitals, 166–9
Sisters of the Holy Sacrament, 8, 141, 144–5, 148–9, 150–1, 158–61, 165, 167, 169, 171–3; beginnings, 144–5; founding sisters, 148–9; widows, 151; demands for improved structures, 158; work in hospitals, 159

Soissons: dépôt de mendicité, 179; diocese, 50, 73
Spéliat, Marie, 148, 149, 158

Tarbes: diocese of, 50
Tenin, Dr Jacques, 162
Teutonic Knights, 47, 49, 64
Theriault, Pierre, 129
Thierry de St-Brieuc, Mme Rouxel de, 152
Thiers: hospital of, 84–5
Thorigny: hospital of, 58, 84
Thouars, 168
Tosserand, Louis, 127
Toulon, 74
Toulouse: archbishop of, 177; city, 60
Tournai, 52
Tours, 50, 73
town and village institutions: thesis on decline, 6–7; Edict of Moulins (1566) ordering towns and villages to care for own poor, 23–4; criteria for re-establishing suppressed hospitals (1693–1705), 70–1; competition between potential regional centres, 77–9, 95–6; convincing local elites to support hôpitaux-généraux, 110–12; curé and local elites, 114; Pontorson tries to re-establish control of its hospital, 122–3; power of local elites, 123–4; elites solicited by church and crown officials, 132–3; internal disputes over Malestroit hospital, 171–2; local resistance to reforms, 206–7
Tréguier: hospital, 58, 62; monastery, 88
Turgot, Anne-Robert-Jacques, contrôleur général, 9, 10, 131, 176–9, 181, 188–9, 206
twenty-fourth of the tithe (Dauphiné), 23–5, 35, 87–8, 113–14, 116